HERBAL MEDICINE IN TREATING GYNAECOLOGICAL CONDITIONS

HERBAL MEDICINE IN TREATING GYNAECOLOGICAL CONDITIONS
Herbs, Hormones, Pre-Menstrual Syndrome and Menopause

*Hananja Brice-Ytsma
and Adrian McDermott*

AEON

Aeon Books Ltd
12 New College Parade
Finchley Road
London NW3 5EP

Copyright © 2020 by Hananja Brice-Ytsma and Adrian McDermott

Photographs © 2020 Peter Jarrett

The right of Hananja Brice-Ytsma and Adrian McDermott to be identified as the authors of this work has been asserted in accordance with §§ 77 and 78 of the Copyright Design and Patents Act 1988.

All rights reserved. No part of this publication may be reproduced, stored in a retrieval system, or transmitted, in any form or by any means, electronic, mechanical, photocopying, recording, or otherwise, without the prior written permission of the publisher.

British Library Cataloguing in Publication Data

A C.I.P. for this book is available from the British Library

ISBN-13: 978-1-91159-770-4

Typeset by Medlar Publishing Solutions Pvt Ltd, India

www.aeonbooks.co.uk

CONTENTS

FOREWORD — vii

INTRODUCTION — xi

CHAPTER ONE
How the body produces oestrogen and progesterone — 1

CHAPTER TWO
Principles of herbal treatment of gynaecological problems — 49

CHAPTER THREE
Key herbs containing isoflavones and flavonoids — 91

CHAPTER FOUR
Key herbs containing steroidal saponins — 117

CHAPTER FIVE
Actaea racemosa (widely known as *Cimicifuga racemosa*) and *Vitex agnus-castus* — 135

CHAPTER SIX
Paeonia lactiflora and *Glycyrrhiza glabra*   165

CHAPTER SEVEN
Herbs, HRT, and the menopause   181

CHAPTER EIGHT
PMS: common myths   215

CHAPTER NINE
Some other gynaecological conditions   253

NOTES   *261*

INDEX   *327*

FOREWORD

I have been in practice for over 30 years and been teaching for more than 20 years. Over that time, I kept hearing from students as well as practitioners that gynaecology, and specifically hormonal issues, are so complicated and confusing. Repeatedly, I had to educate practitioners, students and patients on misinformation about oestrogens/phyto-oestrogens etc., and other herbs that influence different hormones. The internet and magazines are full of false information, especially related to the phyto-oestrogens, seemingly implying they can do the same as endogenous oestrogens.

Before I started personally focusing more on gynaecology and hormones, I must admit I was very confused as well. It was pretty common among herbalists in cases that had anything to do with gynaecology that one just used the hormonal herbs (i.e. *Vitex agnus-castus*, or *Cimicifuga racemosa*, occasionally *Trifolium pratense*).

Luckily enough, as most herbs, in the end, are unlikely to take control (as opposed to the pill), but rather support healthy functions, one is unlikely to go far wrong.

However, more than 25 years ago, I was asked to do a lecture on hormonal herbs to a student group and thought I had better get to understand the subject fully. There is nothing like teaching! I ended up fascinated by the subject, and amazed at the effects that herbs have and the multitude of mechanisms they work with in the body. Now, in the end, ironically, I do not really describe their actions so differently to how I did before I went on this journey. But I found that by understanding the how's and why's of the herb, understanding the different hormones involved, and their metabolism, I was able to explain it so much better to my patients, and with that found that the whole treatment was so more effective. At that point, what started off seeming so complicated turned out to be actually quite straightforward.

There are some real basics one always needs to go back to in treatment of most conditions. Granted, there might be quite specific herbs that have a good reputation for specific conditions, but even with hormones one still needs to work on the key aspects of assimilation, elimination, integration, and circulation.

There are some other things that I kept hold of during the years of teaching:

1. Traditional usage of a particular herb, which usually points to years of observation and clinical use by herbalists in the past, gives us the general pointers. Before we became so-called more 'scientific', the power of observation was crucial!
2. Research gives really useful insight into some of the herbs.

Very often, a herb still baffles scientists, which is always fun, as they know from clinical trials something is safe and effective, but cannot figure out the mechanism by which it works. Classic examples are *Hypericum perforatum* and *Cimicifuga racemosa*. Much of the research is *in vitro* and *in vivo*, something that does not necessarily translate well into clinical use, but does find its way into textbooks as 'facts'. This so much truer in the case of phyto-oestrogens, and it is where much of the misinformation comes from.

Hananja Brice-Ytsma

I had the privilege of working as a clinical tutor alongside Hananja for a number of years, and more recently as a colleague at Heartwood Education, and have enjoyed many discussions with her, and with students, over the principles of herbal treatment. In particular, I am fascinated by the way that science has come from rather undermining herbal treatment to broadly supporting it now that there is a change of emphasis from the 'magic bullet' to solutions that may be synergistic and multifactorial.

So, being able now to contribute to this book has been a privilege and a pleasure, and an excellent opportunity to review the issue, whether science and herbal medicine are somehow merging or whether they are neighbours who at long last are on speaking terms.

The fundamental difference between the viewpoints of pharmacological science and traditional herbal medicine is made very clear within a broadly supportive pharmacological review of the role of herbs (Ginseng, Astragalus, and Echinacea) in cancer therapy. In the end, herbal medicine looks from the standpoint of the individual patient and a customised formula.

> It would certainly be possible to study standard multicomponent agents in randomised trials. However, as individual responses to herbal extracts may vary, it seems reasonable to conclude that such variations would only increase with the increasing complexity of the herbal mixtures.[1]

This quote was specifically about Chinese herbal formulae but it applies equally, or perhaps even more strongly, to western herbal medicine. Herbal medicine has been learnt through experience and tradition, incorporating subtle observation and rich detail. Herbalists practice in a medical community that necessarily uses a common language of diagnosis, management or prognosis, and the language of scientific medicine and pharmacology are essential to that, but they need to be relevant. Medical research follows a model of scientific experimentation that requires standardised preparations and modern diagnostic categories. To dismiss as irrelevant or unscientific everything that does not fit this conceptual framework is to lose the value of the tradition and the work of the people who created it. To bridge this gap, research methods need to fully incorporate the idea of individualised treatments using formulae that are not and cannot fully be standardised.

Our attitude is that the dialogue is fascinating and useful, but we remain firmly in a model that is eclectic, critical, and holistic in approach. Modern research is no longer in denial of this viewpoint, and this book aims to elucidate how current trends in biomedicine give us some very useful pointers. We cannot be definitive because the research is always in progress, so we are somewhat in the position of trying to sweep clean the path while it is still snowing, but we do hope that at least parts of the path are a little more discernible nevertheless.

Adrian McDermott

INTRODUCTION

Who is this book for?

This book is for students and practitioners of herbal medicine or other medical disciplines that use medicinal herbs. There have been significant changes in understanding in recent decades about the interrelationships between the nervous, endocrine, and immune systems, challenging previous thinking about the actions of herbs. At the same time, research typically confirms many traditional indications of medicinal plants. We try as far as possible to try to resolve that paradox: it is clearer than ever that the plants are effective but how they work is still to a great extent a matter for speculation. This is particularly true for reproductive physiology, which is just about as complex as things get.

What is this book for?

Medical herbalists have generally done an excellent job in helping women with gynaecological problems. The question is, as this field is very complex and has been the subject of a great deal of recent research and consequently new insights, is there something that could be done better still? Obviously, that is a question that a practitioner will answer for themselves, but the hope is that this book will help those that think the answer might be 'yes', in particular helping with:

- How recent findings about the immune, nervous, and endocrine systems provide a sound basis for nutritional, lifestyle, and herbal treatment.
- Principles behind the interactions between diet, lifestyle, hormones, and the nervous and immune systems.
- Giving clear, reliable explanations to patients that will enable them to manage the ever-increasing amount of health information they will encounter and give them well-placed confidence in your management plan.

Myths about oestrogenic or progestogenic herbs are widespread, and most herbalists will know the more obvious ones. But it is also useful not only to know this but to be able to offer clarification, which means understanding the complexity of the picture that makes such oversimplifications tempting. The mark of understanding something well is to be able to explain it simply, so we want to enable, as far as possible, to enable practitioners to do this in order to enable patients to engage in an effective treatment plan whose rationale they understand.

What is not covered in this book

This book is about the principles of treating gynaecological problems, and a guide to the main herbs used. It also looks at the two most common presenting complaints in this area that most practitioners will encounter, namely PMS and the menopause. That, we hope, will still make it generally useful. We did not want this volume to be a one-stop manual for all women's problems because (in our experience) one tends to easily lose the overall picture in such a comprehensive work. Our aim has been very much to keep in mind this overall picture that applies to gynaecological problems, but in restricting the main discussion to PMS and the menopause, to use these presentations as an illustration of the principles, and as a way to make their practical application clear.

We do cover, in brief, at the end of the book, a few other diagnoses that are common and not always easy to treat: PCOS, endometriosis, uterine fibroids, and fibrocystic breasts, hopefully in enough detail to be practically useful. These and other conditions will be looked at in much more detail in a companion volume. What we will also cover in that book is the consultation and management in human terms—what is of diagnostic importance, issues of psychological and sexual health—and, although it will not be a general herbal, it will discuss herbs that are of general help without being specifically hormonal (i.e. have anti-inflammatory, circulatory or nervine properties).

Some general principles of herbal treatment

Is there a state of perfect health? Bodies constantly adapt and compensate for stresses, so it is perhaps better to think of the body working well, harmoniously rather than being in a particular state. Team sports might be a useful analogy, so just as stronger players compensate for weaker ones, so functions in the body that are not working optimally will cause compensation reactions elsewhere, but there is a risk that they will themselves get injured or exhausted if they have to do all the work. Disease may be thought of as a point of compensation that becomes obvious as it impinges on normal activity and something feels wrong.

The principles of herbal treatment of almost anything are reasonably simple in outline: alleviate symptoms, lighten the stress so that the degree of compensation need not be as extreme, and tonify organs under chronic stress. That is probably so vague as to be almost useless practically, and it needs spelling out, so let's take the case of hypertension. If blood pressure is high to the point that the patient notices it and seeks help, there are three direct symptomatic measures: smooth muscle relaxation, diuretics, and relaxants. But are the kidneys getting the blood flow they need, and if not, is it because the endothelium of their arterioles is 'sticky' and too permeable, and might that might be because the balance of prostaglandins is wrong, or that the gut is letting in too many pro-inflammatory compounds, or the adrenals are producing more glucocorticoids, or the vagus is not active enough, or there is insulin resistance, or too much sympathetic nervous system activation with too little exercise and sleep, or is it actually a picture in which all of the above play a part? The interconnections are manifold and the potential points of intervention, too. So the principles need to be applied with good knowledge of the interconnections between the pathophysiological factors, in order to decide which points of support or intervention are likely to be most important.

In terms of long-term restoration of health, herbal medicine typically treats the gut and the liver first, then the circulation, then the nervous and hormonal system, and then the problem; the reason being that one treats the neuroendocrine system by treating the liver and circulation, and one treats the liver and circulation by treating the gut. There is no hard separation between treating one system and treating another. To give one example: if blood pressure is high due to the kidneys working less well than they should, the simple addition of flaxseed to the diet will do much just by itself. It will help the gut microbiome repair the integrity of the gut wall. That in turn will decrease the load on the liver, resulting in increased clearance of potentially inflammatory substances and a consequent reduction in the level of pro-inflammatory cytokines. These cytokines affect the lipids in the blood and the tendency to inflammatory processes in the endothelium, to which the kidney vasculature is particularly susceptible. The actions of flaxseed go further than this, however, as they are a useful, balanced source of essential fatty acids. Essential fatty acids will also adjust the balance of prostaglandins away from the 2-series and towards the 3-series. A healthier gut microbiome also affects the balance of neurotransmitters and decreases food craving. This example does not begin to address the whole range of potential points of intervention but just points out the way that one single part of therapy can play a role at many levels of physiological function.

Treating gynaecological problems

How the body's biochemistry is interlinked is increasingly understood, and this underpins the rationale of traditional herbal medicine in treating the whole person, but in a coherent, structured way. In gynaecological problems, the order of initial priority is essentially the same as for this example of high blood pressure, which is a problem that actually appears commonly along with the menopause: treat the gut, the liver, the circulation, and then the nervous and endocrine systems. Again, it is not a sequential order so much as one of the priorities in terms of unloading the pressures. Longer-term, the idea is to use subtle means, and if the system is too noisy, the signal is unlikely to produce a response. The endocrine system is very sensitive and easily upset by stresses. Perhaps the most important is the health of the gut. It is not only important in terms of assimilation but also in terms of the elimination of metabolised hormones. Gut health also affects the functioning of the herbal medicines themselves as many of the phyto-oestrogenic constituents of plants are in the form of glycosides, and the active aglycone will not be bioavailable without fermentation by well-functioning gut flora. It also affects the load on the liver and in turn the composition of the blood and the activity of the immune system.

Of course, symptomatic treatment using herbs with straightforward actions, such as sage for hot flushes, may be quite effective at first and hugely important for the daily quality of life and confidence in the treatment while the unloading and improved compensation takes place.

Explanation to the patient

Attention to nutrition and the digestive system is clearly necessary from the outset; but it is equally necessary that the patient understands the point of it; otherwise, they may feel that they are being sent down a blind alley. Changing the background physiology is normally a matter of months, and that engagement is crucial for the treatment to be sustained for long enough, so it is necessary to be able to explain in simple terms why the lifestyle, dietary, and herbal changes are necessary.

Whole person treatment

This is covered in Chapter 3 in more detail, but it is worth looking at the following list at this point as Chapters 1 and 2 will point out how some of the key plants used both nutritionally and in herbal treatment fit into this strategy:

1. **Reduce the load:**
    Diet: Pre and probiotic, irritants, balanced, trigger foods
    Gut: Microbiome and rhythm (vagotonic input)
    Stress: Sympathetic nervous system not constantly dominant, review use of stimulants
    Immune system: Decrease inflammatory responses in the body
    Sleep: Quantity of sleep, quality
    Liver: Tonics and restoratives to detoxify more effectively

2. **Adjust neuroendocrine balance:**
   Phyto-oestrogenic herbs and other herbs with hormonal effects
   New research has helped shine a light on neuroendocrine interrelationships—for example, the effect of sleep and exercise on serotonin levels confirms the importance of traditional advice. Serotonin likewise has effects on oestrogen receptors, and *Cimicifuga racemosa* has serotonergic activity (See Chapter 2 for the role of serotonin, and Chapter 5 for the serotonergic effects of *Cimicifuga racemosa*). So, this gives a rationale for treatment of menopausal complaints that is now much better (though still only murkily) understood than previously. In other words, there is much new information on the many plants traditionally used for hormonal complaints, some prescribed since ancient times, and this can not only confirm but also refine their application.

3. **Increase resilience:**
   Essentially, the aim is to have a patient who finishes treatment because it is no longer needed, not only because symptoms are now absent or manageable but because the symptoms are not expected to return. The class of herbs labelled 'trophorestorative' is used to establish the health of the digestive, circulatory, nervous, and immune systems so that, provided that a healthy lifestyle and diet are followed, active intervention using herbal medicine is no longer, or is minimally, necessary.

Tradition and science

That the strengths of traditional herbal treatment are now strongly supported by current research creates a great opportunity for practitioners. The traditional rationale of herbal treatment is justified by science in many ways, in terms of these interconnections, complexity, synergy, and so on. This also means that, provided there is sufficient knowledge of scientific medicine, the treatment rationale can be explained to other medical colleagues and to patients who are under their care at the same time as being treated by the herbalist.

CHAPTER ONE

How the body produces oestrogen and progesterone

*Debunking myths about oestrogenic
and progestogenic herbs*

What is often said

1. Conditions are either oestrogen- or progesterone-related, not both
2. Phytoestrogens always have an oestrogenic effect, and so contraindicated and even dangerous in breast cancer (e.g. soya promotes breast cancer)
3. For each particular hormonally-related condition, there is a specific herb indicated for it because it has a specific hormonal action

The reality

These myths all share the same misunderstanding that hormones have fixed actions and plants directly mimic individual hormones. This is at best only partially true, but hormones constitute just part of a signalling system in which the signals interact with each other and are also subject to feedback, so the same substance may have different effects depending on the time of life and the general picture of nervous and hormonal function. Both oestrogen and progesterone levels, and their effects are interdependent to an extent, and one can affect receptors for the other. The endocrine system as a whole also interacts with other communication systems (the nervous system and the immune system in particular). Many other substances can affect sex steroid receptors, and they can affect other transmitters, a phenomenon often referred to as 'cross-talk' (an engineering term originally for phone lines, where one call picks up signals from another).

Phyto-oestrogenic plants, too, do not normally have a single effect, subtly influencing more than one factor in this neuroendocrine picture. Partly this is because they contain more than one active substance, of course, but it is also that each substance may affect more than one pathway, and affect receptors in different ways depending on the balance and concentration of hormones, for example before and after the start of the menopause.

But do not despair. Although a complete picture of all of these interactions may be impossible, the outlines are often broad and definite enough to indicate how herbs influence hormonal conditions, so long as we have a reasonable understanding of the metabolism and effects of oestrogens and progesterone. We need to begin by looking at the production of the different types of oestrogens, their role in the body, and the existence of different oestrogen receptors.

We also will get a sense of what can be known and what will remain uncertain because of excessive complexity. That picture supports the sense of a general influence rather more than of a magic bullet, and that is something herbalists are very much at home with!

Introduction to sex hormones

The function of the hormone system in women is orchestrated by the endocrine system, notably the hypothalamus, pituitary gland, adrenals, and ovaries. From the fact that overriding control rests with the hypothalamus and pituitary, in intimate connection with the rest of the brain, it is clear why the endocrine system is affected by experiences and emotions; for example, when menstruation ceases as a result of stress or trauma. There are also multiple interrelationships between the biochemical pathways that produce hormones in the adrenals and the ovaries, and so we will try to approach the picture from bottom to top, starting with those glands.

HOW THE BODY PRODUCES OESTROGEN AND PROGESTERONE

Sex hormones, derived from cholesterol, are steroidal. Cholesterol is absorbed from the gut from nutrients in the diet and also synthesised widely, predominantly in the liver. Steroid hormones share the same central part of the molecule with their cholesterol precursor, and they share the ability to pass through cell membranes and bind to nuclear receptors, sometimes the same receptors but with different effects. Production shares some common biochemical pathways, as you can see from Figure 1.1. The differences between them hormones are slight but crucial.

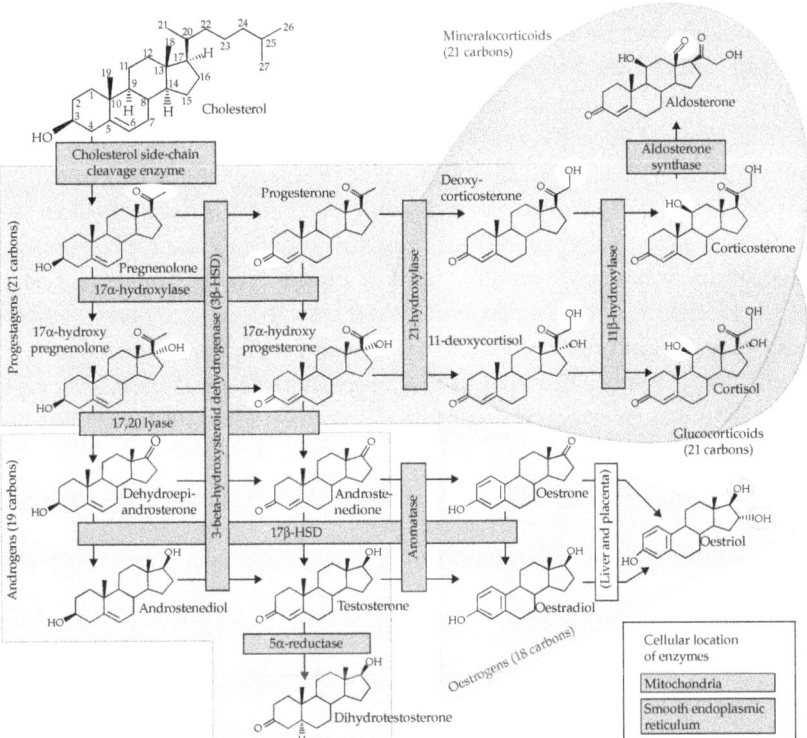

Figure 1.1: Full overview of the production of steroid hormones from cholesterol (mainly in the adrenals and in the case of sex hormones also in the gonads).
Adapted (UK English spellings applied) from: (2014). 'Diagram of the pathways of human steroidogenesis'. WikiJournal of Medicine 1 (1). DOI: 10.15347/wjm/2014.005. ISSN 20018762.

Production of oestrogens, testosterone, and progestins

To understand the production of steroid hormones (steroidogenesis), we first have to look at the function of the adrenal gland, specifically the adrenal cortex, where cholesterol is first converted to pregnenolone. Pregnenolone is then the precursor for all steroid hormones in both the liver and the gonads, as shown in Figure 1.1. Three aspects of this diagram are worth looking carefully. The first is that progesterone and the less active 17-α hydroxyprogesterone are intermediates on the pathway to the production of androstenediol, testosterone, glucocorticoids, and aldosterone. The result of being an intermediate in so many pathways is that progesterone has a half-life in the tissues of just 5 minutes, so what is critical is having a constant supply, whether that be from the corpus luteum in the ovary during the second half of the menstrual cycle, or from a progestin-only contraceptive implant or pill.

The adrenal cortex is under the control of adrenocorticotrophic hormone (ACTH), produced by the anterior pituitary, itself under the influence of the hypothalamus. ACTH is released under conditions of stress, and so stress may also directly affect progesterone levels. ACTH increases the production of pregnenolone and of progesterone but also increases the conversion of progesterone to glucocorticoids, so actually progesterone levels tend to decrease while cortisol and corticosterone increase.

A second feature to notice is that androstenedione is reversibly converted to testosterone, and oestrone is converted to oestradiol by the enzyme 17-β HSD. Oestradiol is the most biologically active of the oestrogens and predominates before the menopause except during pregnancy when oestriol is produced.

The third thing worth noticing at this point is the way that the oestrogens are produced in the tissues from either androstenedione or testosterone by the process called aromatization (so-called because the ring formed by carbons 1–6 in the androgens is converted to a resonant or aromatic structure in the oestrogens). It is not necessary to remember all the structural details or the pathways, but familiarity with the main features of Figure 1.1 will help greatly in contextualizing and understanding the rest of the discussion here.

Androstenedione and aromatization

As mentioned, androstenedione, produced in the adrenals and the ovaries, is the common precursor of oestrogens and testosterone. Levels initially rise in the adrenals in pre-puberty at age 6–8 in a phase called 'adrenarchy', in which changes in learning abilities and behaviour (in boys, especially) are quite marked, and then much more as puberty begins and the hypothalamus and puberty recruit the ovaries, too. Production of androstenedione in the ovaries is under the control of the gonadotropins produced by the anterior pituitary.

Aromatization of androstenedione to oestrone and testosterone to oestradiol is catalysed by an enzyme called P450 aromatase. Around 50% of oestrogen production before the menopause occurs in the ovaries, as oestradiol, by this pathway. After the menopause, most oestrogen is produced in the tissues in the form of oestrone, from androgens.

Glycyrrhiza glabra and *Paeonia lactiflora* in combination increase the conversion of androgen to oestrone by stimulating aromatization (so the combination is useful to use in androgen excess situation such as PCOS).

The main oestrogens

The three main oestrogens, oestradiol, oestrone, and oestriol, have marked differences in biological activity, with oestradiol being the most active.

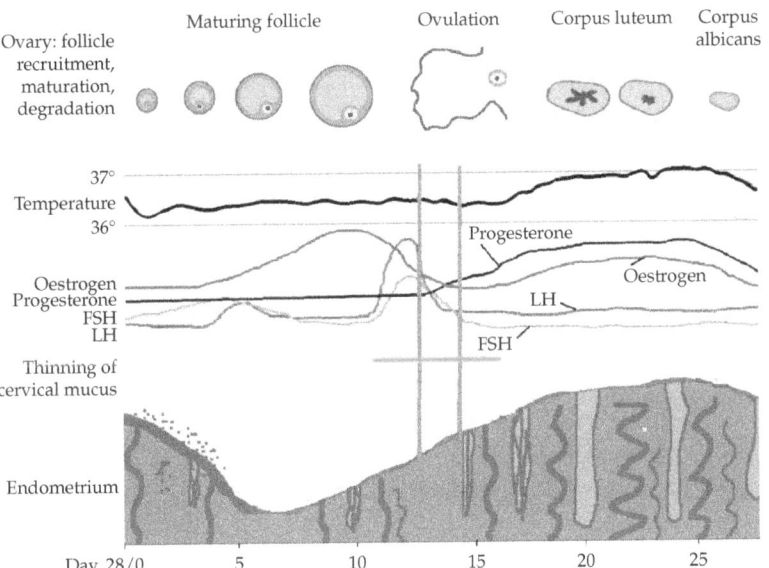

Figure 1.2: Levels of pituitary (FSH, LH) and ovarian hormones during the cycle, together with the development of the follicle and changes in body temperature and in the endometrium.

Follicle-stimulating hormone (FSH), another hormone from the anterior pituitary gland, stimulates the production of androstenedione during the first half of the menstrual cycle as the follicle grows (see Figure 1.2). Through aromatization, oestradiol thus rises in the first part of the cycle and peaks a few days before ovulation. Just before ovulation, there is a surge in FSH and luteinizing hormone (LH) levels. LH promotes ovulation and the conversion of the follicle into a corpus luteum, which secretes both oestrogen and progesterone until the corpus luteum degenerates in the second half of the cycle.

The menstrual cycle, the endometrium, mucus, and temperature

- Under the influence of oestrogen, the endometrium thickens during the first half of the cycle, and in the second half, progesterone promotes the formation of blood vessels in the endometrium.
- Body temperature increases after ovulation, broadly in line with progesterone levels, and the change in temperature can be used as a rough guide to ovulation and fertility.
- Cervical mucus becomes less viscous, with the consistency of raw egg white, from 2 days before ovulation until 2 days after.

After the menopause

As mentioned above, after the menopause most oestrogen production comes from the periphery in the form of oestrone from aromatization of androgens, but the small amount of oestrogens still produced in the ovaries appears to be much more important than used to be generally realised as loss of bone mass is particularly severe following ovariectomy as compared with the normal postmenopausal state.

Other ovarian hormones

The full range of hormones excreted in the ovaries includes not only oestrogen, progesterone, and androgens, but also:

- Inhibin, important for signalling to the pituitary to inhibit FSH secretion
- Activin and relaxin (prior to giving birth).

Oestrogen sources: main points

- Androstenedione, derived from pregnenolone and produced during the follicular phase of the menstrual cycle, is not very biologically active but is the precursor for both oestrone and testosterone in the ovaries and peripheral tissues.
- Conversion from androstenedione to oestrone (the weaker oestrogen) and from testosterone to oestradiol uses the P450 aromatase enzyme.
- Aromatization also occurs in hair follicles, skin, brain, bone, bone marrow, muscle, and fatty tissue.
- Postmenopausal women derive almost all their oestrogen (oestrone) from the aromatization of androgens outside of the ovaries.
- Very thin women may be partially deprived of this secondary source of oestrogen and may thus develop menopausal symptoms early. A body weight 15–20% below average may cause menstruation to stop.
- Excessive levels of exercise can decrease aromatization so ballet dancers and marathon runners may be at risk of osteoporosis despite doing a lot of exercise that would be expected to increase bone density.
- Low oestrogen levels may lead to an erratic menstrual cycle, reduced fertility, vaginal dryness, and decreased bone density.
- Oestradiol and oestrone are interconvertible. The other oestrogen is oestriol, which is mainly around during pregnancy.
- The potency of the different oestrogens is variable, and this variability differs between tissues, but oestradiol is by some way the most potent.

Oestrogen levels and their effects: metabolism, excess and treatment

Oestrogen's various roles in the body

Small amounts of oestrogens have a powerful effect. The development of secondary sexual characteristics, with growth in height, increase in body fat around the abdomen, hip and breasts, and the growth of uterine muscle and endometrium, are well-known examples. But oestrogen actually has many more physiological effects—steroid hormones in general pass easily through membranes, being lipid in nature themselves, and trigger a wide range of gene transcription events in many tissues: this gene response is dependent on the subtype of oestrogen receptor, co-regulators, exposure time, and amount of oestrogen, so it is both pervasive and subtle.

General effects of oestrogen

- Stimulates proliferation wherever there are oestrogen receptors, and thus leads to thickening, elastication, and lubrication of tissue in the vagina and vulva
    - Reduced oestrogen, as in the menopause, leads to vulva losing collagen, fat and water-retaining ability so flattens, thin, dry and loses tone. The vagina shortens and narrows, and the wall of vagina thins and become less elastic and paler in colour, leading to vaginal dryness, vaginal discharge, and dyspareunia.
- Makes skin and blood vessels elastic and resilient.
- Mucosal tissues such as the bladder and the lungs depend on oestrogens for secretions and elasticity
    - Hence postmenopausal women can be more prone to bladder infection or suddenly develop hay fever.
- Maintains bone strength.
- Affect nerve structure and functions in many ways (will be discussed in more detail in the section on neuroendocrine interconnections)
    - Potentiates the growth of nerves and nerve cells.
    - Supports blood flow to the brain.
    - Prevents the formation of reactive oxygen species and helps the brain use glucose.
    - Supports memory and cognition.
    - Improves mood and reduces the negative effects of stress.

Oestrogen levels tended to be lower in premenopausal women with hot flushes than those without. This picture is clearly not the whole story as after the menopause (and also during puberty) there are low oestrogen levels, but not, as a rule, hot flushes. During pregnancy, too, hot flushes can be present, but oestrogen levels are very high. One suggestion is that there is an imbalance in the beta-endorphins and other opiates in the brain which may influence temperature regulation, causing a withdrawal of opioids and triggering hot flushes. This is interesting as Cimicifuga and Vitex have effects on opioid receptors.

Common misconceptions

In general, when oestrogen is implicated in gynaecological problems, it is in terms of excess or deficiency. For example, in oestrogen-dependent cancers, one of the main targets is oestrogen excess. The idea is in some ways useful, but it can lead to frustrating and ineffective interventions. A more detailed understanding creates an opportunity for more nuanced, effective therapy.

The bigger picture

Firstly, it is important to realise that menstrual and menopausal syndromes are not entirely due to hormones and that the whole system is involved, including the nervous and digestive systems and in particular the liver (which would surprise few herbalists). Furthermore, there are not only different oestrogens but different receptor types, whose distribution and density vary over time. The next two sections try to present a more in-depth overview.

Oestrogen is metabolised in ways that depend, among other things, on lifestyle and gut flora, and the oestrogen metabolites have different actions in the body, so that clearance can also be a major factor. One particular implication of this is for oestrogen-dependent gynaecological cancers, where different oestrogens, receptors, and metabolites are responsible for both negative and positive influences of oestrogens.

It's complicated...

This is the most difficult part of this book to understand, and it may be useful to do some re-reading and note taking, perhaps with one or two comments in the margins. It is important to get as much of it as you feel you can because the rest of the book, while easier, does refer to the same concepts quite frequently. Unfortunately, some of the actions referred to will also be invalidated or clarified over time, and so those notes will also need updating from time to time!

Making it simpler

Oestrogen production and metabolism are really complex, but when they broken down into their component parts, they becomes much easier to understand. So far, we have looked at oestrogen production, but there are three other important factors influencing the activity of oestrogens, namely:

- Oestrogen metabolism and clearance, and how it may be supported or disrupted
- Environmental oestrogens and phyto-oestrogens
- The two types of oestrogen receptors

These factors are often mentioned in terms of oestrogen dominance or deficiency, and although these concepts are perhaps a bit overgeneralised, they are useful concepts in the management of hormonal conditions.

Oestrogen metabolism

Sticking to the basics

This section will be very detailed, and seem self-contradictory in places, so apologies in advance for that. The reason is that many substances, particularly flavone-rich plants, tea, and cruciferous vegetables, both speed up and slow down the metabolism of oestrogens by influencing the different pathways in opposite ways. This information is not always completely reliable, but much of it (for example regarding flavones and sulfotransferase (SULT)) is consistent. At the end of this section, we give a summary of these influences and some general guidelines for treatment, to give it practical relevance, so the detailed breakdown is really for a general background to that practical advice.

Preamble: how oestrogens are converted and carried

The body can produce oestrogens from cholesterol via various pathways, as we saw. Oestrogens are also then metabolised and removed from circulation, which has a major impact on their blood level and is one of the main factors in successful treatment. When herbs or foods are given with the aim of introducing substances with a hormonal effect, the effect on the body is entirely a matter of what the body does with the substances. In general, herbal treatment needs to adopt the idea of the organism as active and interactive. In neuroendocrine therapy, this is especially true.

It is not just how hormonal substances are metabolised that influences their relative concentrations but how they are interconverted (e.g. androgens to oestrogens) and how they are carried in the body by sex hormone binding globulin (SHBG). This binds to sex hormones, making them unavailable to the tissues, so the amount of free SHBG in circulation is critically important to the availability of hormones.

Three major stages of oestrogen metabolism

Oestrogens are mainly metabolised in the liver and excreted via bile or urine. There are three main phases, the first two in the liver, the third via the gut or kidneys.

In the liver

Phase 1: hydroxylation by CYP450 enzymes

This phase introduces a hydroxyl group (–OH) onto oestrogen, making it more hydrophilic and more readily removed by the kidneys or excreted in bile. The liver uses the same process to deal with toxins and drugs (although some of the CYP enzymes are mostly extrahepatic). Phase 1 is catalysed by enzymes: the cytochrome P450 (CYP450) enzyme group, found on the membrane system of hepatocytes.

The process can cause oxidative damage within cell systems because of the formation of reactive, electrophilic molecules, and it is important that Phase 2 metabolism can keep up with Phase 1 metabolism.

Phase 2: conjugation (methylation, sulfation, glucuronidation)

Products of Phase 1 detoxification need to be detoxified by Phase 2 reactions, using methyl groups, sulphate groups, or glucuronides. Phase 2 metabolites are water soluble and unreactive and excreted primarily in the bile or in the urine.

Clearance

Conjugated oestrogens are eliminated either via the urine or via the bile and subsequently excreted via the bowel, meaning that the liver and the gut are both important targets for herbal treatment.

Metabolism of hormones (in refernce to oestrogens)

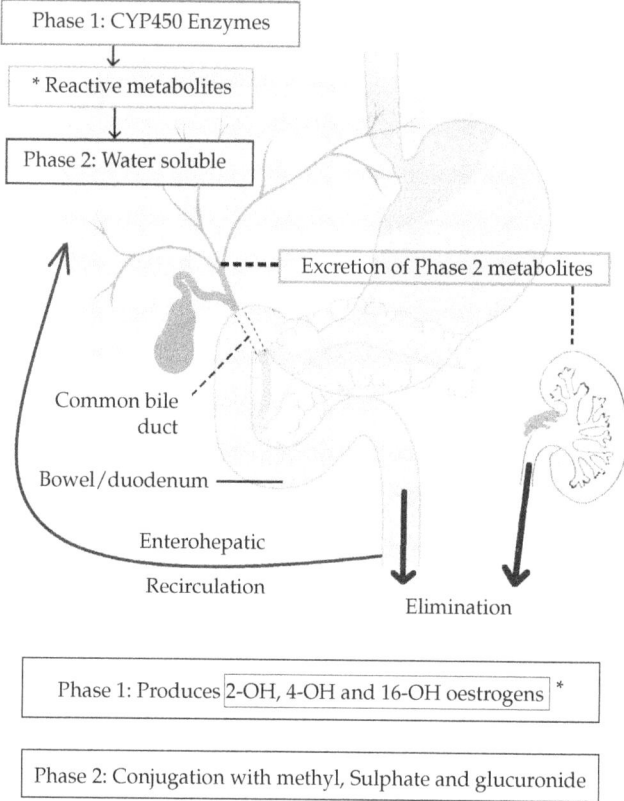

Figure 1.3: Metabolism of hormones, production of inflammatory intermediates, and enterohepatic recirculation.

The three stages are discussed in detail below and shown in Figure 1.3.

Phase 1 metabolism: hydroxylation

Phase 1 produces a range of oestrogen metabolites, grouped together as the:

- 2-hydroxyoestrogens
- 4-hydroxyoestogens
- 16-hydroxyoestrogens

The ratio depends on which of the CYP450 enzymes in individuals leads to differences in the levels of each of those metabolites.

2-OH Oestrogens

Conversion to 2-OH oestrogens is catalysed by CYP 1A1, and CYP 1A2 (Cytochrome P450 1A1 and 1A2). These enzymes are responsible for metabolizing many other compounds (for example, CYP 1A2 is responsible for metabolising caffeine).

The 2-OH oestrogens have a low binding affinity for the oestrogen receptor (ER) and are widely seen as 'good oestrogens', with non-oestrogenic and anti-oestrogenic activities. They inhibit cell growth and are associated with normal cell differentiation and apoptosis.

So far, there is insufficient data to confirm the role of oestrogen metabolites as predictors of breast cancer, but it seems likely that 2-OH oestrogens tend not to promote and may inhibit development of oestrogen-sensitive cancers whereas the 4-OH and 16-OH metabolites tend to promote it.

It is important to bear in mind that all the products of Phase 1 metabolism are intermediates and are normally converted rapidly to their corresponding Phase 2 metabolites. That conversion can be affected by various nutrients (as shown in Table 1.1).

Table 1.1: Detailed look at nutrients affecting Cytochrome P450 1A1 and 1A2 enzyme activity

Effect on enzyme	Substance(s) or other factors
CYP1A1 inducers	*Clinical studies:* • Cruciferous vegetables, indole–3-carbinole (brassica vegetables)[1,2] • Resveratrol[3] (found in grapes, wine, peanuts, soy) • Normalizing body weight,[4] exercise[5,6]
CYP1A1 is mainly extrahepatic	*In vivo experiments:* • Green and black tea • Curcumin (0.1% of the diet) • Soybeans (100mg/kg)

(Continued)

Table 1.1: Continued

Effect on enzyme	Substance(s) or other factors
CYP1A1 inhibitor (*in vivo*) could reduce CYP1A1 overactivity (so are a modulator)	• Garlic, rosemary • Astaxanthin (algae, yeast, salmon, trout, shrimp) • Fish oil, Omega 3,[7] flaxseed[8] • Black raspberry, blueberry, ellagic acid (high in berries, pomegranate, grapes, walnuts, black currants) • Black soybeans (1g/kg) • Turmeric (diet of 1% turmeric) • Theaflavins (20mg/kg)
CYP1A2 inducers	***Clinical studies:*** • Cruciferous vegetables[9–11] ***In vivo experiments:*** • Green and black tea • Chicory root • Astaxanthin (algae, yeast, salmon, trout, shrimp)
CYP1A2 inhibitors possibly diminish excessive CYP1A2 action (modulation).	• Apiaceous vegetables[12] (carrots, fresh celery, parsnips, dill and parsley) • Quercetin 500mg[13] (apple, apricot, blueberries, yellow onions, kale, green beans, broccoli, black tea, chilli powder) • Daidzein (400mg)[14] • Grapefruit[15] ***In vivo experiments:*** • Kale, garlic, chamomile, peppermint, dandelion, and turmeric.

2-OH oestrone will be methylated to 2-methoxyoestrone (which seems to slow tumour growth by inhibiting angiogenesis); 2-OH oestradiol is similarly converted to 2-methoxyoestradiol, which has significant anti-tumour properties.

Interpretation needs to be careful, however, because isolates might be different to foods, and some substances have a biphasic effect, i.e. opposite effects depending on the quantity.[16]

4-OH oestrogens

The 4-OH oestrogens are produced by CYP 1B1 enzymes and rapidly converted to DNA-damaging quinones. CYP1B1 is expressed in high frequency in various human cancers, but not in normal tissue. High circulating levels of 4-OH oestrogens also cause oxidative metabolism of oestradiol and oxidative DNA damage. Phase 2 metabolism of 4-OH oestrogens creates 4-methoxyestrogens which prevent that damage.

So, there is good reason to suppose that the inhibition of CYP 1B1 could be a very useful therapeutic measure, particularly if Phase 2 is not adequate to remove the 4-OH oestrogens quickly.

Table 1.2: Details of nutrients affecting Cytochrome P450 1B1 enzyme activity

Effect on enzyme	*Substance(s) or other factors*
CYP 1B1 inducer (*in vivo*)	• Curcumin • Cruciferous vegetables • Ginseng
CYP1B1 inhibitors (*in vivo* and *in vitro*)	• Quercetin, green tea • Chrysoeriol[17] (rooibos tea and celery) • Avoidance of polycyclic aromatic hydrocarbons[18]

16-OH oestrogens

The 16-OH oestrogens (produced as a result of the action of enzymes CYP 2C and 3A4) are considered to be more strongly oestrogenic than oestradiol and associated with excess cellular proliferation, DNA damage, and carcinogenicity. These levels are found to be higher in the presence of chemical contaminants, such as environmental oestrogens.[19]

Obesity, low thyroid function, and pesticide exposures are associated with higher levels of 16-OH oestrogens. However, as always, the picture is not 100% 'this is good, and that is bad': in South Asian women this metabolite is associated with increased protection from osteopaenia (one of a number of differences in enzyme pathways).

Table 1.3: Details of nutrients affecting Cytochrome P450 3A4 enzyme activity

Effect on enzyme	Substance(s) or other factors
CYP3A4 inducer	• Curcumin, hyperforin
	• Environmental oestrogens
CYP3A4 inhibitor *(clinical studies)*	• Grapefruit,[20] resveratrol[21]
	• Garden cress[22]
	• Soybean[23]
CYP3A4 inhibitor *(in vivo studies)*	• Kale[24]
	• Myricetin[25] (onions, berries, grapes, red wine)
	• Green and black tea

Experimental studies have suggested a link between concentrations of individual metabolites or the ratio of specific metabolites to the risk of breast cancer, and in particular that a decrease in the urinary 2/16α-hydroxyoestrone ratio could be a risk marker for breast cancer.[26] A systematic review did not support the hypothesis, however, noting the presence of possibly carcinogenic 4-hydroxyoestogrens as a potential confounding factor.

One can get a bit lost in this maze of different enzymes, and potential dietary inhibitors and stimulants, in which case perhaps the most important message is the traditional one: eat your greens, and vegetables, pulses, teas, berries, and have healthy food as a whole in one's diet! Perhaps the main thing to note is the action of green tea and resveratrol (e.g. in grape skins) in particular in inducing CYP 1A1 and inhibiting CYP 1B1 and CYP 3A4 enzymes, so shifting the balance towards the 2-OH metabolites. It is also perhaps worth noting that most of the metabolites, particularly of the CYP 3A4 pathway, are very short-lived if the liver is generally working well, as the reactions are tightly coupled with Phase 2 conjugation, which detoxifies these intermediates.

Phase 2 conjugation

Products of Phase 1 metabolism need to be detoxified by Phase 2 reactions, which add methyl groups, sulphate groups, or glucuronides.

Phase 2 metabolites are relatively unreactive, being water soluble, and are excreted primarily in the bile or in the urine.

1. Methylation

Catechol-O-methyltransferase COMT (a Phase 2 enzyme) conjugates hydroxyoestrogens into non-genotoxic methoxyoestrogens.[27] The activity of COMT depends on gender, age and physiological status, and supporting COMT function may be an important focus of treatment.

Table 1.4: Details of nutrients affecting COMT enzyme activity

Effect on COMT	Substance/factor
Promote COMT activity	Vitamins B_6 and B_{12}, methionine (e.g. in legumes and onions), betaine, folic acid, magnesium
Inhibition of COMT and other methylation enzymes	A high-sucrose diet
Level and type influence the risk of breast cancer and of mood disorders	Genetic variations

2. Sulfation

Sulphotransferases (SULTs) are responsible for the transfer of a sulphuryl group to hydroxyl or amine groups, a process known as either sulfation or sulphurylation. Decreased function of these enzymes can lead to eventual interference with thyroid hormone, oestrogen, and androgen levels.

In the case of oestrogens, sulfation can increase the amount of circulating oestrogens but can also decrease their availability to some tissues, as will be explained below. If inadequate sulphate is in the diet, there will be a smaller total amount of circulating oestrogen.

Sulfation of oestrogens is reversible. Thus, for tissues with sulfatase capabilities, circulating sulfated oestrogens effectively form a pool of oestrogens, as these tissues can hydrolyse them to release free oestrogens, while for other tissues the sulfated oestrogens cannot be utilised. So, tissues with high levels of sulfatase may have elevated oestrogenic effects even though blood levels of free oestrogens are normal. Soy isoflavone supplements are said by some to increase locally available oestrogens in breast and other tissues as they lower SULT levels and so may decrease the total pool of circulating oestrogens that are sulphated.

3. Glucuronidation

UDP-glucuronosyltransferases (UGTs) add glucuronides to the Phase 1 oestrogen metabolites to make them soluble and allow them to be cleared by the kidneys or the bile. In the gut, certain bacteria produce beta-glucuronidase, breaking down the glucuronide molecule (deconjugation) and allowing the oestrogen to be reabsorbed as it becomes more lipid-soluble, a phenomenon known as enterohepatic recirculation.

Table 1.5: Details of nutrients affecting SULT enzyme activity

Effect on SULT	*Substance/factor*
Induction	Caffeine[28] and retinoic acid[29] (the bioactive form of vitamin A) (*in vivo studies*).
SULT inhibitors (but there is conflicting evidence)	Wine, anthocyanins and flavonols, citrus fruits, synthetic food colours (especially red), apple and grape juice, catechins, epigallocatechin gallate, quercetin, curcumin, resveratrol, flavonoids (apigenin, chrysin, fisetin, galangin, kaempferol, quercetin, myricetin, naringenin, and naringin), certain phyto-oestrogens (daidzein, genistein), and caffeic acid. Xenoestrogenic compounds often inhibit SULT.
Sources of inorganic sulphate necessary for the production of SULT	Fish, meat, eggs, cheese, lentils, peas, oatmeal, cabbages, leeks, spinach, brazil nuts, almonds, ginger and mustard.

Many studies note that effects are variable depending on both gender and genotype[30] so this means that the effect of diet on UGTs may be a little uncertain—but then again many of these substances have a broad range of effects and so it would be hard to differentiate this particular action in an individual patient.

Elimination

Conjugated oestrogens are eliminated either via the urine or via the bile and excreted via the bowel (note here, the potential of *Taraxacum radix* and other cholagogues and choleretics).

Table 1.6: Details of nutrients affecting UGT and β glucuronidase enzyme activity

Effect on glucuronidation	Substance/factor
Induction	Cruciferous vegetables,[31] resveratrol,[32] and citrus fruits[33] (clinical studies). Some of this stimulating effect is restricted to individuals with low baseline enzyme levels or activity, suggesting that some phytochemicals may be modulators. Possibly also dandelion,[34] rooibos tea, honeybush tea, rosemary, soy, ellagic acid, ferulic acid, curcumin, and astaxanthin (salmon, shrimps) (*in vivo* studies).
Inhibition of reversal (deconjugation) in the gut by β glucuronidase so decreasing reabsorption of oestrogen (enterohepatic recirculation). May help limit cancer risk	Foods containing glucaric acid (broccoli, brussels sprouts, oranges and grapefruit, cherries, apples, and spinach), from *in vivo* research; polyphenol extracts of certain berries (strawberries and blackcurrant).[35]

The gut microbiome is of key importance: a healthy gut flora[36] reduces the activity of beta-glucuronidase (meaning for the practitioner, attention to gut health, diet, and pre- and probiotics).[37] After deconjugation, they are either excreted or reabsorbed back into the bloodstream. Constipation will increase the amount reabsorbed.

Availability of oestrogens

Sex hormone binding globulin (SHBG)

Oestrogen induces production of SHBG, which then binds it and carries it in the bloodstream. Oestrogens bound to SHBG are inactive. Increasing the circulating SHBG thus causes a decrease in the amount of available oestrogen.

Endogenous factors affecting the level of SHBG

- Enterohepatic recirculation may stimulate production in the liver of oestrogen-induced proteins such as SHBG.
- Insulin lowers the production of SHBG, so overproduction of insulin (associated with incipient Type 2 diabetes), can raise the level of free oestrogens.
- Glucocorticoids and growth hormone also lower SHBG levels.
- After the menopause, oestrogen levels are lower and the ratio of testosterone to oestrogen higher. This causes a decrease in SHBG, making what oestrogen there is more available and thereby keeping the low levels of oestrogen functional for longer in tissue.
- Thyroxine and oral oestrogen increase SHBG.
- SHBG in the luteal phase has been positively associated with craving sweet and carbohydrate-rich foods.[38]

Diet, lifestyle and SHBG

- Foods that are high in lignans (for example, flaxseed and sesame) can increase the level of sex hormone binding globulin. A marked increase in serum levels of SHBG have been observed in a phyto-oestrogen-rich diet (soybean and flaxseed) group (clinical study).[39]
- Olive oil consumption is associated with elevated SHBG serum levels.[40]

- Low glycaemic index diets, with low sugar and high fibre content, may be associated with higher serum SHBG concentrations among postmenopausal women.[41]
- Serum concentration of sex hormone binding globulin is inversely related to weight, and according to *in vivo* studies is inversely related to protein intake.[42]
- Greater consumption of total red and fresh red meat and dairy products influences circulating concentrations of SHBG and oestradiol, lowers SHBG levels, and thus increases circulating concentrations of oestradiol.[43]

Table 1.7: Details of nutrients and endogenous factors affecting SHBG levels in the blood

Effect on SHBG levels	Substance or process
Increase—resulting in higher levels of free circulating sex hormones	Enterohepatic recirculation
	Thyroxine and oral oestrogen
	Olive oil
	Low glycaemic index diets, low sugar, high fibre
	Lignans, phyto-oestrogen-rich diet
	Low levels of oestrogen and testosterone
	Obesity
Decrease—resulting in lower levels of free circulating sex hormones	Red meat and dairy products

Aromatase

Aromatase (CYP19) is the enzyme responsible for aromatization of androgens into oestrogens. The enzyme is found in the gonads (granulosa cells), brain, adipose tissue, placenta, blood vessels, skin, and bone. It is also found in endometriosis tissue, uterine fibroids, breast cancer, and endometrial cancer. The effect is not systemic as a rule but makes oestrogen available to these local tissues without the raising the blood level of oestrogen. In the case of osteoporosis, for example, testosterone will stimulate the osteoblastic bone building, while oestrogen inhibits osteoclastic reabsorption.

Factors that inhibit or increase aromatization

Table 1.8: Details of nutrients and endogenous factors affecting aromatase activity in tissues

Increasing aromatization	Inhibiting aromatization
Intake of excess energy and obesity	Cox-2 inhibitors: • omega-3 fatty acids • low-dose aspirin
Insulin (related to sugar intake)	Prolactin
Gonadotropins	Anti-Müllerian hormone
Fatty acid precursors of inflammatory prostaglandins concentrated in red meat (arachidonate), milk, eggs	Many flavones, flavanones, chalcones, and xanthones: • Resveratrol[44] • Flaxseed lignans[45] • White button mushrooms[46] • Grapes and/or wine[47] • *Garcinia mangostana* L. (mangosteen)[48] • Flavonoids, e.g. in Ginkgo,[49] Chrysin, Apigenin[50] • Catechin in green tea[51] • Isoliquiritigenin (in liquorice)[52] Glyphosate (systemic herbicide)

Reducing aromatase activity:
- Adipose tissue has aromatase activity, hence the importance of maintaining a healthy body weight.
- Regulation of insulin and glucose metabolism is important.
- Aromatase activity in fibroids and endometriosis is stimulated by the pro-inflammatory prostaglandin PGE-2, so reducing inflammatory processes is crucial in these oestrogen excess conditions.

Increasing aromatase activity:
- Vitex will increase activity by lowering prolactin levels, and Paeonia and Glycyrrhiza will increase activity via stimulating aromatase as well as by lowering prolactin levels.

Summary of dietary influences on oestrogen metabolism

Table 1.9: Nutritional influences on Phase 1 and 2 metabolism and reabsorption of oestrogens

Substance(s) or other factors	Effect
Cruciferous vegetables, soybeans **Resveratrol** **Green and black tea** Garlic, rosemary Astaxanthin (algae, yeast, salmon, trout, shrimp) Fish oil, Omega 3, flaxseed	CYP1A1 & CYP1A2 inducers, increasing metabolism of oestrogens to 2-OH oestrogen metabolites
Ellagic acid (high in berries, pomegranate, grapes, walnuts, black currants) Possibly apiaceous vegetables, e.g. carrots Possibly **quercetin** (apple, apricot, blueberries, yellow onions, kale, green beans, broccoli, chilli) Daidzein Grapefruit	CYP1A1 & CYP1A2 inhibitors: less conversion of oestrogensto 2-OH oestrogen metabolites
Cruciferous vegetables	CYP 1B1 inducer: more production of 4-OH oestrogens
Ginseng **Green tea**, chrysoeriol (rooibos and celery)	CYP1B1 inhibitors: less production of 4-OH oestrogens
Curcumin, hyperforin	CYP3A4 inducer: more production of 16-OH oestrogens
Grapefruit, **resveratrol** Garden cress, kale, soybeans Myricetin (onions, berries, grapes, red wine) **Green and black tea**	CYP3A4 inhibitor—less production of 16-OH oestrogens

(*Continued*)

Table 1.9: Continued

Substance(s) or other factors	Effect
COMT activity depends on vitamins B_6 and B_{12}, methionine (e.g. in **legumes and onions**), betaine, folic acid and magnesium.	**Increased methylation** of Phase 1 metabolites in liver and tissues
A high-sucrose diet may inhibit methylation enzymes such as COMT.	**Decreased methylation** of Phase 1 metabolites
SULT inducers include caffeine and retinoic acid. Activity is dependent on sulphate (**protein-rich food**, oatmeal, **cabbages**, leeks, spinach, nuts, almonds).	**Increased sulfation** of oestrogen metabolites from Phase 1
Many antioxidant substances have been reported as **SULT inhibitors**, including **quercetin**, curcumin, **resveratrol**, flavonoids and caffeic acid. Phyto-oestrogens (daidzein, genistein). Xenoestrogenic compounds often inhibit SULT.	**Decreased sulfation** of oestrogen metabolites from Phase 1 (some possibly theoretical)
UGTs are induced by **cruciferous vegetables**, resveratrol, and citrus as foods.	**Increased glucuronidation** of Phase 1 oestrogen metabolites
Foods containing glucaric acid (**apples and grapefruit, cruciferous vegetables**) and polyphenol extracts of certain berries (**strawberries** and **blackcurrant**s) may **inhibit intestinal beta-glucuronidase activity** and **decrease enterohepatic recirculation**.	Decreased **enterohepatic recirculation** (may help limit cancer risk) and **reduce excess oestrogen** syndromes.
Resveratrol, grapes, wine Flaxseed lignans White button mushrooms, green tea	**Decrease** conversion of androgens to oestrogen in tissues by **aromatization**

Dietary recommendations for oestrogen conjugation and clearance
- Looking at the table of effects of foods on the CYP450 and Phase 2 enzymes, it looks at first like a mass of contradictions. In particular, many of the antioxidants seem to inhibit the sulfation of metabolites. In reality, the two phases are mostly quite tightly locked, so it is best not to overemphasise the effects of foods, but there are a few key points about metabolism that are very useful:
    - **Cruciferous vegetables** encourage metabolism by CYP1A1 and CYP1A2 enzymes, and so favour the creation of 2-OH metabolites which are generally thought to be the least damaging (but stimulate 4-OH production, too). They induce glucuronidation, inhibit recirculation of oestrogen metabolites and are a useful source of sulphur for sulfation.
    - **Green and black tea** also favour 2-OH production over 4-OH and 16-OH, and green tea inhibits aromatization.
    - The damage caused by Phase 1 metabolites is through oxidative stress. Antioxidants (curcumin, resveratrol and flavonoids) have mixed effects on the various metabolic pathways but have a very wide range of health benefits particularly for the circulatory system and tend to inhibit recirculation—but it is best to encourage a range of different antioxidant foods, so there is no risk of disproportionate inhibition of one particular pathway. Many of these foods decrease aromatization.
    - **Onions, leeks, garlic** are a useful source of sulphur, too, but particularly promote methylation by COMT and are strongly worth recommending.
    - **B vitamins** are important for Phase 2 conjugation.
- Most metabolites can be reabsorbed if they are split and made lipid-soluble so the gut bacteria are extremely important, at least as much as and probably more than the enzymes.
    - **Saturated animal fat** is associated with colonic bacteria that produce enzyme beta-glucuronidase.[53] These then deconjugate the glucuronated oestrogens, leading to greater recirculation of oestrogen, which is probably why high fat intake is related to breast cancer,[54] excessive menstruation, endometriosis,[55] fibroids.
    - **Vegetarians** normally have lower levels of beta-glucuronidase[56] activity in the colon as they have a more varied and friendlier microflora.

- ○ **Dietary fibre** increases elimination as it binds metabolites and leads to lower oestrogen levels—although excessive consumption can lead to low levels of all hormones and to anovulation.[57]

Lifestyle and oestrogen metabolism

- **Body weight:**
  - ○ **Obesity** interferes with ovarian function and is linked to greater conversion of androgen to oestrogen. Obesity also accelerates Phase 1 metabolism of oestrogens.
  - ○ **Higher upper body fat** is linked to reduced SHBG, so oestrogen is more readily available.
  - ○ **Low body mass**: 15–20kg below the ideal causes of interference with the cycle, low fertility, and decreased bone density.
- **Antibiotics** affect the gut flora, as does the contraceptive pill[58] affecting not only enterohepatic recirculation but phyto-oestrogen absorption.
- **Vitamin A deficiency**[59] leads to decreased activity of 3-beta hydrogenase in the ovaries, vital for the production of oestradiol in ovaries, and thus reduces serum oestrogen.
- **Over-exercising**[60] decreases body fat and causes amenorrhoea and low bone density.
- **Smoking**[61] is associated with earlier menopause and a higher incidence of osteoporosis. Smoking lowers progesterone metabolite levels in smokers during the luteal phase, leads to the elevation of FSH and shortening of the follicular phase, and to inadequate corpus luteum function. This pattern of higher FSH levels and shorter cycles in smokers is also consistent with the observation that smokers tend to experience an earlier menopause. The decreased progesterone and perturbation of FSH both indicate a reason for reduced fertility in smokers.
- **B vitamin deficiency**[62] increases oestrogen levels, perhaps because it is needed for normal liver function.
- **Alcohol**[63] in moderation is related to reduced oestrogen levels, lower incidence of uterine cancer in obese woman, but an increase in breast cancer. Alcohol in the menopause is associated with more severe hot flushes.

Excess oestrogen symptoms and conditions

High oestrogen levels are associated with:

- Menorrhagia (heavier and longer than usual menstruation)
- PMS
- Endometriosis
- Fibroids
- Menstrual irregularities: amenorrhea, abnormal vaginal bleeding
- Fibrocystic breast disease
- Breast and endometrial cancer

It is important to note that even relatively high levels of oestrogens are not reliably detected in a single blood test.

Endogenous and iatrogenic causes of excess oestrogens

Exposure of tissues to oestrogen in women nowadays is much higher on average than in previous ages. For one thing, although the age of menopause has not changed, menarche starts earlier. In 1840, it was at 16.5 years on average, and in 1990 it was 12.8 years.

The cause is probably food availability, as the mean weight when periods start is 47.8kg. This is not the only reason that women today have more menstrual periods than their ancestors; the main one is the amount of time spent in pregnancy and lactation, and it has been estimated that in previous centuries most women had only 20% or so of the number of menstrual cycles that would be normal today.

Environmental oestrogens

Xenoestrogens are oestrogen-mimicking compounds found particularly in cosmetic products, pesticides, and plastics,[64] binding to oestrogen receptors. We are exposed to these environmental oestrogens throughout our lives, even before birth, as they are not only part of our household environment in the form of fragrances, foodstuffs, and packaging, but also in the water and air as a result of industrial processing and incineration, particularly of waste. These ubiquitous oestrogenic compounds may be another factor, alongside food availability, responsible for reducing the age of menarchy and increasing the risk of oestrogen excess illnesses. They are also strongly implicated in the decline of male fertility not only of humans but also of fish and mammals.

Being lipid-soluble, xeno-oestrogens accumulate over the years in fatty tissue and tend to be higher in people who consume lots of meat.[65] Pesticides, for example, can mimic oestrogens, and levels of DDT and persistent organic pollutants have been found to be higher in fibroid tissue than in normal tissue.[66]

Pharmaceutical oestrogens (hormone replacement therapy and the contraception pill) also find their way into the environment. Singly, xeno-oestrogens may have little effect, but a combination of environmental oestrogens can exert effects 1,000 times more potent than any individual compound.

When assessing diet and lifestyle, it may be practical to regard substances that disrupt hormonal metabolism as environmental oestrogens, as well as those with direct oestrogenic effects.

Ways to avoid environmental oestrogens (as far as possible):

- Eat organic fruit and vegetables to avoid pesticides, herbicides, and fungicides (wash food with a biodegradable, non-toxic solution if not organic).
- Use glass or ceramic containers to store food, do not leave food or drink in plastic containers (worse if left in the sun).
- Don't buy food wrapped in plastic, do not cook or buy ready-made meals in plastic containers.
- Avoid buying food and drink in plastic or Styrofoam containers.
- Avoid tinned foods.
- Do not heat food in plastic containers.
- Do not use clingfilm, especially avoid cheese and fatty foods in clingfilm.
- Replace chemical-based household cleaning products with natural products (e.g. lemon juice, baking soda, vinegar).
- Buy hormone-free, organic meat, and dairy, avoid fat on meat or poultry where the chemicals accumulate.
- Avoid food and drink with artificial additives.

Source	Substance and mode of action	Effect
Cows' milk and other dairy and meat products	Cows lactate during the latter half of pregnancy when there is a high concentration of oestrogens in blood, and thus in the milk.	Meat, milk and cheese intake has been associated with breast cancer. Milk and cheese are also linked with a raised risk ovarian and uterine cancer.[67]
Cigarette smoke	Methylnitrosamino-pyridyl-butanone (**NNK**) stimulates ER α and β receptors; cotinine, a nicotine metabolite, is an aromatase inhibitor.	NNK is associated with lung adenocarcinoma particularly in women, via CYP 450 1B1.[68] Cotinine decreases oestrogen end increases testosterone levels.[69]
Traffic emissions chemicals	Polycyclic aromatic hydrocarbons (**PAH**) are oestrogen ligand active compounds present in polluted air.	Affect oestrogen homeostasis.[70]
Industrial emissions and industrial products: processed food, nickel/cadmium batteries, pigments, and plastics[71]	**Cadmium, arsenic and heavy metals**: lower progesterone levels and bind to ER α.	Cadmium has been linked to renal cancer in people with a particular ER α polymorphism.[72]

(*Continued*)

Source	Substance and mode of action	Effect
Plastics and cans	**Styrene** and its metabolites bind to ER α.	Styrene has been associated with breast cancer risk (men and women).[73] Transplacental exposure to low levels of styrene may lead to the disturbed development of male reproductive organs.[74]
Aluminium-containing antiperspirants	**Aluminium salts** are a metalloestrogen.[75]	May be a risk factor for the development of breast cancer.
Cosmetics, such as lipsticks and moisturisers; food preservatives	**BHT** (butylated hydroxytoluene) is thought to mimic oestrogen.[76]	May prevent expression of male sex hormones,[77] resulting in adverse reproductive affects.
Cosmetics and nail polish	**DBP** (Dibutyl phthalate), a plasticiser, now banned in the EU from this use.	DBP can enhance the capacity of other chemicals to cause genetic, developmental defects, changes in the testes and prostate and reduced sperm counts.[78] Suspected endocrine disruptor as it interferes with hormone function, and toxic to reproduction as it may cause foetal harm and impair fertility.[79]

HOW THE BODY PRODUCES OESTROGEN AND PROGESTERONE 31

Fragrance in cosmetics and household products such as detergents, softeners and cleaning products	**DEP** (diethyl phthalate) is suspected of interfering with hormone function, causing reproductive and developmental problems.[80]	Phthalates have been linked to reduced sperm count in men and reproductive defects in the developing male foetus (mother exposed during pregnancy), among other health effects.[81]
Preservatives in cosmetics, very widespread	**Parabens** penetrate the skin and are suspected of interfering with hormone function.[82]	Detected in human breast cancer tissues,[83] suspected of interfering with male reproductive functions.[84]
Cosmetics to soften, smooth and moisten: hair products, deodorant creams, moisturisers and facial treatments	**Siloxanes**: cyclotetrasiloxane, cyclopentasiloxane, cyclohexasiloxane and cyclomethicone are endocrine disruptors.[85]	May impair human fertility.
Antiperspirants, cleansers and hand sanitisers, cosmetics, soap, toothpaste, deodorants Also in household products, toys, mattresses, toilet fixtures, clothing, furniture fabric, paints, laundry detergent, facial tissues, and cosmetics	**Triclosan** (5-chloro-2-(2,4-dichlorophenoxy) phenol is a broad-spectrum antibacterial that can pass through skin, and through mucosa of the gastrointestinal tract and mouth. It is suspected of interfering with hormone function (endocrine disruption).	The extensive use of triclosan in products may contribute to an increase in the prevalence of antibiotic-resistant bacteria. Triclosan does not readily degrade. Several studies have found it in urine, serum, and breast milk.[86] Triclosan may play a role in cancer development, possibly due to oestrogenic effects or due to its ability to inhibit fatty acid synthesis.

(Continued)

Source	Substance and mode of action	Effect
Polycarbonate (used to make CDs, spectacles lenses, water bottles and many other consumer products requiring a clear plastic) and resins such as the material used to line food cans to prevent corrosion. May be present in plastics marked with recycle codes 3 or 7	Bisphenol A (**BPA**), and polychlorinated biphenyls (**PCBs**) are endocrine disruptors and bind to ER α and β. Now banned from production or use in specific products, such as baby bottles,[87] they are otherwise still in widespread use. Can leach into foods; lining of cans and food containers and bottles made from certain plastics especially when heated or abraded by cleaning.	Associated with breast and prostate cancers, genital defects in males, early onset of puberty in females, obesity and behavioural problems such as attention-deficit hyperactivity disorder. They are metabolised quickly, and there is some debate as to how strong a cumulative effect BPAs have, but it is certainly best to avoid using them with hot foods or environments, e.g. microwaves or the dishwasher as the plastic may break down over time and allow BPA to leach into foods.
Flame retardants in soft furnishings	Polybrominated diphenyl ethers or **PBDEs**.	Have been measured in human milk.[88]
Pesticides	Many different ones exist, and affects hormonal dysregulation in many ways, and disrupt the hormonal function of the female reproductive system and in particular the ovarian cycle.	Epidemiological studies suggest exposure to pesticides is associated with menstrual cycle disturbances, reduced fertility, prolonged time-to-pregnancy, spontaneous abortion, stillbirths, and developmental defects. Also, occupational exposures to pesticides appear to have adverse effects on female reproduction.[89]

- Use natural, chemical free cosmetics. Avoid nail polish and nail polish removers. Use organic soaps and toothpaste, and naturally-based perfumes.
- Avoid artificial solvents.
- Use natural pest control.
- Avoid birth control pills and conventional oestrogen replacement therapy (ERT, HRT).
- Do not use spermicide.
- Avoid surfactants found in many condoms and diaphragm gels.
- Avoid exposure to new carpets.
- Avoid fabric softeners, use simple laundry and dish detergent with less chemical.
- Avoid exposure to gases from copiers and printers, carpets, etc.
- Use a high-quality water filter in your home.
- Avoid phthalates in cosmetics.
- Use products that do not list 'perfume' or 'fragrance' as an ingredient.
- Products marketed as 'fragrance-free' or 'unscented' may nonetheless contain fragrance ingredients, so try to find brands you can trust.

Excess oestrogens: a summary of possible causes

- Environmental oestrogen effects (pesticides in foods, plastics, e.g. clingfilm wrap, especially on fatty foods).
- **Relative excess**, i.e. particularly where progesterone is low.
- Diet and lifestyle:
    - Saturated animal fats (higher β-glucuronidase: increasing recirculation).
    - Refined carbohydrates: low fibre leads to constipation and more recirculation of the endogenous oestrogens; high-sucrose content can lead to suppression of COMT.
    - B_6 Deficiency: the liver is not able to metabolise oestrogen and thus increases the susceptibility of breast, and uterine tissue, to the effects of oestrogen.
    - Obesity leads to more conversion of androgen to oestrogen.
    - High upper body fat reduces SHBG, increasing the number of free oestrogens.

- Metabolic syndrome increases insulin levels, which also lower SHBG.
- Lack of exercise increases the level of circulating oestrogens.
- Unhealthy gut flora decreases phytoestrogen accessibility and increases the recycling of endogenous oestrogen.

Medical causes should also be eliminated, particularly

- Ovarian tumours
- Aromatase excess syndrome (familial hyperoestrogenism)
- Liver cirrhosis

Oestrogen receptors, and phyto-oestrogens

Working with new research findings about hormonal herbs

As the level of precision in molecular research increases, the complexity of knowledge increases. The scientific principle involved here is the inverse relationship between accuracy and precision: the vaguer you are, the less likely you are to be wrong. But as tools available to scientists improve, previous scientific statements start to appear overgeneralised. New cell and receptor subtypes and details of their biochemical interrelationships are emerging all the time, but this can mean that the overall picture is hard to see.

Given our long familiarity with herbs that have effects on hormonal activity, it is tempting to rewrap existing ideas in new terms. For example, it has been assumed that Vitex is a progestogenic herb, and must increase LH or interact with progesterone receptors. This is widely stated by health websites and practitioners, and it 'feels' true. Likewise, we may be tempted to talk about black cohosh having a balanced effect on oestrogen receptors. In both cases, these explanations seem plausible but are wrong. The balance of evidence for a long time now has been that Vitex suppresses LH, FSH, and testosterone production, so while Vitex is a very useful herb for luteal phase deficiency, and can indeed correct progesterone deficiency, the story is more complex. In the case of black cohosh, there are lots of interactions with neural pathways, but no effect has been found so far on oestrogen receptors.

But just because the old explanations are now not valid anymore, it does not mean the herbs stopped working or that we should have less faith in them. In the end, the truth about herbs does emerge: traditional knowledge is increasingly validated, but not necessarily in the way we expect. Learning both sides, i.e. the history and the research, gives us an opportunity to offer patients and the wider public the benefit of our training and understanding to differentiate what is reliable from what is not.

The next sections discuss a useful distinction about the oestrogenic activities of herbal medicines. Firstly, they have effects on different types of oestrogen receptors, which explains why they can be oestrogenic without promoting some of the more harmful effects of oestrogen, and secondly, oestrogenic plants may be useful in treating both oestrogen excess and deficiency conditions.

Two oestrogen receptors (ER)

So far, we have looked at the role of diet and lifestyle on the production and availability of hormones. To understand the roles of phyto-oestrogens and other herbs, we also have to look at the two types of oestrogen receptors and the difference in their actions.

The main oestrogen receptors are intracellular, and they switch on gene expression in the nucleus. The two types, alpha and beta, are both widely distributed in the body, but there are differences in their distribution. The relative expression of the two types varies with the quantities of the different oestrogens, and also the amount of progesterone. Here is a brief guide to what is currently understood.

Oestrogen is a trophic (or growth-producing) hormone in certain tissues (breast and endometrium). In other tissues such as bone liver, endothelium, skin, brain, the alpha and beta receptors (ERα and ERβ) can have either an agonist or antagonist effect, allowing oestrogen to act as either growth or suppressor of growth. The two receptor types are both opposite and complementary. Oestrogens may stimulate or be agonistic in one tissue, and be depressant or antagonistic in another.

The differences between ERα and ERβ

Table 1.10: Characteristics of the two types of oestrogen receptors

ERα	ERβ
Expressed in ovarian cancer lines and oestrogen receptor node-positive breast cancers.	Expressed preferentially in normal breast and ovarian tissue.
Expression of ERα in breast tissue is usually low.	Most strongly expressed in the ovary, prostate, bladder, and lung.
Activation of alpha receptors leads to uterine proliferation.	The brain, bone and intestinal mucosa are also rich in beta receptors. ERβ protects against breast cancer development, promotes greater bone density, gives cardiovascular protection and helps reduce menopausal symptoms.

Oestrone has a high affinity for ERα. Thus, it is possibly more active in the breast, endometrium, and ovaries. It has less effect on ERβ found in bone, brain, and endothelium, which are often the target for HRT, and if oestrone is used for HRT it requires higher doses of oestrone to be effective. Oestradiol is more effective than either oestrone or an oestrone-containing combination.

Phyto-oestrogens and PhytoSERMs

Myths about phyto-oestrogens

Despite phytoestrogens and flavonoids being a major part of human diets throughout history, there have been stories that they are bad for you, should be avoided in endometrial or breast cancer, and can make the contraceptive pill ineffective. So, how much truth is there in this? The simple answer is, little if any.

This kind of statement effectively says that human experience tells us less than generalizing from a small set of scientific statements. The fact is that there is just too little known to do this, and trying to generalise rules from a limited body of work often leads to either overconfidence (e.g. the development of corticosteroid treatments or HRT) or paranoia, which continually sees new rules about how much and what kind of fats, carbohydrates, and so on are bad for us, and often a combination of the two that led people into over-refined diets and excessive consumption of hydrogenated or trans fatty acids. Establishing the whole picture takes a huge amount of work, and in the case of phyto-oestrogens, this work is still very much in its infancy, but trusting nature is generally a good principle as it got us this far.

Phyto-oestrogens are plant substances that have an effect on oestrogen receptors. They are found in plant-based foods: grains, seeds, legumes, where they are important for growth and maturation of plants. They are highest in sprouting plants.

In the diet, they are of the most benefit consumed early in life (before puberty) but there are still benefits from taking them later. To understand more about what they do in the body we need to look briefly at the different types of oestrogen receptor.

Phyto-oestrogenic compounds

There are four classes of phyto-oestrogenic compounds; one type tends to predominate in a particular species or family of herbs.

- Phenolic phyto-oestrogens (see Table 1.11 below)
- Triterpenoid saponins
- Steroidal saponins
- Resorcylic acid lactones

All four of these categories of phyto-oestrogens are also strictly speaking xeno-oestrogens, and all of them have some influence in our environment. However, only the first three are normally used therapeutically, as resorcylic acid lactones are produced by moulds, often of cereal crops, whereas the others are found in both foods and medicinal herbs themselves. Phyto-oestrogens may exert oestrogenic or anti-oestrogenic effects depending on the endogenous oestrogen concentration, meaning that they are SERMS (selective oestrogen receptor modulators).

PhytoSERMS

- In a **high oestrogen environment** endogenous oestrogen is displaced, so excessive activity of oestrogens is damped.

- In a **low oestrogen environment**: there is a net oestrogenic effect because the effect of phyto-oestrogens, though weak, at least causes some oestrogen receptor activity (and if there the tissue concentration of phyto-oestrogens is high, the number of receptors activated can mean a significant oestrogenic effect).

There is undoubtedly more to this picture. Many health benefits may be *not* due to oestrogen receptors, but rather to effects on enzymes, protein synthesis, cell proliferation, angiogenesis, calcium transport, lipid peroxidation, cell differentiation, and more. But the direct effects on receptors are important, nevertheless.

Table 1.11: Nutritional and herbal sources of phyto-oestrogens

Phenolic phyto-oestrogens are phytoSERMS, mainly interacting with ER β receptors, and are found in many vegetables, beans and pulses.		
Isoflavones:	genistein, formononetin, daidzein, and glycosides	mainly found in the leguminosae soy, red clover
Lignans:	source of enterodiol and enterolactone	flaxseed (also sunflower, pumpkin and sesame seeds)
Flavones:	apigenin	parsley, celery, thyme, celeriac, chamomile, onions, lemon balm, and oranges
	luteolin	broccoli, parsley, green pepper, thyme, celery, chamomile.
Flavanons:	naringenin, 8-prylnaringenin	Hops (also stimulate ER α)

(*Continued*)

Table 1.11: Continued

Flavonols:	kaempferol	apples, citrus fruits, grapes, red wine, onions and leeks; tea, Ginkgo, St. John's wort, pinto beans
	quercetin	fruits and vegetables
Coumestans:	coumestrol binds strongly to both oestrogen receptors	split peas, pinto beans, lima beans, alfalfa and clover sprouts

Steroidal saponins are thought to have amphoteric effects on oestrogen levels, often found in plants traditionally used for menstrual problems.

Wide range of substances in monocotyledonous angiosperms; some are oestrogenic	Dioscin (-> diosgenin) Trillarin (-> diosgenin) Chamaelirin, diosgenin Tribestin, protodioscin Asparacosides, shatavarins	*Dioscorea villosa* *Trillium erectum* *Chamaelirium luteum* *Tribulus terrestris* *Asparagus racemosus*

Triterpenoid saponins are mostly not phyto-oestrogenic but have a wide range of physiological effects, and often affect the nervous and endocrine systems.

In many traditionally anti-inflammatory and adaptogenic herbs	Ginsenosides Eleutherosides Glycyrrhizin Actaein	*Panax ginseng* *Eleutherococcus senticosus* *Glycyrrhiza glabra* *Cimicifuga racemosa*

Phenolic phyto-oestrogens

Phenolic phyto-oestrogens mainly interact with ER β receptors, and include the following plant constituents:

- **Lignans**: flaxseed (and to an extent sunflower, pumpkin and sesame seeds) is a rich source of the lignans enterodiol and enterolactone.
- **Isoflavones**: genistein, formononetin, daidzein, and glycosides mainly found in the leguminosae, e.g. soy, red clover.

- **Flavones**: apigenin (parsley, celery, thyme, celeriac, chamomile, onions, lemon balm, and oranges), luteolin (broccoli, parsley, green pepper, thyme, celery, chamomile).
- **Flavonols**: **kaemfperol** (apples, citrus fruits, grapes and red wine, onions and leeks, tea (*Camellia sinensis*), *Ginkgo biloba*, St. John's wort, pinto beans), **quercetin** in fruits and vegetables.
- **Flavanons**: naringenin, 8-prylnaringenin (in hops).
- **Coumestans**: coumestrol (split peas, pinto beans, lima beans, alfalfa and clover sprouts).

Phenolic phyto-oestrogens as phytoSERMs[90]

- Most isoflavones & lignans preferentially bind to β-receptors. ERα binding has been also shown *in vivo*, but requires ingestion of enormous amounts.
- **Genistein**: β affinity, some α affinity (*in vivo*).
- **Coumestrol**: binds as strongly as 17β-oestradiol to *both* human oestrogen receptors *in vivo*. Consumption of coumestrol is linked to infertility in horses.
- **5-OMe-genistein** and **formononetin** show significant binding to ER-α (*in vivo*).

Steroidal saponins

- Similar in structure to steroidal hormones (oestrogen, progesterone, androgen, cortisone).
- Used by pharmaceutical companies to produce steroid hormones, progesterone and cortisone.
- Soapy: tinctures containing saponins are foamy when shaken.
- The saponins cause irritation in the back of the throat.
- Traditionally used for menstrual problems.

Herbs containing steroidal saponins

- *Dioscorea villosa*
- *Trillium erectum*
- *Chamaelirium luteum*
- *Tribulus terrestris*
- *Asparagus racemosus*

Gut bacteria separate the sugar molecule from the steroidal sapogenin, the best-known example being diosgenin, and then a proportion of the sapogenin is absorbed.

Diosgenin-rich herbs are traditionally used for improving fertility, and helping to regulate the menstrual cycle. This is probably not due to effect on ER-β, but on the Hypothalamus-Pituitary-Ovary axis, by initiating ovulation. Post-ovulation the corpus luteum increases oestrogen and progesterone (and improves the oestrogen/progesterone ratio).

Triterpenoid saponins

Triterpenoid saponins are found in many traditionally anti-inflammatory and adaptogenic herbs, including *Panax ginseng*, *Eleutherococcus senticosus*, *Aesculus hippocastanum*, and *Glycyrrhiza glabra*. In terms of hormonal activity, the most notable is black cohosh, *Cimicifuga racemosa* and its triterpene glycoside, actein, which (without actually binding to either type of oestrogen receptor) has at least three different actions:

- Anti-proliferative action, and anti-tumour activity
- Helpful in menopausal symptoms
- Dopaminergic activity, which would lead to lowering prolactin levels, and might also explain reduction of hot flushes and the anti-tumour activity
- Activity in other neural pathways; serotonergic, opioidergic
- Thought to have an inhibitory effect on the pituitary LH secretions

Resorcylic acid lactones

This is a final category, which we might also think of as xeno-oestrogens, as they are phytoestrogens formed by the kinds of moulds that are often responsible for cereal crop contamination.

Progestogens

Progestogens are a class of hormones that bind to progesterone receptors. There are three: progesterone, pregnenolone, and 17 α-hydroxyprogesterone, progesterone itself being by far the most potent. As the name oestrogen means 'promoting oestrus', i.e. menstruation, the name progestogen means 'promoting gestation', i.e. pregnancy. Progesterone is produced to some extent in the adrenal glands but mostly in the ovary in the luteal phase of the menstrual cycle after ovulation, triggered by LH, so that pregnancy is supported if the released ovum is fertilised.

A common mistake is to believe that progesterone alone is produced by the corpus luteum, and oestrogen by the growing follicle. It is true that the follicle produces oestrogen but the corpus luteum produces both hormones, and so the luteal phase is important in both progesterone and oestrogen deficiency.

The role of progesterone

The main role of progesterone in gynaecology is to stimulate the growth of secretory tissues, namely the breast and endometrium. In particular, progesterone prepares the endometrium for the egg to be implanted and develop. It inhibits muscular contractions of the uterus, as this would lead to reject the adhering egg.

If fertilization occurs, the corpus luteum will function for another 7 weeks during the pregnancy (this is where Vitex could help to maintain early pregnancy). The implanted fertilised egg will then form the placenta (the placenta is part of the embryonic tissue, not part of the uterus), and this takes over the production of progesterone during the period of pregnancy. If there is no pregnancy, the corpus luteum involutes to become the corpus albicans and levels of progesterone and oestrogen drop. The growth of the uterine lining then stops, and menstruation follows.

Apart from inhibiting uterine contractions, progesterone:

- Stimulates glycogen production and increases the viscosity of cervical mucous.
- Stimulates production of blood vessels in the endometrium to enable it to support the embryo.
- Stimulates production of glandular structures that can secrete sugars.
- Increases basal body temperature.

Other actions of progesterone

Progesterone also has activities in a wide range of other tissues:

- Glandular changes in the breast that enable milk secretion.
- Competes with androgens for binding sites in the body so, if progesterone is low, androgens increase as in menopause/PCOS (facial hair, loss of scalp hair).

- Stimulates aldosterone secretion indirectly via renin and angiotensin system (which may lead to salt and water retention—commonly seen before menstruation).
- Helps prevent cancer and benign tumours as it counterbalances oestrogen effects (this, however, can change after menopause, where it can increase some oestrogenic effects).

Pregnenolone, the precursor of other steroid hormones such as the glucocorticoids, oestrogen, and testosterone, is involved with various metabolic processes. Pregnenolone assists the body in maintaining stable blood sugar, reducing inflammation, and withstanding stress.

Along with pregnenolone and dehydroepiandrosterone (DHEA, an androgen that is a precursor of androstenedione and androstenediol), progesterone belongs to an important group of endogenous steroids called 'neurosteroids'. These have an important role in brain function and are also produced by glial and other brain cells. Through its metabolite allopregnanolone, progesterone has anxiolytic, analgesic, sedative, and anaesthetic properties. In the brain, allopregnanolone acts as a neuromodulator, interacting with gamma-amino butyric acid (GABA) receptors (one of the main receptors inhibiting neurotransmission). Lower levels of allopregnanolone are found in some cases of PMS.

Metabolism of progesterone

As mentioned at the beginning of this section, progesterone is rapidly converted to other hormones. It is also metabolised in the liver, initially mostly through the action of reductase enzymes which convert carbonyl groups (carbon attached to oxygen by a double bond) to hydroxyl ones (where the oxygen is attached by a single bond, the other bond being with hydrogen). CYP3A4, the enzyme responsible for converting oestrogens to their 16-OH metabolites, is also responsible for 70% of this Phase 1 conversion of progesterone. The transformed progesterone molecule is then either sulphated or glucuronidated in the same way as oestrogens and thus removed either through the intestine by way of bile secretion or through the urine.

Because of the many pathways for conversion of progesterone, it is active only for a very short time in the body, generally about 5 minutes.

Causes of progesterone deficiency or progesterone resistance

As progesterone production is mostly tied into the menstrual cycle, anovulation means that hardly any progesterone is produced. Conditions associated with anovulation include PCOS, hypothalamic amenorrhoea, and hyperprolactinaemia (so progesterone deficiency is not necessarily the prime target of treatment). Progesterone is also often diminished after childbirth or termination, miscarriage, stopping oral contraceptives, or breastfeeding, and again at both menarche or approaching menopause.

Other irregularities in the cycle may be that the corpus luteum does not secrete enough progesterone, or does not produce it for long, or that a follicle develops but does not rupture—a possible cause of infertility in endometriosis. Excessive prolactin can prevent ovulation, leading to inadequate progesterone production and thus an abnormal menstrual cycle and shorter luteal phase. Many of these conditions are associated with a luteal phase defect—a term used primarily in reference to causes of infertility (inadequate development of the endometrium in the secretory phase of the menstrual cycle) and referring to a luteal phase of 11 days or less.

Progesterone deficiency might also suggest other causes to the practitioner, including hypothalamic-pituitary axis failure leading to insufficient production of FSH or LH or both. Stress and the interplay with other hormones are also possible causes of inadequate production. In adrenal exhaustion, less pregnenolone is produced, resulting in lower production of all steroid hormones. As with oestrogen, women who do excessive exercise or are underweight will generally also produce less progesterone.

It may also be that progesterone receptors are not sensitive enough, leading to under-stimulation by progesterone in the endometrium, breast and elsewhere. The lack of progesterone receptivity may lead to cyclic breast pain (for example, prolactin causes abnormal tissue response to progesterone). PMS, too, has been associated with decreased responsiveness to progesterone receptors.

Progesterone and oestrogen often work in tandem, so that the progesterone is in effect being swamped by oestrogen in cases of oestrogen excess.

A few pages ago, it was mentioned that Vitex probably does not enhance LH levels, and is not directly progestogenic. However, two common causes of progesterone insufficiency—luteal phase defects and progesterone receptor resistance—are commonly associated with prolactin, and Vitex does suppress prolactin release by being dopaminergic, and so it is after all certainly one of the main herbs indicated when progesterone insufficiency is suspected.

Oestrogen and progesterone

The expression of particular oestrogen receptor types is induced by the presence of oestrogen, and oestrogen-like molecules, e.g. tamoxifen. The receptors are down-regulated by progesterone, as progesterone receptors are preferentially expressed, so in this way oestrogen and progesterone can have a see-saw type of effect.

Oestrogens and progesterone are in a state of dynamic balance that varies between tissues. In the endometrium, oestrogen receptors are high in number during the follicular phase, and low or absent in late luteal phase after the progesterone receptors appear. In other tissues, e.g. breast, progesterone receptors are expressed throughout the menstrual cycle, potentially functioning to suppress oestrogen receptors, suggesting that the two tissues may respond differently to progesterone stimulation. They may also respond differently in the postmenopausal state than in the premenopausal state.

Effects of progesterone deficiency

- PMT
- Dysfunctional bleeding patterns
- Cyclic breast disorders
- Endometriosis, fibroids
- PCOS
- Inadequate transformation of the endometrium during the secretory, luteal phase, which can result in
    - Unexplained infertility
    - Repeated miscarriage

Detecting progesterone deficiency or resistance

Progesterone levels vary throughout the cycle and repeated blood tests might be needed to establish deficiency, particularly if the cycle is irregular. However, this will not reveal progesterone resistance. The main indicators, apart from blood and urine tests, are the length of the luteal phase and the whether the symptoms (e.g. tension, irritability, anxiety, mood changes) exist mainly in that phase. Basal temperature rises slightly during ovulation (this is reliable 77% of the time). To gauge length of luteal phase, body temperature should be checked daily and then the number of days counted from ovulation to the onset of menstruation. Fewer than 11 days from ovulation to the period are suggestive of luteal phase defects.

Laboratory tests include

1. Urine test, blood test or scan to check ovulation.
2. Blood test: usually 7–9 days after ovulation: deficiency is indicated if progesterone is below 10nmol/millilitre is low (but as stated the blood test is not always reliable).
3. Endometrial biopsy (but this needs to be repeated several times to be conclusive).

Main principles of treatment for progesterone deficiency

The main context where progesterone abnormalities arises is menstrual problems, and so treatment here overlaps with, and is greatly extended by, the section of the book on PMS. Other conditions will be covered in-depth in the second, companion volume on a wider range of gynaecological problems including endometriosis and fibroids. Below is a very basic set of principles just as a brief overview.

If the follicle develops but does not rupture, progesterone levels are lower, this is potentially an indication for treatment with steroidal saponins, especially *Chamaelirium luteum*.

Other irregularities in the cycle may be that the corpus luteum does not secrete enough progesterone, or does not produce it for long. In such cases both *Vitex agnus-castus* and Paeonia and Glycyrrhiza combination tend to increase the activity of the corpus luteum by inhibiting prolactin production.

Stress and/or interplay with other hormones suggest nervines, adaptogens, *Vitex agnus-castus*, and perhaps also *Cimicifuga racemosa*.

- Faulty progesterone receptors (*Vitex agnus-castus*).
- The list of generally indicated herbs also includes Paeonia and Glycyrrhiza combination, and those containing steroidal saponins.

- Flaxseed, B_6 and vitamin E.
- Stress management.
- Weight control, diet, avoid excessive exercise.
- Check for other conditions.

In the case of relative progesterone deficiency, i.e. too much oestrogen, the main principles are those highlighted for oestrogen excess as given earlier in this chapter.

Patient-friendly summary

Throughout this book, we try to give some simple explanations and guidelines at the end of each chapter, partly as a useful summary and reminder, but mostly to provide material that assists explanations of treatment to patients.

- Reproductive hormones are made by the female body in the adrenal glands and the ovaries.
- In later years they are also made in different tissues by conversion from androgens such as testosterone in skin, muscle, fat, and other tissues.
- The balance of hormones varies at different times of life and also in relation to stress and diet.
- Oestrogen is necessary for brain health, mood, the health of the skin and blood vessels, and bone density.
- Over-exercising and eating too little will deprive the body of oestrogen it needs.
- Generally, women's bodies are exposed to far more oestrogen over a lifetime than used to be the case, and many substances in the environment also have oestrogenic effects, particularly strong-smelling artificial chemicals and soft plastics.
- Oestrogen excess conditions are common, and include:
  - Endometriosis
  - Fibroids
  - Heavy or abnormal menstrual bleeding
  - PMS
  - Fibrocystic breast disease
  - Breast and endometrial cancer.
- The key principles to follow to bring oestrogen levels into a normal range involve avoiding environmental oestrogens, keeping oestrogen

availability in the body in balance and making sure the elimination process works properly.
- Environmental oestrogens affect men's reproductive health powerfully by disrupting testosterone production: sperm count and quality need to be assessed whenever infertility is a concern for a couple.
- High vegetable and low meat consumption tend to keep more oestrogen in a bound state, so it does not reach high levels in tissues.
- Elimination of hormones happens mostly after processing by the liver, and there are two phases to this processing—ideally, they should be closely coordinated so that the process is completed, and the substances can be excreted
  - Some foods, particularly vegetables in the cabbage family and onion family, help the second phase of metabolism.
  - Refined carbohydrates, being overweight and a lack of B vitamins (particularly B_6) decrease the elimination of oestrogens; whole grain foods are helpful.
  - Some hormones are reabsorbed into the blood from the gut after excretion, particularly if the bowel flora is not healthy, and may cause oestrogen excess.
- Oestrogen excess and deficiency can both be helped by phytoestrogenic plants such as flaxseeds and soy products, as well as plants such as wild yam, as they have some oestrogenic effects and work like substitutes for the body's own oestrogen. When oestrogen levels are high, they have a balancing influence and when low, a compensating influence.
- Many of these herbs need a healthy gut flora to work properly—flaxseeds, in particular, are conducive to gut health, too, and are one of the best sources of omega-3 oils.
- Some plants, such as Vitex and black cohosh, work on a different principle, not affecting oestrogen or progesterone directly but via links with the nervous system.
- Vitex in particular helps with low progesterone production, a common cause of infertility and other hormonal problems, by lengthening the second half of the menstrual cycle.
- Progesterone deficiency is often relative to oestrogen excess and is helped by the same general measures.

CHAPTER TWO

Principles of herbal treatment of gynaecological problems

There is nothing unique about the general principles of treating gynaecological problems compared with other kinds of presentation. The person needs treating as a whole, restoring general health, and using the therapeutic encounter, herbs, diet, lifestyle, and exercise to do this. Nevertheless, some *aspects* of treating the whole person do need special attention. In the last chapter, we looked at the hormonal picture as this obviously needs to be understood well enough to have a clear idea of what effect treatment may have on hormones. This chapter explores the principles of whole person treatment in general, and specifically how it affects the hormonal picture.

For some readers, it may seem like a lot of detail with only a short set of concrete treatment suggestions. The idea of the book is really to help practitioners understand the principles in order to put those principles into practice. Here we review physiological principles that lie behind systematic and comprehensive treatment of menopausal complaints and PMS presented in later chapters (treatment of a wider range of commonly presenting gynaecological problems is also discussed briefly at the end).

For other readers it may feel like we are missing out all kinds of useful details, e.g. listing inflammatory cytokines or receptors and their interactions. Our aim has been to give enough to be a useful text that is easy to refer to in practice, and a solid basis for further exploration. The end of chapter references will often take you to review papers that give a wealth of such detail.

The most important thing is to have a good overview of the connections between the digestive system, inflammation, and the brain, so we include a short introduction to brain neurotransmitters, and a brief discussion of herbs with hormonal functions. What will emerge again and again is how frequently new scientific findings confirm long-standing principles of herbal practice, as well as suggesting new possibilities. Even when, as is often the case, science explains what we know from practice, it is useful in giving practitioners and patients alike increased confidence in the treatment, and ideally a useful way to construct and explain treatment rationales.

Neuroimmunoendocrinology and systematic treatment

We generally set out a single set of therapeutic guidelines, with variants, for the conditions under examination. We do not expect people to follow them exactly but rather give them as suggestions, as there are various ways of working and each case will be different. Regarding these ways of working, rationales of practice typically follow one of three lines. Some are drawn to a humoral picture and look at symptoms first and foremost as indicators of humoral imbalance within the whole body, manifested in specific organs. Others, advocates of functional medicine, are more likely to think pharmacologically and physiologically and view symptoms in terms of physiological challenge and compensation, trying to remove the challenge as far as possible and fine-tune the compensation to minimise knock-on effects. Others may treat systematically, in terms of 'a healthy mind in a healthy body', aiming for ideal functioning of organ systems based on general indicators of their health rather than specific signs with humoral or biochemical significance, trying to establish general health following standard practices and deal with organ imbalances according to the symptoms.

There are points in favour of all of these approaches: humoral medicine connects to the emergence of the European model of practice that is a cousin of Unani Tibb doctrines, arising ultimately from Graeco-Roman medicine via Galen. This particular orientation helps practitioners to see herbs portrayed in historical texts through the eyes of their authors.

Functional medicine takes full account of the pharmacological effects of herbal and nutritional interventions, using the language of modern science rather than the language of the humours. The systematic approach relates both to the principles of Salerno or Hippocrates and to the Physiomedicalist impetus that popularised herbal medicine in the US and the UK in the nineteenth century using much of the medical language of that time, which is based on tissue and organ states and a general picture of vitality: astringing, relaxing, restoring and so on. These are not separate ways of understanding but different standpoints or orientations.

Describing the approaches in this way may make rather too much of their differences, and many practitioners take something from each. But it is worth bearing in mind methodological differences, and important when it comes to discussions of the basis of treatment. The outlook of this book is somewhere in between systematic and functional. There are three reasons for this. The first is that general guidelines are genuinely useful, and there has to be in any case some standardization of approach as a starting point. The second is that the language of our time depends on modern scientific terms, even though they may lack the holistic emphasis of previous ones. The third is that basic principles of healthy eating, digestion, exercise, and mental attitude long espoused by herbalists are becoming part of mainstream medical research, so there is a wider dialogue in place that confirms and informs that dialogue. In particular, recent research discussed in this chapter reveals valuable insights into the links between the gut biome and how it affects blood chemistry, immune, endocrine, and neural functioning.[1]

The possibilities of psycho-neuro-endocrino-immunology (PNEI)

The general change in outlook in conventional medicine stems from the growth of the discipline, over recent decades, of psychoneuroimmunology, now sometimes called psycho-neuro-endocrino-immunology. The key idea is seeing these systems as an interconnected entity whose job is to respond to changes in the environment. The advantage of seeing things in this way is that these undeniable interconnections are properly acknowledged, and need to be factored in. The disadvantage is that all of these systems are complex enough when treated individually, and suddenly got a lot more so!

There is an implicit temptation to seek a kind of theory of everything that needs constantly updating to add new bits as more details of epigenetics (how gene expression is controlled) and gut health become major foci of research. But the search for a medical theory of everything is perhaps not what is needed so much as an open framework in which interconnections can be explored, and that openness includes the possibility of generalisations such as the traditional medical ideas of the temperaments and vital force.

The digestive system

In the chapters about treating PMS and menopausal problems, we repeatedly suggest that the first phase of treatment is to relieve the stress on the body by helping digestion and reducing inflammation. It is hard to overstate the importance of doing this.

There is abundant research currently on the importance of the gut microbiome in maintaining health. A wide variety of useful bacteria will crowd out those that are unfriendly and prevent the damage that the latter cause to the tight junctions between epithelial cells that allow inflammatory compounds to enter the bloodstream.

Looking after the microbiome

Prebiotics are substances that favour a healthy biome, and probiotics supply gut-friendly bacteria. To take prebiotics first, soluble fibre found in fruits, vegetables and whole grain cereals provide a variety of substrates, particularly oligosaccharides, that form substrates for fermentation by healthy gut bacteria. Probiotics generally contain lactobacilli and other bacteria that are directly introduced into the gut rather than just the conditions that favour them.

Detailed discussion of prebiotics and probiotics lies outside the scope of this book and is generally familiar to practitioners being, in essence, a matter of eating plenty of fresh organically grown fruit and vegetables, with variety (using the colour spectrum to support the nutrition of a wide range of bacteria). Lacto-ferments such as kimchi and sauerkraut have both prebiotic and probiotic functions and encourage bacterial diversity, which is the main indicator of a healthy gut biome. They are quite easy to make at home now that jar lids with one-way valves to release carbon dioxide and not allow in oxygen are widely available and patients may very much enjoy the sense of involvement in their treatment that creating these ferments provides.

How healthy gut epithelium helps hormonal balance

A healthy microbiome will decrease the amount of deglucuronidation and hence the recycling of metabolised oestrogens and other hormones, and increase the deconjugation of phyto-oestrogens provided by a wide range of fruits and vegetables, particularly flaxseed and soy. Many of the herbs we use for hormonal effects, for example all those containing saponins or other glycosides (in fact, the majority) depend on bacteria breaking the glycoside bond for their absorption, and this, too, depends on a healthy gut flora. There is a big overlap between foods that are healthy in general and those that help with oestrogen deficiency (or excess—and are also thus indicated in conditions of relative progesterone deficiency).

Table 2.1 gives a summary list of these foods that is probably a useful basis for general recommendations. For a more detailed plan, a full list of foods can be found in Chapter 1—it is a very good idea to make your own dietary advice sheets from both lists.

It is important not to hurry. Diet is a matter of habit and, as building habits is hard, patients can become demotivated or feel guilty that they are struggling. Getting symptomatic improvement will be very motivating, and so it is best to prioritise and to treat diet as a work in progress. Adding soy or flax (to be discussed in the next section) may

Table 2.1: Foods to support metabolism of oestrogens

Stimulating Phase 1 detoxification (see Section 1 for a full list, including the other oestrogen metabolites):
Foods to encourage Phase 1 metabolism of excess oestrogens to -2OH oestrogens: • Brassicas • Soy beans, turmeric (curcumin), omega 3/oily fish, flaxseed • Grapes (resveratrol) • Garlic • Green or black tea
Phase 2 detoxification (may be more important than Phase 1 as it allows elimination of oestrogen and other metabolites):
Methylation: • B6 and B12 • Methionine (legumes, onions)

(Continued)

Table 2.1: Continued

- Betaine, folic acid and magnesium (green leaves, whole grains, and beetroot)

Sulfation:
- Caffeine
- Vitamin A
- Flavonoid- and anthocyanin-rich foods (yellow, orange and red foods)
- Phyto-oestrogenic daidzein (legumes) and genistein (soybeans)

Glucuronidation:
- Brassicas
- Grapes (resveratrol)
- Soy beans, turmeric (curcumin)

not be that inspiring, so recipes and the encouragement to experiment with lots of interesting tastes and colours is also important. The sense of satiety is somewhat helped by the fact that most of the healthy foods are bulky. But what may help most is to realise that improvement in diet is self-rewarding: as gut health improves, the change in gut bacteria actually cuts food craving and makes healthier foods more appealing, so the emphasis should be on the flora first.

The biome and general health

Is research interest in the microbiome a bit of a fad? The evidence seems to be very much that it is not. The background to this surge of interest is, as in other areas we have been looking at, a greatly increased research capabilities, in this case due to genome sequencing methods that can assess biome diversity without having to grow bacterial cultures. The results are likely to change biological thinking permanently.

The theory is not only of individual bacterial richness. Recent thinking is even that microbiome and host evolve together, and we should think of ourselves as 'holobionts', i.e. that each is effectively a community, and not only that, but our make-up as individual communities (if that makes sense) is also influenced by, and influences our social behaviour—when we shake hands, the theory goes, we are offering to share gut biomes and in effect saying that the other person's biome is worth sharing to the extent of taking a risk over catching an infectious disease. Given the relationship between the biome and nervous and immune system, that seems quite plausible.

A rich flora dominated by beneficial bacterial species prevents invasion of the epithelium by harmful bacteria and maintains the tight junctions necessary for the integrity of the gut lining. Fermentation of fibre by friendly bacteria provides the short chain fatty acids (SCFAs)—acetate, propionate, butyrate—that encourage the growth of other gut-friendly bacteria by lowering the pH of the gut environment and, being readily absorbed into the blood, have beneficial effects on inflammation throughout the body. One such benefit is improved glucose homeostasis (insulin resistance is now generally seen as part of a general picture of low-grade systemic inflammation).[2] Microbiome diversity is also associated with increased vagal afferent activity to the brain, with beneficial effects on the limbic system, modulating GABA and serotoninergic activity (see next section) and thus improving mood, decreasing anxiety and reducing appetite.[3]

Consumption of refined sugars tends to create an unhealthy gut flora, with a higher pH and less bacterial diversity and increasing absorption of lipopolysaccharides (LPS). If SCFAs are on the side of the angels, LPS are their demonic counterparts, absorbed through the gut lining in obesity, diabetes, and related disorders. Leakage of LPS into the blood triggers low-grade inflammation and affects the liver adipose tissue, and muscle metabolism. In addition, those endotoxins can alter the activity of the enteric nervous system (ENS) as well as the gut-brain axis, again via the vagus nerve, suppressing the release of leptins (which alleviate the sense of hunger) or leading to leptin resistance, and increase the production of ghrelins, which give a sense of hunger.[4]

L-cells and GLP-1

Part of the explanation for the benefit of gut health on other systems is the role of enteric endocrine cells secreting hormones such as peptide YY and glucagon-like peptide (GLP-1). These have broadly similar effects. To take GLP-1, which is probably at present the most well studied, it is produced by L-cells in the gut epithelium when SCFAs bind to receptors on the L-cell. It improves glucose tolerance, increases the sense of satiety and is cardioprotective and anti-inflammatory, as shown in Figure 2.1. GLP-1 is just one part an emerging story of 'cross-talk' between gut, nervous system, endocrine system and immune system.

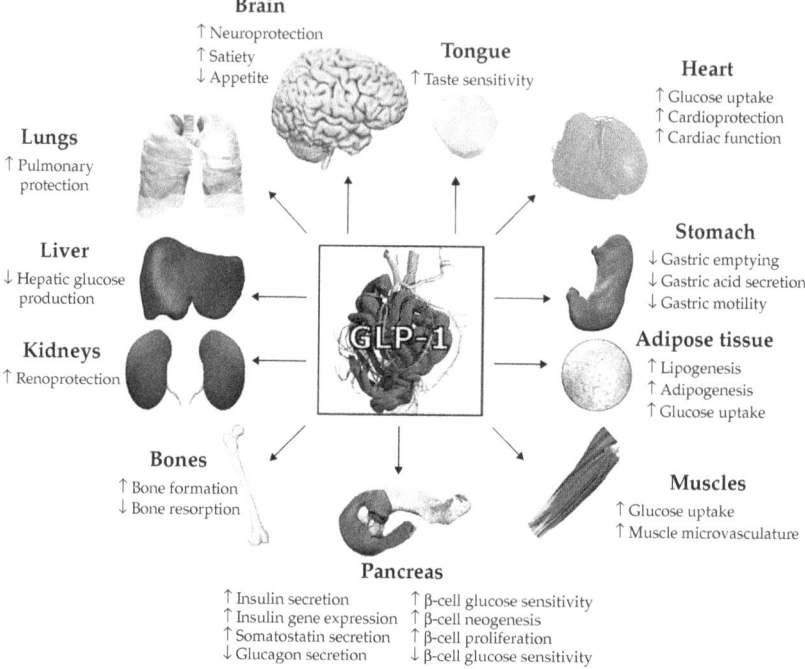

Figure 2.1: The many physiological actions of GLP-1 from https://en.wikipedia.org/wiki/File:FunctionsOfGLP-1.png.

It is an excellent example, however, of the importance of gut health to the endocrine and immune system.[5]

What is also worth mentioning is that the gut-brain axis is a two-way street with the gut of course responding to the activities of the sympathetic and parasympathetic nervous system, as well as sending feedback to the brain via the vagus nerve.[6] Bitter herbs are traditionally seen as liver tonics but it is now thought that their activity may be more to do with stimulating the parasympathetic nervous system in a way that encourages a healthier gut biome, which then creates a much lighter load for the liver. In contrast, a period of prolonged activation of the sympathetic nervous system triggers more sugar production in the liver and muscles and decreases secretions and blood supply to the gut, and also increases gut permeability. This increases the load on the liver and tends to decrease the variety of the gut flora and increase the ratio of the firmicute group of bacteria to the bacterioidetes group,[7] and this change in ratio is commonly regarded as being associated with pro-inflammatory markers, although this is something of a generalization as some members of each group are friendly and some not.

Endocannabinoids

The endocannabinoid system is the focus of a great deal of research, though it is at present difficult to say how much is relevant to our topics, i.e. gut and gynaecological problems, although that is likely to change. The endocannabinoid receptors (CB1 and CB2) and their endogenous ligands are involved in numerous biological processes, particularly in determining receptor sensitivity and the production of neurotransmitters throughout the body, and have a key role in the regulation of energy homeostasis, inflammation and gut-barrier function.[8] CB1 are found particularly in the brain but also widely in the enteric nervous system. Increased activity in CB1 receptors is generally associated with increased permeability of the gut, increased inflammation, craving for high calorie foods and metabolic syndrome.[9] CB2 receptors are predominantly associated with the immune system and have a generally anti-inflammatory function. Plant compounds of various kinds stimulate CB2 receptors, particularly the alkylamides in Echinacea,[10] and β-caryophyllene, found in volatile oils of plants such as rosemary, cloves and hops, and so these may be useful as both general anti-inflammatories.

The role of the liver

If the tight junctions of the gut epithelium have been lacking in integrity for any length of time, the liver will have been exposed to a major toxicological challenge. So the liver may need support after a period of prolonged stress, particularly if alcohol consumption is moderate or high, and particularly also in smokers (or following antibiotic use, of course). Liver restoratives such as milk thistle will be useful if there is a suspicion that the liver has been overloaded, but bitters are likely to generally suffice by reducing the load (provided that other dietary recommendations are being followed, too). Abstinence from alcohol is also very important for the first few weeks if the liver appears to have been overloaded. Dandelion root would be near the top of most people's lists for a general liver tonic, and its inulin content is also likely to play a part in decreasing inflammation and stabilizing blood sugar.

EFAs

Omega 3 EFAs are involved in neurogenesis, signal transduction, and neurotransmission in the brain. Levels in a typical western diet have declined substantially over time, and as the ratio of omega-3:omega-6 is important, ensuring a good dietary intake is important to prevent inflammatory disease of all kinds. Apart from the well-known oily fish, which obtain it from algae, there are numerous plant sources, and hempseed oil and, even more so, flaxseeds, are excellent sources.

Docosahexaenoic acid (DHA) is important for the maintenance of normal neurological function in the brain: hippocampal DHA levels decrease with age and in Alzheimer's disease. Both DHA and eicosapentaenoic acid (EPA) have antioxidative, anti-inflammatory, and anti-apoptosis effects, protecting neurons. Dietary omega 3 polyunsaturated fatty acids also alter the levels of opioid peptides in plasma,[11] thus aiding relaxation and a sense of wellbeing.

The nervous system

The main brain neurotransmitters: GABA and glutamine

As mentioned, the nervous system and the endocrine system are tightly coupled, and nervines and activities that help to alleviate prolonged sympathetic nervous activation will also directly help both the gut and the liver, as will herbs that have a vagotonic effect. None of this is, of course, very new, but it is striking how far this is now this is becoming scientific orthodoxy.

Regarding the link between the nervous system and steroidal hormones, there will be much more detail in the PMS section of this book, as this syndrome has led to much of the research, but it is worth introducing some of the main neurotransmitter systems here. While the autonomic nervous system two neurotransmitters, acetylcholine for the parasympathetic nervous system and noradrenaline for the sympathetic, the brain has vastly more. They occur in three main classes, the amino acid ones such as aspartate, glutamate and glycine, to which class can be added GABA. Glutamate and GABA form an excitatory/inhibitory pair in the brain. Glutamate is the main excitatory neurotransmitter in the central nervous system, and GABA has calming, sedative effects and its receptors are the main target of benzodiazepines. Aspartate and glycine in the spinal cord are likewise paired as excitatory/inhibitory pair.

Prolonged use of benzodiazepines results in habituation via adaptation of the receptors. Habituation is something of a general rule with psychoactive substances, and perhaps most bioactive compounds. Benzodiazepines are an extreme example, however, and withdrawal is liable to produce symptoms worse than the ones originally treated. Receptors may also increase in number and/or sensitivity to GABA when it is short supply, so its functions are to an extent self-adjusting. GABA activity (or lack of it) seems to be strongly implicated in premenstrual dysphoria.

GABA is most highly concentrated in the substantia nigra and globus pallidus of the basal ganglia, followed by the hypothalamus, the periaqueductal grey matter ('central grey') and the hippocampus. The GABA concentration in the brain is 200–1,000 times greater than that of acetylcholine or the monoamines dopamine, serotonin, and noradrenaline.

Dopamine, serotonin, and noradrenaline

Many gynaecological problems are associated with states of stress, both in terms of cause and effect. In general, herbs that are known to be calming and uplifting in their actions thus have an effect on both mind and body. It is interesting in this respect that Vitex, Cimicifuga, and Hypericum are all useful in menopausal and/or premenstrual syndromes associated with stress and all of them have an influence on either dopamine, melatonin or serotonin function.

The monoamines are the main steering neurotransmitters of the brain, affecting learning, disposition of attention, mood, and much more. Dopamine and noradrenaline are closely related catecholamines, noradrenaline being synthesised in the brain from dopamine, which itself is produced from the amino acid phenylalanine or its product tyrosine. Serotonin is produced from L-tryptophan, like melatonin.

Dopamine affects many physiological functions, including gastrointestinal motility, pituitary hormone release, voluntary movements, motivation, and higher cognitive processes. It is the main positive reward hormone—the one that says 'go for it now' and 'YES!!!'.

There are four main dopaminergic tracts in the brain:

1. The nigrostriatal tract from the substantia nigra to the corpus striatum accounts for most of the brain's dopamine, and loss of neurons here is main pathological feature of Parkinson's disease.

2. The tuberoinfundibular tract from the hypothalamus to the pituitary stalk, which inhibits the release of prolactin.
3. The mesolimbic tract from the ventral tegmental area to many parts of the limbic system, highly involved in reward, motivation and addiction.
4. The mesocortical tract from the ventral tegmental area to the neocortex, particularly the prefrontal area, also involved in reward, motivation and addiction.

The mesolimbic pathways are very much involved in cognition and reward, and overactivity here is strongly implicated in florid schizophrenia. Dopaminergic activity is strongly affected by oestrogen, and also by Cimicifuga and Vitex, whose actions are thus indicated in treating hyperprolactinaemia.

Serotonin is in some ways complementary to dopamine, yin to its yang, if you like, being associated with finding non-violent paths to satisfaction. A vivid way to think of this is to imagine being locked in a room with high windows that one can see out of only by standing on the bed. If the mattress is too low, one needs to jump up and down or stay in the dark. The function of dopamine would be rather like making the mattress springy so that one can jump and see out. The function of serotonin would be to raise the bed so that one can look out without having to jump. It's an odd analogy, but it does in a way help to picture why both transmitters are important and have a reciprocal relationship.

Low levels of serotonin and high levels of dopamine are both associated with violent behaviour and addiction,[12] and particularly with poor perfusion of the prefrontal cortex and increased subcortical activity, specifically in the amygdala (which is involved in emotional memories and responses, and social engagement), associated with deficient control of negative emotion by prefrontal serotonergic activity. This local abnormality may predispose people to emotional dysregulation and aggressive behaviour, whereas more global serotonin deficiency is linked more with depression.

Serotonergic pathways in general are stimulated by selective serotonin reuptake inhibitors (SSRIs), and also markedly by MDMA (ecstasy). Habitual use of MDMA causes atrophy in learning and motivational pathways and is associated with long-term depression and cognitive impairment, and it is probably worth being sceptical about long-term use of SSRIs. As you can see from Figure 2.2, oestrogen and progesterone receptors are closely associated with areas of

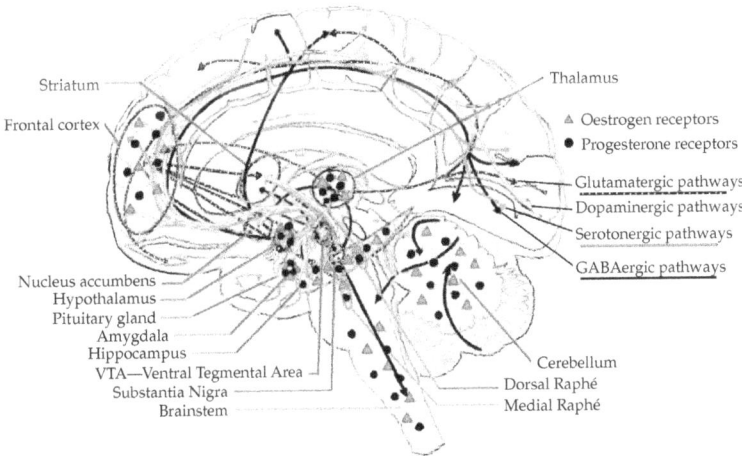

Figure 2.2: The spatial relationship between oestrogen and progesterone receptors and areas of the brain and neural pathways associated with motivation, learning and cognition.

dopaminergic and serotonergic innervation. Many of these areas are important for perception (e.g. thalamus), learning, and reward (VTA, hippocampus, prefrontal cortex) as well of course physiological functioning (pituitary and hypothalamus) and explain why dysregulation of hormonal function causes a distressing array of neurological and psychological symptoms.

Tryptamine can also be derived in the body from tryptophan and itself is thought to have neuromodulatory effects, shifting activity from noradrenergic pathways to serotonergic and dopaminergic ones in the brain. A number of Acacia species contain tryptamine and have a history of hallucinogenic use. Both tryptophan and tryptamine are implicated in improving immune surveillance in the gut epithelium, and their metabolism in the gut depends on a healthy microbiome. Tryptophan-rich foods include nuts, seeds, tofu, cheese, red meat, chicken, turkey, fish, oats, beans, lentils, and eggs.

Noradrenaline is the other main monoamine, and is synthesised from dopamine. It used to be the main target of antidepressants, either tricyclic or monoamine oxidase inhibitors, until SSRIs took over as the treatment of choice through having fewer contraindications and less obvious adverse reactions. Being related to adrenaline, noradrenaline is similarly involved in alertness and readiness for action.

The level of complexity involved in the interactions between the transmitter pathways, endocrine function and gut microbiota is huge and knowledge is partly speculative in any case. The main points are really that the function of the monoamine pathways in the brain is closely tied to having a healthy gut flora, but that stress itself causes problems with the gut flora.

Dopamine and prolactin

Any process (e.g. some prescription medication) that disrupts dopamine secretion or interferes with the delivery of dopamine may cause hyperprolactinaemia. Likewise, some medications can cause hyperprolactinaemia: for example, tricyclic antidepressants, monoamine oxidase inhibitors, serotonin reuptake inhibitors, opiates and cocaine, and several anti-hypertensive medications. In the menopause, high prolactin levels will tend to decrease oestrogen levels by suppressing aromatase activity, and in the reproductive years will tend to reduce both oestrogen and progesterone levels by leading to luteal insufficiency.

Prostaglandin E1 (PGE1), derived from dietary essential fatty acids, is able to attenuate the biological actions of prolactin, so deficiency of prostaglandin PGE1 could exaggerate the effects of prolactin. Prolactin inhibits testosterone secretion in men. Vitex at low doses tends to increase prolactin secretion and at higher doses it inhibits it, so this may explain why a Vitex is known as 'monk's pepper' or 'chaste berry'—even a little of it was enough to temper a man's ardour.

Endogenous opioids, the hypothalamic-pituitary-adrenal (HPA) axis and cortisone

High levels of endorphins are a normal stress response, and tend to suppress the HPA axis—an effect that may be lost in long-term stress as tolerance to the endorphins then leads to a blunting of the cortisol response, and this is one potential link between PMS and stress.

Cross-talk between steroid hormones and effects on the immune system

A central feature of the menopause is an increase in the level of adrenaline in response to low oestrogen, along with a general increase in cortisol production and decrease in insulin sensitivity. Adrenaline can also cause downregulation of triiodothyronine (T3) receptors. When adrenaline is continuously elevated, the body tries to balance by lowering oestrogen and thyroid hormone, so this, coupled with tissue desensitization to T3, can exacerbate low oestrogen levels and also lead to functional hypothyroidism. Both oestrogen deficiency and hypothyroidism can cause a loss of energy, depression and bone demineralization.

Cross-talk is a phenomenon in which receptors can receive inputs from other endogenous substances apart from their primary ligand. One example is that progesterone can upregulate the activity of oestrogen at oestrogen receptors. Cross-talk is common in steroid hormones and particularly sex hormones. These steroid receptors include oestrogen receptors ERα and ERβ, androgen receptors, glucocorticoid receptors, progesterone receptors, and mineralocorticoid receptors. When steroid hormones pass through cell membranes, they bind to these nuclear receptors to form transcription factors (i.e. switches that increase or decrease the activation of sections of DNA). So there is a plethora of pathways by which steroids influence the production of different proteins such as epidermal growth factor, insulin, IGF-1 (insulin-like growth factor) and cyclic AMP, and these have an impact on inflammatory disease and on the growth of cancers.[13] Oestrogen levels also influence immune protein production, with menopausal women, compared to premenopausal controls, showing elevated levels of cytokines including interleukins IL-6, IL-2 and IL-4, and C-reactive protein (CRP). Elevated CRP and IL-6 (a common pro-inflammatory cytokine) are both raised in Alzheimer's disease and it is thought that they make the blood-brain barrier more permeable to systemic inflammatory mediators.[14]

Circulatory and immune systems

The effect of herbal medicine on the circulation is to a great degree just one aspect of improved tissue state generally, particularly the balance of inflammatory and anti-inflammatory processes in the body. The dietary suggestions made above have a detoxifying and anti-inflammatory effect and should decrease glycation of the endothelium of blood vessels. Flaxseeds and soy also have beneficial effects on blood cholesterol and blood sugar, and to an extent blood pressure, as does improving the health of the gut. Perhaps the most important factor to add to this, in terms of the circulation, is to take regular exercise. Again, more detail is beyond the scope of this book, but that is not to underestimate the benefit of exercise, both in terms of strengthening the heart and improving the flexibility of the arterial network, and in terms of aiding relaxation.

Of course, that does not mean that specific circulatory herbs are not required, for example *Ginkgo biloba*, *Crataegus* spp. or *Achillea millefolium*, and likewise venous and lymphatic herbs. These are perhaps best used to in response to specific indications: an anti-inflammatory diet combined with regular exercise and neuroendocrine support should itself be trophorestorative to the circulation over time.

A broadly similar principle applies to the immune system, too. A fruit and vegetable-rich diet (along with other additions noted above) not only favours the growth of a healthy gut flora but also contains a variety of phytochemicals with anti-inflammatory and antioxidant functions, particularly flavonoids, polyphenols, and polysaccharides. What are thought of as anti-inflammatories and immune herbs broadly overlap in function and are probably best thought of as immunomodulatory, the canonical example being *Echinacea purpurea* (alkylamide-rich preparations).[15] Detailed discussion of immunomodulatory herbs (beyond brief lists in the specific treatment sections) is beyond the scope of this book but it is worth noting that many are also antimicrobial, an excellent example being the plants containing berberine, which give a helping hand to re-establishing healthy gut flora.

The importance of exercise and sleep

Regular exercise has been shown to delay the onset of Alzheimer's disease and other neurodegenerative diseases, speed recovery from neurological trauma and alleviate stress and psychological disorders. The effects have been attributed to increased metabolic capacities and antioxidation, but in addition exercise tends to increase the production of monoamine neurotransmitters, notably serotonin, with a positive effect on learning, mood, and cognition.[16] In premenstrual women, exercise has also been noted to decrease prolactin, oestrogen, and progesterone levels.

Exercise is particularly important in older patients, who often show exaggerated and prolonged inflammatory response to tissue injury and illness—this may be partly because of sluggish circulation and elimination.[17]

At this point you will not be surprised to read that regular exercise also increases the diversity of the microbiome, particularly in lean individuals.[18] A number of causes can be theorised for this—a shift in general metabolism, reduction in stress, and better perfusion of the gut at rest (secondary to improved blood flow and increased haemoglobin levels).

General wellbeing

Research into exercise and diet is increasingly coming to the conclusion that it is not any particular factor in isolation, but all taken together with the mental attitude of enjoying diet, exercise, and also, company. Evidence suggests that older people who interact more often with the people in their communities have gut microbiomes resembling those of younger individuals. Recently, the relationship between social stressors and the microbiome has been experimentally established, suggesting that acute or chronic exposure to a social stressor can significantly modify the community structure of the gut microbiome.[19]

Psychological health

One thing that practitioners need to bear in mind, of course, is that the patient comes expressing their experience of discomfort and this almost always has a personal, psychological component. The discomfort may be related to their feeling of not being at home in their body or in the world around them. Not all of that may be fully treatable by the herbalist, and so it is important to realise the limits of treatment at any given time, and not to take responsibility beyond what can usefully be offered. The fact of presenting oneself for treatment with a practitioner may itself be a major contributor to the healing process and reveal to the patient, perhaps over time, what other steps they may wish to take, steps in which the practitioner may be more a helpful ally than an expert.

Specific indications and systematic therapeutics

What emerges from so many aspects of the current scientific view of the interconnectedness of body systems is that it is perfectly plausible for a plant medicine to have actions across multiple systems, either because the receptors that respond to phytochemicals are widely distributed, or because it contains a variety of active principles, or because actions in one system have repercussions in another. The view, too, that the body has to be regarded as a complex, single entity rather than a collection of interlocking parts, is supported by the sheer complexity of interactions and the fact that many of them are interdependent.

A detailed review of the effects of herbs on the systems of the body lies beyond the scope of this section, as this is not a general herbal. But that does not mean that the actions of herbs are not still central to the therapeutic intervention: in relaxing, tonifying, and stimulating organs, herbs have both targeted and system-wide effects, and often very dynamic ones, reflecting in many cases their functions in the plants to protect them from diseases and parasites. The idea of a plant having specific indications, for example being indicated for migraine associated with an irritable bowel, is also now increasingly plausible in conventional scientific terms rather than raising the question 'but which one is it really good for?' The sense that a herb particularly suits one type of person is also evidently not at all unreasonable: although it is hard to investigate scientifically, there are good grounds to believe in it.

The model we of treatment we are presenting is mostly systematic, i.e. improving the health of the nervous, endocrine, immune, cardiovascular, and digestive systems in a general sense, recognizing that these are not really separate systems but just useful categories to organise the approach. It is certainly possible to think in terms of using highly targeted therapeutics if one is certain enough that this particular biochemical process is the key, but we have so much support for general principles that a great deal of therapeutic success lies in applying them using plants, food, exercise and lifestyle support in a synergistic fashion. In effect, modern research increasing reveals what practitioners have for a long time seen for themselves, and it helps both explain and refine treatment at the same time.

Patient-friendly summary

- All the systems of the body are interconnected, an insight that is finally and increasingly supported by modern scientific research:
  - A healthy microbiome aids mood, memory and concentration
  - A healthy microbiome decreases food cravings and sugar highs and lows
  - A healthy digestive system aids the detoxification work of the liver

- Liver and gut health decrease general inflammation in the body
- General inflammation is linked to healthy blood lipids and blood sugar
- Disturbances affecting one hormone also affect others
- Hormonal health requires effective elimination in the gut
- Hormonal health is necessary for the brain circuits involved in attention, motivation and mood
- How to support gut health:
  - Lots of vegetables, particularly root vegetables; multicoloured diet
  - Flaxseeds, beans, pulses are microbiome-friendly
  - Fermented foods—kimchi, sauerkraut, home-made lacto-ferments
- How lifestyle helps:
  - Exercise and being sociable both increase microbiome diversity
  - Exercise has anti-inflammatory effects and helps to maintain healthy blood sugar and lipids
  - Exercise helps re-establish healthier brain chemistry to assist with attention, motivation, and mood
  - Sleep is important for both anti-inflammatory effects in the body and for healthier brain chemistry necessary for attention, motivation and mood
- Endocrine and brain health
  - Enough tryptophan-rich food (nuts, seeds, tofu, cheese, red meat, chicken, turkey, fish, oats, beans, lentils) to support gut health and brain function (serotonin and melatonin for calmness and sleep health)
  - Soy and flaxseed in the diet
  - Foods rich in B vitamins also support brain function
  - Cabbage family and onion family help with elimination (more elsewhere on this)
- Anti-inflammatory diet and lifestyle
  - Anxiety, depression and hormonal problems are all linked to pro-inflammatory processes in the body (metabolic syndrome) which can cause diabetes, heart disease and cancer
  - Most of the advice given above is aimed at helping with this one aspect of physiological function because it is the biggest cause of many kinds of chronic ill health
  - In addition to the general advice for gut health and general lifestyle, omega-3 EFAs are needed for immune system health, either with oily fish supplementation or with flaxseed or hempseed oil

Phytoestrogen-rich loaf: this is a dense, rich and moist 'cake'

Ingredients
- 100g soya flour
- 100g rolled oats
- 100g whole meal wheat flour
- 100g cracked linseeds, or put them in liquidiser to crack (linseeds do get rancid quickly so need to use fresh)
- 400g dried fruit; e.g. current, raisins, cranberries, dates, apricots (chopped)
- 150g mixture of sunflower seeds, sesame seeds, flaked almonds lightly toasted (could also add nuts, e.g. walnuts, chopped)
- 2 tbsp honey
- 2 tsp ground ginger
- 2 tsp cinnamon
- 4–5 stem ginger pieces, in syrup—chopped
- 650–750ml soya milk

Instructions
Preheat the oven to 190°/fan oven 170°

Mix all the dry ingredients into a large bowl, along with the chopped stem ginger. Mix in soya milk and honey and leave to soak for half an hour.

Line a small loaf or round cake tin with baking paper, and add the mixture, if to should drop easily from spoon. If too dense mix some more soya milk.

Bake for about an hour, use a knife to check if ready: it should come out clean.

Take out of the tin and leave to cool.

This can freeze well if you want to have some spare in future. Can be toasted or eaten straight.

Flaxseed (Linum usitatissum)

Introduction to one of our most useful plants

If you are looking for one universal recommendation for helping with oestrogen deficiency or oestrogen balance in gynaecological disorders, taking a good amount of flaxseeds daily is probably as close as it gets, given their overall contribution to bowel and immune health, and their phyto-oestrogen content in the form of lignans, whose moderating effect can be useful both before and after the menopause. It used to be thought, for example, that all phyto-oestrogens were contraindicated in oestrogen-dependent tumours, but flax seeds actually increase the effectiveness of tamoxifen in breast cancer.

History

'*Usitatissimum*' means 'really useful', probably due to the plant's triple role as a textile, a source of oil, and an animal feed. This plant has been cultivated throughout recorded history, the fibre (linen) used in both textiles and paper, being both long and durable. Flaxseeds and woven cloth have been found in Egyptian tombs.

Flax has been used as a medicine since ancient times: Hippocrates recommended the seeds for abdominal pain and Theophrastus their mucilage as a cough remedy. Hildegard von Bingen advised using flax meal in hot compresses for the treatment of both external and internal ailments.

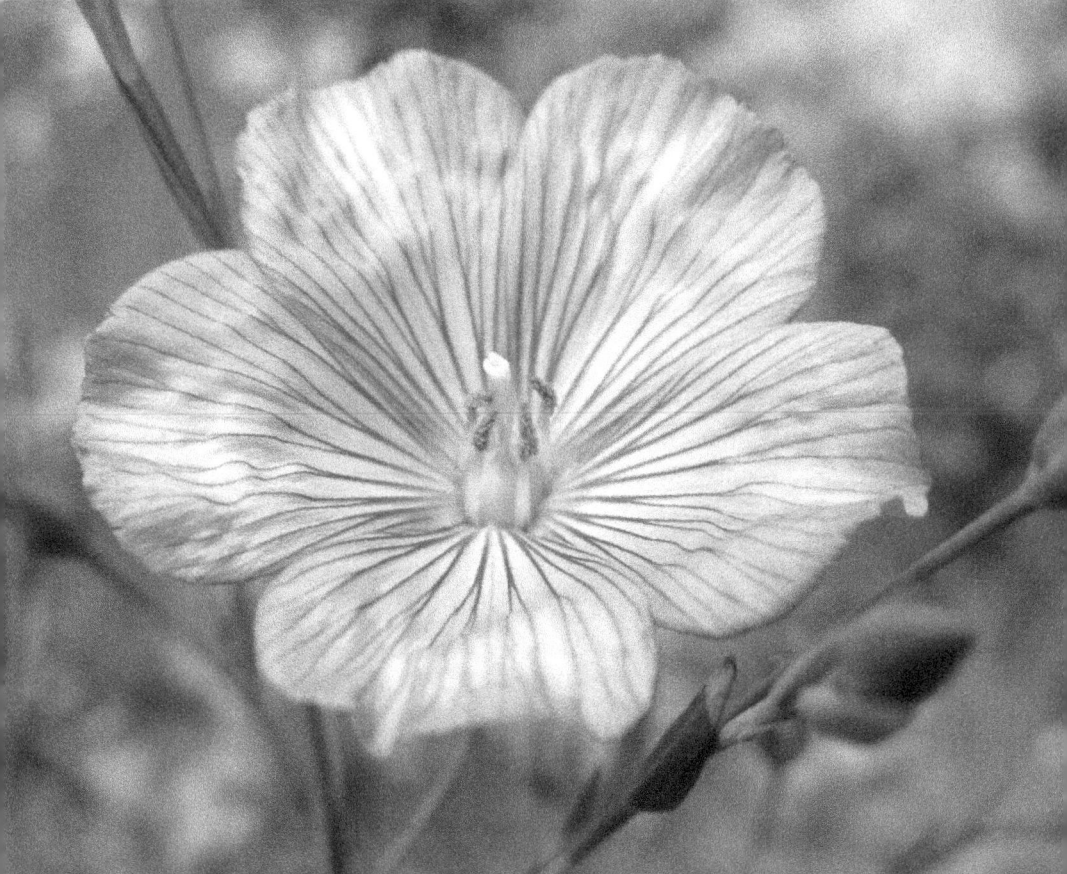

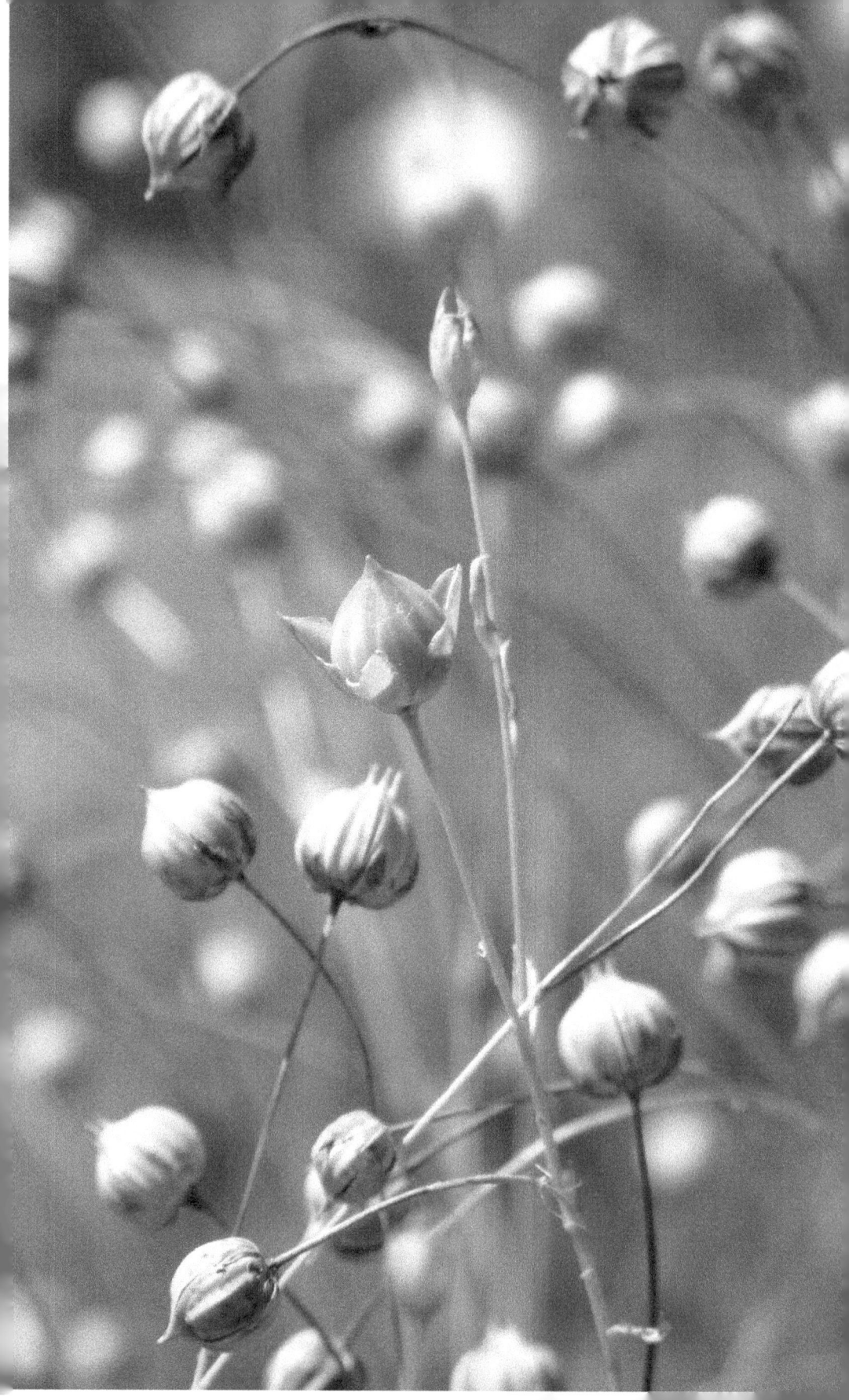

The seeds, likewise, long used for oil, are known as flaxseed when used for food for human consumption, and linseed when used in industry or for animal feed.

Modern biochemical research has confirmed that flax seeds are as just as useful medicinally, as they combine three important factors: mucilage that benefits the bowel and its flora, something that herbalists have always seen as a first point of treatment; an ideal balance of essential fatty acids; and lignans that on conversion in the gut are taken up into the plasma and have SERM and other properties. All three of these factors benefit cardiovascular health, create an anti-inflammatory terrain in the body, and are anticarcinogenic. Thus, it seems likely that taking the seeds is a much better policy than taking isolated extracts. It is remarkable how often the synergies in unprocessed plant material work in this way.

To get the full benefit of the seeds, the intake has to be high enough, so not just a small sprinkling on breakfast cereal but a couple of tablespoons a day is ideal. The fatty acids are subject to spoiling, so it is important to keep them cool and dark and in an airtight container.

It is important to take the seeds with enough water, as otherwise they can swell in the bowel and cause discomfort or even obstruction. This is true for all soluble fibre: to have its full benefits, it must be given with enough liquid.

Constituents of flax seeds

1. **α-linolenic acid (ALA), oleic, linoleic, palmitic and stearic acids.** Its ω-6: ω-3 fatty acid ratio of approximately 0.3:1[20] is thought to be the perfect balance for human consumption. In most foods containing EFAs the proportion of ω-6: ω-3 is much higher.

   Flaxseed oil is easily oxidised by light and contact with air, so it needs to be kept in a dark, cool container and opened as infrequently and for as short a time as possible.

   ω-3 fatty acids have many health benefits related to their anti-inflammatory properties, as they are involved in the synthesis of the anti-inflammatory 3-series. Consumption of ω-3 fatty acids from fish oils and krill lowers blood markers of inflammation such as C-reactive protein, interleukin 6, and TNF-alpha. EPA also competes directly with pro-inflammatory arachidonic acid and thus inhibits synthesis of the pro-inflammatory 2-series prostaglandins, so its anti-inflammatory effect is partly because of this.

Their effects are very widespread, particularly for the cardiovascular system, reducing cardiovascular disease, hypertension and atherosclerosis and improving vascular function. But their effects extend to reduction in the risk or severity of diabetes, cancer, arthritis, osteoporosis, autoimmune and neurological disorders.[21]

To get the full benefit of the seeds, the intake has to be high enough because isoflavonoid absorption is limited, and ω-3 fatty acids need to be converted in the body to the long-chain forms (EPA, DHA found in fish oils) to be converted to prostaglandins, and this conversion is relatively inefficient.

2. **Soluble (mucilage gums) and insoluble dietary fibres (cellulose and lignin).** As these are water soluble, they make flaxseeds a gentle bulk laxative, improving elimination and helping stabilise blood glucose levels and lower blood cholesterol.
3. **Vitamin and mineral content**: Flaxseed is a good source of vitamins A, C, and E, and minerals especially calcium, magnesium, phosphorus. It has a high potassium content.
4. **Lignans**. Lignans are phenolic compounds (derived from phenylpropanoid precursors) that are usually small and soluble. They are not to be confused with lignin, the insoluble fibre often seen alongside cellulose in plants, which strengthens cell walls and seeds and is responsible for tough, woody tissue (lignum means 'wood').

Flaxseed lignans are **secoisolariciresinol diglucoside** (**SDG**), and **matairesinol**. They are transformed in the body by bacterial action in the gut into **enterodiol** and **enterolactone** which can then be absorbed into the blood (these words are easier to remember when one recalls that 'entero-' signifies the gut, as in 'gastroenterology').

Lignan pharmacokinetics and actions

- **Uptake**: enterolactone and enterodiol are absorbed from the large intestine following conversion of SDG by bacteria in the colon. Thus, the phyto-oestrogenic effect of flaxseed lignans depends on a healthy gut flora—the fermentation that splits them enables the uptake and so determines serum levels.[22]
- **Metabolism**: enterolactone and enterodiol are conjugated with glucuronic acid or sulphate in the liver, and leave the body via faeces, or are then deconjugated again by gut bacteria (see Chapter 1 for more

PRINCIPLES OF HERBAL TREATMENT   73

details on the metabolism of oestrogen) and reabsorbed. Some are excreted in the urine.
- **Main pharmacological effects of SDG metabolites are**:
  - Oestrogenic or antiestrogenic (SERM)
  - Antioxidant
  - Hypotensive, cardioprotective
  - Hypoglycaemic, hypocholesterolaemic
  - Anti-cancerous, reducing angiogenesis

Lignan hormonal effects based on laboratory studies and clinical trials

Results of human trials using lignans

- Increased sex hormone binding globulin synthesis (SHBG) therefore less oestrogen is available in the body[23,24]
- Reduced risk of breast, prostate, and other hormone-sensitive cancers[25]
- Lignan phyto-oestrogens may have a protective effect against incontinence in postmenopausal women[26]

In vitro: Lignans have demonstrated inhibition of

- Aromatase[27]
- 5-α-reductase[28] (the enzyme responsible for converting testosterone into dihydrotestosterone, the more biologically active and potent form)
- 17-β-hydroxysteroid dehydrogenase activity[29] necessary for production of testosterone and oestrogens which might explain the association flaxseed consumption with reduced risk of breast, prostate and other hormone-sensitive cancers

General results of clinical studies using flaxseed as a dietary supplement

- Decreased menopausal frequency of hot flushes and improved quality of life.[30,31] Not all clinical trials have been convincing, however, and this may be due to use of lower doses compared to studies that found a positive effect on menopausal symptoms.

- Reduced serum levels of 17-β-oestradiol and oestrone sulphate.[32]
- Increased prolactin levels in postmenopausal women.[33]
- Oestrogen metabolites: an increase in the urinary ratio of 2-hydroxyoestrogen to 16-α-hydroxyoestrone.[34]
- Testosterone biosynthesis decreased in a case study of a patient with PCOS, who had reductions in androgen levels and hirsutism.[35]
- A favourable, but not clinically significant, effect on blood cholesterol though no significant change in BMD (bone mineral density) or other symptoms in healthy menopausal women.[36]
- Increased level of ω-3 fatty acids in plasma and some effect on apolipoprotein metabolism in healthy menopausal women.[37]
- Efficacy similar to oral oestrogen-progesterone for mild menopausal symptoms, lowering glucose and insulin levels in hypercholesterolaemic menopausal women (however, in that trial only hormone replacement therapy significantly improved cholesterol profile and favourably modified markers related to cardiovascular health in these women).[38]
- Eating a muffin containing ground flaxseed (25g daily for 3 months) significantly reduced symptoms in women with severe cyclic mastalgia.[39]

Anti-tumour activity of flaxseeds

The main focus of research into lignans is their beneficial effect on breast cancer. Epidemiological research shows that lower plasma levels of lignans are commonly found in women with breast cancer. Vegetarian women, who have higher concentration of lignans in plasma and urine than omnivorous women, tend to have lower rates of breast cancer and the lower incidence of breast, colon, and prostate cancer in Finland is thought likely to be attributable to high consumption of rye bread, whose lignan content is also relatively high.

Flaxseed also inhibits the formation of colon, breast, skin, and lung tumours *in vivo*,[40] and lignans appear to be generally effective in reducing growth of cancerous tumours, especially hormone-sensitive ones such as those of the breast, endometrium and prostate. They also seem to be generally effective against new tumour development. Both flax seed and SDG are protective against chemical-induced carcinogenesis of the liver *in vivo*.[41] Once again, the benefits of flax are probably synergistic, as alpha-linolenic acid (ALA) has also been found effective in reducing growth of established tumours *in vivo*.[42]

The main anti-tumour factors looked at have been reduction in cell proliferation and angiogenesis, and an increase in apoptosis via modulation of the oestrogen receptor (ER)- and growth factor- signalling pathways.[43] However, flaxseed has also been shown to lower circulating levels of insulin and insulin-like growth factor 1 (IGF-1). Higher levels of insulin and IGF-1 stimulate cell proliferation and protect DNA-damaged cells.

Another reason for the effectiveness of the lignans is likely to be that they raise endostatin levels. Endostatins are secreted by blood vessels in response to tumour development, and they inhibit angiogenesis and increase apoptosis.

Breast cancer

Observational studies with flaxseed and lignan intake have shown that urinary excretion or serum levels are associated with reduced breast cancer risk, particularly in postmenopausal women, reducing all-cause mortality without reducing tamoxifen effectiveness.[44] Ground flaxseed significantly reduced markers of tumour cell proliferation in women newly diagnosed with breast cancer.

Alongside tamoxifen

From *in vivo* studies, neither flaxseed at the level of 10% of the diet nor the lignan equivalent to that quantity of seeds interfere with the effectiveness of tamoxifen but rather increase it, while 4% flax seed oil increases Trastuzumab/Herceptin (2.5mg/kg) effectiveness.[45] Flaxseeds are not the only type of phyto-oestrogenic plants of benefit in breast tumour treatment, going against the often-quoted idea that phyto-oestrogenic plants are contraindicated.

In vitro: additive effects when used with tamoxifen for inhibiting breast cancer tumour cell proliferation and inducing tumour regression in oestrogen receptor-positive breast cancer models.[46]

Tamoxifen increases endostatin levels both in women *in vivo* and in cultured breast biopsies, while flaxseed in the diet of healthy premenopausal women increased the extracellular endostatin in breast tissue significantly.[47,48]

Other mechanisms involved in flax seed's anti-tumour activity in breast cancer

- Decreased cell proliferation and angiogenesis, and increased apoptosis through modulation of:
  - oestrogen metabolism
  - oestrogen receptor signalling pathways
  - growth factor receptor signalling pathways[49]
- Stimulation of SHBG synthesis in the liver and inhibition of aromatase enzyme activity in pre-adipose cells may inhibit growth of hormone-dependent cancer cells.[50]
- Increased urinary ratio of 2-hydroxyoestrogen to 16-α-hydroxyoestrone.
- Reduced insulin-like growth factor I (IGF-I) plasma level concentrations, a factor associated with increased breast cancer risk.

Altogether, the evidence is strong that flax seed and its components are effective in the risk reduction and treatment of breast cancer, and safe for consumption by breast cancer patients.

Prostate cancer

- Flaxseed supplementation also inhibits cancer cell growth and reduces tumour angiogenesis in patients with prostate cancer.[51]
- Population research also suggests that intake of dietary lignans is associated with a decreased risk of developing prostate cancer.[52]
- Adding ground flaxseed to a fat-restricted diet reduces prostate specific antigen (PSA) levels in men with prostatic intraepithelial neoplasia (PIN), slowing proliferation of the prostate epithelium, and lowering testosterone levels.
- One could speculate on several mechanisms for the reduction of testosterone levels, including increased production of SHBG and increased excretion in the bowel.

Colorectal cancer

High dietary intake of lignans is associated with reduced risk of developing colorectal cancer[53] and enterolactone and enterodiol have been found to inhibit colon tumour growth *in vitro*.[54]

Other actions of flax seeds

Hypoglycaemic effect

Dietary fibre, lignans, and ω-3 fatty acids are individually all protective against diabetes.[55] Flaxseed has been shown to lower insulin levels in post-menopausal women[56] and decrease the risk of obesity and dyslipidaemia (risk factors for the development of diabetes and insulin resistance).[57]

- Clinical research has shown a reduction in fasting blood glucose, haemoglobin A1C (HbA1C) and markers of inflammation compared to placebo in patients with Type 2 diabetes.[58]
- This is not a universal finding: other studies have found no effect on fasting serum glucose and insulin levels and reported no change after flaxseed supplementation.

Obesity

Viscous soluble fibre slows gastric emptying and prolongs the nutrient absorption phase, increasing bulking in the small intestine and along with it the sensation of satiety. Young, non-obese adults taking flaxseed fibre (2.5g) in a drink or as tablets, 2 hours before a meal, were found to consume 9% fewer calories during the meal.[59] Levels of leptin (a hormone that suppresses appetite) were elevated in animals taking diet supplemented with 10% flaxseed. Changes in leptin expression were strongly and positively correlated with adipose ALA levels and inversely correlated with risk of atherosclerosis.[60]

Clinical trials on cardiovascular benefits and hypercholesterolaemia

Flaxseed preparations reduce total cholesterol and low-density lipoprotein (LDL) cholesterol in people with normal cholesterol levels, patients with hypercholesterolaemia, and patients with peripheral arterial disease.[61] Flaxseed supplementation also reduces platelet aggregation[62] and production of A-1 and B apolipoproteins (indicators of the risk for coronary heart disease).[63] Flaxseed supplementation seems to significantly reduce the risk of developing aortic atherosclerosis.[64] So, as with its anti-tumour effects, flax seems to have a broad range of beneficial effects on cardiovascular disease. Meta-analysis of research concludes that flax seed lowers blood pressure slightly, the effect being greater when it is consumed whole.[65]

Systemic lupus erythematosus (SLE) nephritis

Flax seed is thought to improve renal function by decreasing blood viscosity and serum cholesterol, and reducing inflammatory response.[66]

Haemodialysis patients

In kidney dialysis patients with lipid abnormalities, flaxseed consumption improves these lipid abnormalities and reduces systemic inflammation. Daily use of whole or ground flaxseed can lower serum creatinine[67] and a dietary milled sesame/pumpkin/flaxseed mixture has been found to lower triglyceride, C-reactive protein, TNF-alpha and IL-6 levels and improve glycaemic control, fatty acid profile, and pruritus symptoms.

Osteoporosis

In vivo research has shown a beneficial effect on bone production, but clinical trials have not supported this. Long-term trials would be needed to evaluate this, but research seem to suggest that it does not affect markers of bone metabolism or improve bone mineral density in healthy, postmenopausal women.[68]

Dosage: The typical dosages used in the clinical trials are 10–50g of ground flaxseed. It is easy to use by mixing with yoghurt, or mix into bread mixtures as flour, although the essential fatty acid content will be degraded in that way.

Safety: Flaxseed is safe for most adults when taken by mouth.

Can lead to bloating, gas, abdominal pain, constipation, diarrhoea, stomach ache, and nausea. Higher doses are likely to cause more GI side effects.

Large amounts of flaxseed could block the intestines due to the bulk-forming laxative effects of flaxseed, and thus should be taken with plenty of water.

Patient-friendly summary

- Flax seeds combine three important factors
  - Mucilage that benefits the bowel flora, acts as a bulk laxative and aid to elimination
  - An ideal balance of essential fatty acids
  - Lignans that on conversion in the gut and absorption have oestrogen-balancing (phytoSERM) properties

- The phenolic phyto-oestrogens reduce the level of free oestrogen in conditions related to oestrogen excess
- The seeds are anti-inflammatory because of the combination of essential fatty acids and mucilage
- The level of ω-3 essential fatty acids in the diet is thought to have gone down markedly in the average diet since prehistoric times and is one explanation for the prevalence of inflammatory disease
- Flax seed can help to lower cholesterol and blood lipid imbalance
- It is protective against heart disease
- Flax helps with weight reduction by increasing the release of leptins
- Flax seed may reduce the risk of various cancers including breast cancer and bowel cancer

Soy (Glycine max)

Myths about soy

Soy beans are not really part of the traditional western diet, and so it is natural enough to ask questions about them, particularly as they are not nearly as tasty as some other more recent imports such as avocado or mango. One pervasive myth is that they are processed differently by Eastern Asians and Westerners and so, for example, are contraindicated in breast cancer in Westerners because they only have a protective effect if you are of Eastern Asian origin. This has a tiny element of truth, but is very misleading. It now seems that soybeans have a strongly protective effect if they are consumed regularly earlier in life, but at the same time they still have a protective effect if taken regularly later, helping to prevent recurrence and, like flaxseeds, they also enhance the effectiveness of tamoxifen. Like flax seeds, they are also beneficial for the gut flora and for healthy elimination; however, their essential fatty acid profile is not as balanced.

A further myth is that the isoflavones are better absorbed from fermented soybean products than from the unprocessed cooked beans. The data is inconsistent on this, and this may well depend on the health of the microbiome, which benefits from the oligosaccharide content of soy as it does from that of other legumes.

A final group of myths concerns other presumed side effects, notably that it suppresses thyroid function, interferes with mineral absorption or can have adverse effects on oestrogen-dependent tissues after the menopause. As with most common foods, analysing individual constituents can create an impression of theoretical risks that do not occur in the real world and this certainly seems to be the case with soy, given the very extensive clinical trials it has been subject to in recent years, not to mention its history of consumption as a dietary staple.

History of soy consumption

Soybeans have been a central feature of the diet in China for around 5,000 years, constituting between 20 and 60% of daily dietary protein. They were introduced by Buddhist missionaries to Japan and Korea. Soy sprouts are used in traditional Chinese medicine.

Since their introduction in the eighteenth century, soybeans have never become a major part of the Western diet and this contrast is almost solely responsible for the difference in isoflavonoid content of the diets of the two regions, with European or American diets providing 1–3mg per day of isoflavonoids, as opposed to East Asian diets where this figure is typically 20–80mg.

Epidemiology

In Japan, China, and Korea the prevalence of hot flushes is low among native Japanese women, and the incidence of most cancers that are common in the Western world is also low. It is too much to give soybeans sole credit for the difference but there is good reason to suppose that it is one of the factors responsible. Soybeans have more than one potentially therapeutic effect. Along with other legumes, they are good prebiotics, and as we have seen in the last chapter, prebiotics are of great importance in promoting a gut flora that allows glucuronidated oestrogens to be egested. Fermentation by gut flora is also very important in splitting isoflavonoid glycosides that are present in unprocessed soy beans (along with pharmacologically important glycosides in other plants).

The isoflavonoids in soybeans are the main focus of research interest, but it may be that the effect of isolated extracts is rather different from the effect of whole soybeans or even of processed products such as tofu and tempeh in the diet. The dietary effects are rather variable, presumably because of the differences in the composition of gut flora. This varies not only between individuals but between populations, and understanding in this area is likely to improve a great deal over the coming decades.

Soybean constituents

Soybeans contain (percentage content by weight):

- 35% proteins.
- 20% lipids (essential fatty acids linoleic acid) (omega-6) and α-linolenic acid (omega-3). The Ω-6:Ω-3 ratio between 5:1 and 13:1, so not a particularly good source of Ω-3.
- 30% carbohydrates Contains oligosaccharides (stachyose), which are poorly digested, and in the colon stimulate the growth of bacteria such as bifidobacteria, and thus are seen as prebiotic.[69] Processing reduces or eliminates the oligosaccharide content, e.g. in tempeh, tofu and isolated soy protein.[70]
- 9% fibre.
- Vitamins and minerals: potassium, iron, and calcium. Although soy contains phytate and oxalate, calcium absorption from soybeans is good.[71] Iron absorption is also good as most of it is in the form of ferritin.[72]
- Japanese soyfood natto is produced by fermentation using a strain of *Bacillus subtilis* and is a rich source of vitamin K2.[73]

Isoflavone content of processed and unprocessed soybeans

The isoflavones themselves are genistein, daidzein, glycitein, but in the plant these are present in the form of glycosides, respectively genistin, daidzin, and glycitin. Soy also contains a small amount of coumestrol.

Processing leads to a loss of isoflavones:[74] tofu and protein concentrate contain only a tenth of the original soy bean isoflavone content, but still significantly more than other legumes, or non-leguminous plant foods.

Typical isoflavone contents of soy-based foods per 100g/100ml

- Textured soy protein granules: 110mg (in *isolated* soy protein 80–90% of isoflavones can be lost)
- Roasted soy nuts: 106mg
- Tofu (curd made from hot water extract of soy bean): 31mg
- Cooked soy beans: 31mg
- Tempeh: 31mg
- Soy milk: 13mg

In fermented soy foods (miso, tempeh, and natto), the isoflavones occur as aglycones due to bacteria hydrolyzing the glycosides during the fermentation process, just as they do in the human gut. It has been suggested that isoflavones are better absorbed from fermented soya products because of this: however, studies have had contradictory results, and there is probably a great deal of variability in particular because of the diversity of gut microbiomes and thus the proportion of glycosides in unprocessed soya that are digested.

Isoflavone Pharmacodynamics

As mentioned above, isoflavonoids are inactive when present in the bound form (as glycosides)—the glycosides are then fermented by intestinal flora. As a result, individual variability in colonic microflora influences the amount of isoflavonoids entering the body.

Urinary recovery, which is an indirect measure of absorption, can vary from 15% to 66% for the isoflavones, and is higher for fermented than for unfermented soy products. Followers of a macrobiotic diet (which is normally high in soy and particularly fermented soy products) excreted more than four-fold the amount of urinary phyto-oestrogens compared with lactovegetarians, who in turn excreted double the amount that omnivores did.[75] As you might expect from the positive effect of oligosaccharides on benign gut flora, the presence of fibre correlates positively with urinary excretion of isoflavones.

Hormonal effect of isoflavones

Isoflavones bind to ERs (the binding is weak compared to oestrogen) but can still have a major effect due to their concentration in the body. Circulating levels of isoflavones after ingestion of approximately two servings of soy foods can be high compared to the endogenous oestrogen.[76] They bind preferentially to, and transactivate, ER-β.

RCTs have shown that a soy-rich diet can be helpful in menopausal symptoms such as hot flushes, although there are some contradictory results. There is meta-analysis support for the use of isoflavones for hot flushes, reduced their frequency and severity, with 40mg total isoflavones derived from whole soybeans providing the required amount of genistein.[77] A systematic review of 47 studies[78] using isoflavone-rich soy products showed the following effects:

- In premenopausal women, a decrease in FSH and LH, and an increase in the length of the menstrual cycle of 1.05 days.
- In postmenopausal women, there was a possible increase in oestradiol.

Potentially a weak effect on the hypothalamic-pituitary-gonadal axis in women.

Isoflavones and fertility

A positive effect has been found for isoflavones on live birth rates during infertility treatment[79]

- In cases of unexplained infertility, with a timed intercourse cycle and clomiphene citrate and phytoestrogens (120mg/d during cycle days 1–12), the clinical pregnancy rate was higher and there was increased endometrial thickness.
- In women undergoing infertility treatment using IVF along with a daily isoflavone supplement (1,500mg/d), the pregnancy/delivery rate was nearly double that of women receiving placebo, and again an increase in endometrial thickness was noted.
- In a prospective cohort study with mean total isoflavone intake of 3.4mg/day from consumption of soy foods and infertility treatment with Assisted Reproductive Technology, there were positive associations with live births, clinical pregnancy and fertilization rates, although no increase in endometrial thickness was noted.
- *In vivo*: improvements in gamete interactions were noted and soy consumption appeared to negate the adverse reproductive effects of the endocrine disruptor bisphenol A.[80]

Protective effects on bone density

In the osteoblastic cell line, ER-α is the predominant oestrogen receptor type, and as noted above, soy isoflavones interact more with this receptor. Studies investigating the effect of soy on bone density have shown greater enhancement from soy as a whole food than from isolated isoflavonoids. In epidemiologic studies in women, soy intake was associated with a one-third reduction in fracture risk[81] and soy-milk consumption has been associated with a lower risk of developing osteoporosis in postmenopausal women. One clinical trial including osteopaenic women also showed that isoflavones favourably affect bone turnover and/or BMD.[82] Interestingly, moderate doses of isoflavones (50–100mg/day) appear to be more efficacious for promoting bone health than higher doses.

Soy isoflavones and cancer protection

In addition to the hormonal effect of the isoflavones, soy has anti-proliferative activity through a variety of mechanisms:

- Inhibition of tumour invasiveness
- Inhibition of cell cycle progression
    - Anti-angiogenesis and antioxidant effect
    - Tyrosine kinase inhibition (tyrosine kinase has many signalling functions in cells, one of which can be to trigger tissue growth, and so it can also promote cancers)

Breast cancer risk

One of the ways in which soy may be protective against oestrogen-promoted cancers is once again its stimulation of β-receptors. So, this is not a straightforward oestrogenic or anti-oestrogenic effect, but the balance of activity of the two main receptor types.

The impact of soy food intake on breast cancer risk has been investigated extensively, particularly as it was at first thought to increase the risk. Most studies seem to suggest that early exposure leads to lower incidence of breast cancer. A meta-analysis of 18 epidemiological studies found that soy intake might be associated with a small reduction in breast cancer risk. The data suggest that for soy to reduce risk, consumption must occur during childhood and/or adolescence, but high soy protein intake during adulthood was protective against breast cancer among women who had not much soy during adolescence.[83,84] The degree of protection against breast cancer was similar to that observed from early pregnancy.[85] As with hot flushes, genistein seems to be particularly important, as it is associated with a higher amount of differentiation among breast epithelial cells, a marker associated with lower breast cancer risk. Longitudinal studies indicate that isoflavone supplements do not affect breast tissue density in premenopausal women and may decrease density in postmenopausal women.

Breast cancer treatment and prognosis

In treating breast cancer, soy has been found safe to take alongside tamoxifen, even enhancing its effect. Epidemiologic data also suggest that soy intake enhances the efficacy of tamoxifen, with a tamoxifen and soy combination offering twice the reduction in carcinogenesis provided by tamoxifen alone.[86] There are two ways in which soy can actually lower oestrogen levels, firstly that soy consumption correlates with inhibition of enzymes involved in oestrogen biosynthesis, and secondly that it stimulates production of SHBG, lowering the amount of free oestrogen available to tissues.

Soy intake improves the prognosis when breast cancer has been diagnosed. A meta-analysis involving over 11,000 women with breast cancer found that soy consumption was associated with statistically significant reductions in breast cancer recurrence, a benefit seen equally in Asian and non-Asian women.[87]

Endometrial cancer

There are differences in the effects of soy intake on endometrial thickness, with North American trials indicating a decrease in thickness and Asian trials an increase, but meta-analysis shows an inverse association between soy intake and the risk of endometrial cancer for both Asian and non-Asian women.[88] In premenopausal women with non-atypical endometrial hyperplasia, genistein (54mg/day) improved symptoms after 6 months to approximately the same degree as norethisterone.[89]

Prostate cancer

In population studies of Asians, higher soy consumption is associated with as much as a 50% reduction in prostate cancer risk,[90] and in prostate cancer patients isoflavone exposure slows the rise in PSA levels.[91]

Genistein seems to be mainly responsible for this chemopreventive effect through binding to ERβ. ERβ is expressed in prostate epithelial cells and is important in cellular homeostasis, as well as being anti-proliferative, pro-differentiative, and pro-apoptotic.

Other cancers

- In gastric cancer, high tofu consumption is associated with a better outcome.
- Studies found no change in mammography and vaginal maturation from daily administration.[92]

Renal disease

Preliminary evidence indicates that soy protein places less stress on the kidneys than other high-quality proteins. Meta-analysis involving patients with chronic renal disease has found that dietary soy protein decreased serum creatinine, serum phosphorus, inflammation (assessed by CRP) and proteinuria in pre-dialysis patients. Where renal function is compromised, serum phosphorus levels often become abnormally high, so it appears that replacing animal protein with soy protein would be very helpful.[93]

Depression

There is good evidence that soy intake has an antidepressant effect around and after the menopause, which certainly makes sense given the effect of oestrogen on the nervous system. It is comparable to chemical antidepressants and can be used alongside them—below are some of the findings of clinical research:

- In postmenopausal women, genistein has been shown to reduce depression.[94]
- In peri- and postmenopausal women, isoflavones 25mg reduced depressive symptoms and reduced anxiety.[95]
- Isoflavones (100mg) reduced depressive symptoms in clinically depressed postmenopausal women and are comparable to Zoloft (50mg/day) and Prozac (10mg/day). A combination of Zoloft and isoflavones resulted in a greater reduction in symptoms than the other three individual treatments.[96]

PRINCIPLES OF HERBAL TREATMENT   87

The effects of oestrogen on skin health are mentioned in the previous section, and we might also note the common ectodermal origin of skin and nerves; several trials suggest that isoflavones help to reduce wrinkles[97–99] (which might itself help with self-esteem peri- or postmenopausally).

Circulation

Soy consumption has been shown to be inversely associated with the risk of stroke and CHD,[100] and soy has a number of cardioprotective effects. C-reactive protein is an indicator of inflammation, and a risk marker and predictor of CVD, and in postmenopausal women with elevated CRP,[101] soy is associated with a decrease. Consumption of 47g/day of soy has been shown to decrease serum concentration total cholesterol, LDL-cholesterol and triglycerides, and to increase HDL, with a greater response to soy protein in hypercholesterolaemic compared to normocholesterolaemic individuals.[102] One hypothesis is that peptides formed from the digestion of soy protein upregulate hepatic LDL receptors.[103]

Soybean isoflavones have also been shown to improve vascular endothelial function (also related to developing CHD) in postmenopausal women with impaired endothelial function.[104] The effect is attributed to the anti-inflammatory effects of isoflavones. A systematic review found reduced arterial stiffness in people taking soy products. Soy is also mildly hypotensive according to meta-analyses, reducing systolic and diastolic blood pressure by approximately 2.5 and 1.5mmHg respectively.[105]

Side effects

Menopause and menarche

Although total protein intake and animal protein intake are associated with earlier menarche and the development of early pubertal characteristics,[106] a cross-sectional study found that soy intake was unrelated to the age of onset of menarche.[107] The European Food Safety Authority (EFSA) concluded that in postmenopausal women, isoflavones do not adversely affect breast, thyroid, and uterus. Similarly, in respect of the endometrium, a review of 25 clinical studies measuring endometrial thickness and histopathological changes concluded that isoflavones have no adverse effect.[108]

It is important to bear in mind that isoflavones cannot be equated with oestrogen, nor soy foods should with isoflavones. The soybean, like all foods, is a collection of many biologically active molecules, and it is a major part of much of the world's diet.

Thyroid function

Although, based on *in vitro* and *in vivo* research,[109] the isoflavones could theoretically lead to depletion of iodine, clinical trials have shown no effect for soy consumption on thyroid production a review in 2006 of 14 clinical trials concluded neither soy foods nor isoflavones adversely affect thyroid function in euthyroid men or women.[110] Subsequent studies have since come to similar conclusions. In people taking thyroid medication, soy protein could increase the amount required (as is the case of other drugs) by interfering with the absorption of levothyroxine, but as thyroid medication is supposed to be taken on an empty stomach this should not actually happen.[111]

Mineral uptake

Phytates can block uptake of minerals, but less so if eaten with meat or fish or in fermented products such as miso.[112] Recent research shows that the uptake of calcium and iron from soya products is good,[113] and a high phytate diet can reduce the negative effect of phytate on non-haem iron absorption among young women with sub-optimal iron stores,[114] so again this risk seems theoretical rather than real.

Allergy to soy

Soy can be somewhat difficult to digest, and its content of trypsin inhibitors can affect protein digestion.[115] But only few trypsin inhibitors are left behind after processing so usually digestion is not affected.

Conclusion

The big thing to reassure people about is that consumption of soya foods and other plant-based phenolic phyto-oestrogen is safe and beneficial in many ways. Population and clinical studies involving adults suggest benefits are associated with approximately two to four servings per day, typically providing 15–60mg/day.

On the other hand, supplementation with isoflavonoids, using synthetic ipriflavone, which provides 200–600mg/day of isoflavonoids a quantity near to impossible to take in a diet, is much more questionable.

To summarise very briefly, soy, like flax, is a good source of fibre and beneficial to the gut biome, something that is needed to absorb the isoflavones from unfermented beans and products as they are contained in the form of glycosides. The isoflavones, in particular genistein, have a wide range of anti-inflammatory and hormone-balancing effects, interacting particularly with beta oestrogen receptors, helping with hot flushes and other menopausal symptoms, having protective effects against gynaecological and other cancers, as well as being cardioprotective and useful in kidney disease. This, like flax seeds, is clearly a dietary addition with the greatest benefit in the menopause, but actually for women throughout life.

Patient-friendly summary

- Asian diets contain nearly 20 times as much soybean content as western diets, and a correspondingly greater amount of isoflavonoids.
- Soy beans are nutritionally useful as they are prebiotic because of their oligosaccharides, and quite mineral rich (iron, calcium).
- Isoflavones are available from fermented soya products (miso, tempeh and natto), but these are not necessarily better sources than beans.
- Soy isoflavones have a moderating effect on oestrogen levels in the reproductive years and slightly lengthen the menstrual cycle.
- Soy isoflavones interact mostly with the oestrogen beta receptors which help maintain bone density after the menopause but do not increase the risk of breast or endometrial cancer.
- Soy seems to be generally cancer protective and particularly for breast cancer after the menopause; it also reduces the risk of recurrence.
- Soy also appears to be protective against endometrial carcinoma.
- Soy helps with menopausal hot flushes (to an extent).
- Soy is also recommended to improve fertility.
- Soy has anti-inflammatory effects and helps improve blood lipid profiles, so it reduces the risk of heart disease and strokes.

CHAPTER THREE

Key herbs containing isoflavones and flavonoids

Red clover, Trifolium pratense

The name in Latin literally means 'three-leaved of the meadow', which defines clover pretty well. Like soy, it is a leguminous plant rich in isoflavones, and one of the most intensively researched in that respect. But it also has a long history of traditional use in the west in both agriculture and medicine.

Theophrastus in around 370 BCE described its use as a soil fertiliser, and this use remained common: fields of cultivated clover were described by Albertus Magnus in 1270, too. It is now known that the legumes are nitrogen-fixing plants containing symbiotic bacteria called Rhizobium within nodules in their root systems and releasing the ammonia when the plants die or are harvested with their roots being left behind.

History

America's nineteenth century Eclectic physicians[1-3] refer to red clover mostly as an alterative, a general deobstruent in chronic skin diseases and an antispasmodic, useful in some cases of whooping cough and for

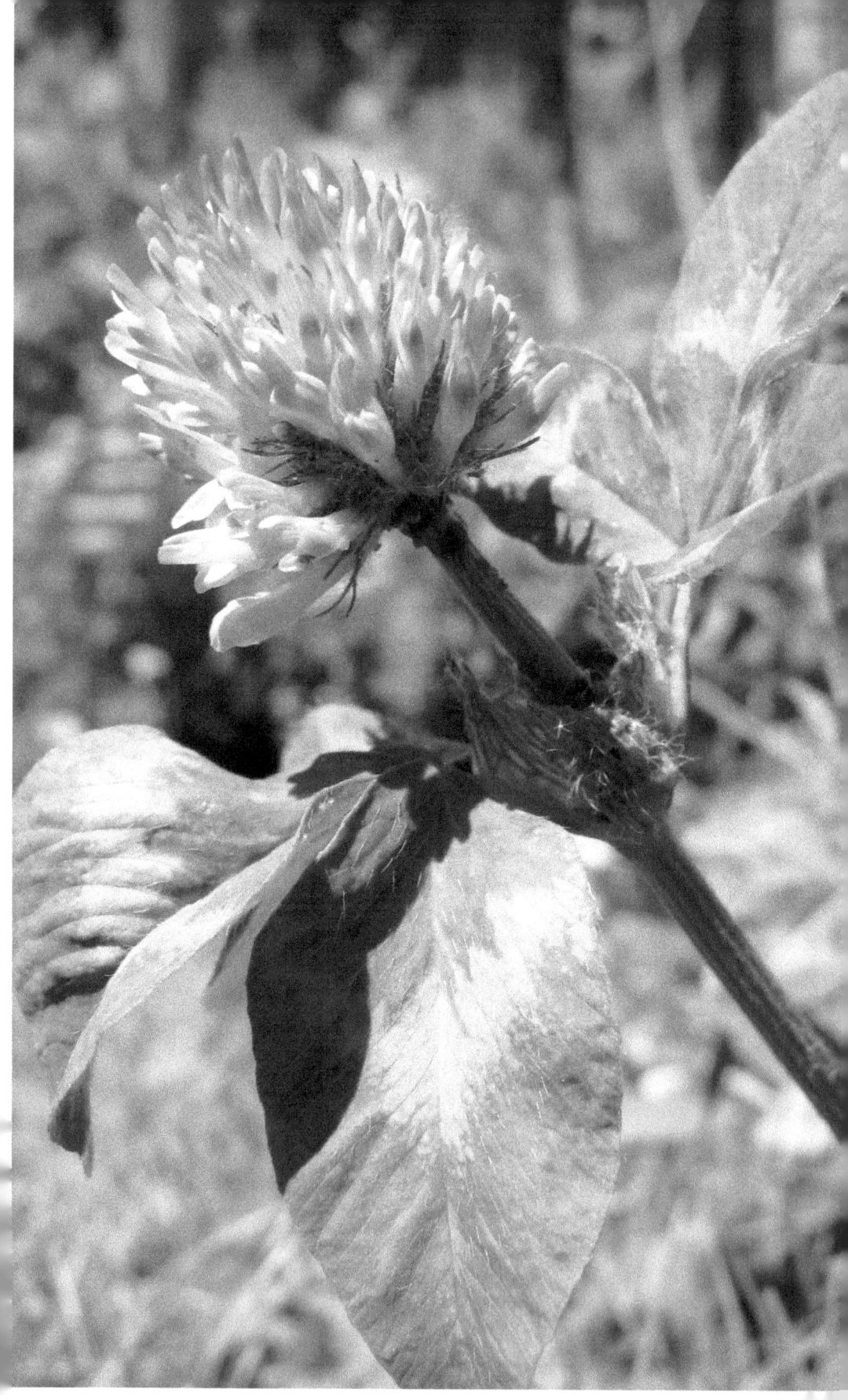

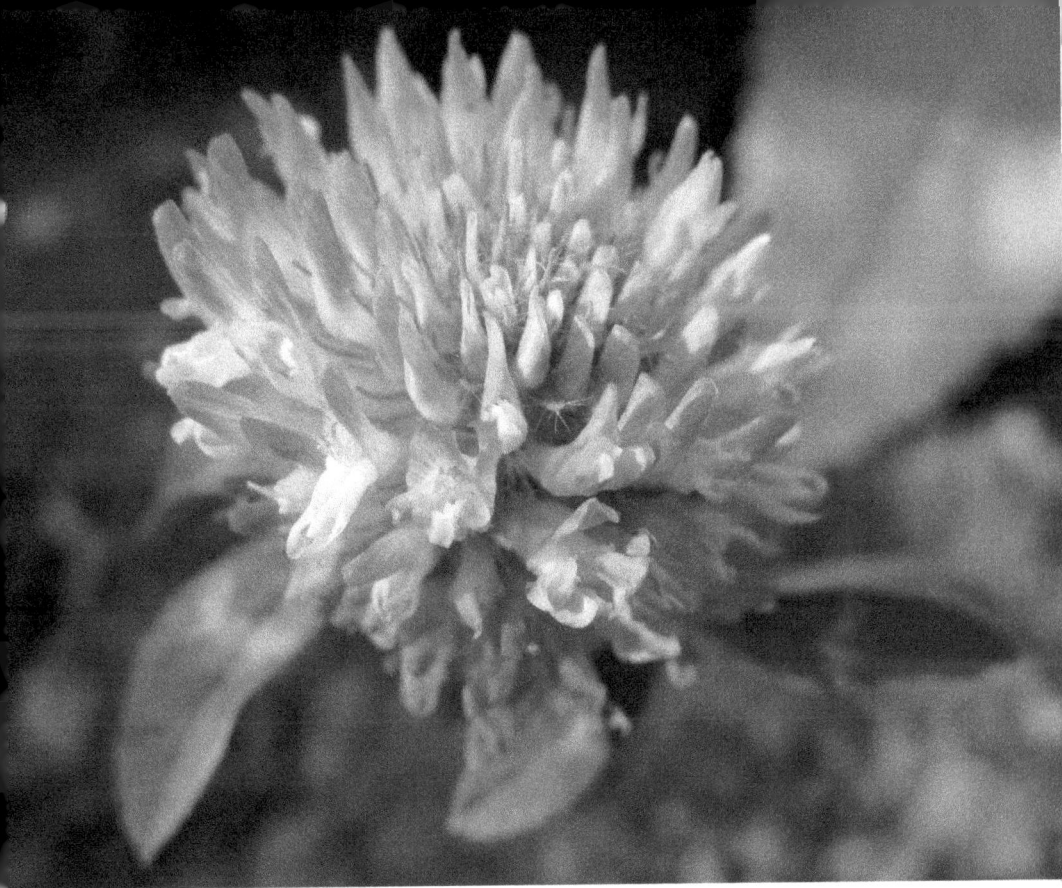

the cough accompanying measles, but not effective in all cases. It was also used as a soothing remedy for dry, irritable, spasmodic cough, bronchitis, and tuberculosis.

Red clover was applied externally for indolent ulcers and cancers and taken internally over a prolonged period for malignant neoplasms to retard their growth. It was a major ingredient in the Hoxsey formula, devised in the 1940s and still used in some cancer clinics. This treatment for cancer (added buckthorn) is somewhat similar to Trifolium compound in King's American Dispensatory 1898 which also includes *Stillingia sylvatica*, *Arctium lappa*, *Phytolacca decandra*, *Cascara amarga*, *Berberis aquifolium*, *Podophyllum peltatum*, *Xanthoxylum carolinianum*, and potassium iodide. It was used for syphilis, scrofula, chronic rheumatism, glandular and various skin affections.

Red clover became of medical interest when in the 1940s, Australian sheep grazing large quantities developed 'clover disease' extensive lesions on the reproductive organs (cystic endometrial hyperplasia) leading to permanent infertility. It was suggested that red clover was acting as a contraceptive but studies since have been contradictory in relation to sheep fertility. However, the idea of oestrogenic activity resulted in the herb becoming investigated as a possible treatment for menopausal symptoms.

There was no tradition of this usage, but this is not very surprising, the idea of the menopause being a medical condition rather than simply a transitional phase in life, as we would see menarche, and there are plenty of herbs for symptomatic treatment of hot flushes, for example, including hops and sage. Aside from this, menopausal women probably formed a smaller proportion of the population in previous centuries and most of them were probably adhering to many of the recommendations made for adjusting to the menopause—more exercise, more whole grains and less fat, sugar and refined carbohydrates—because this was how most people lived.

Constituents

Isoflavones in the flowering tops: biochanin A, formononetin, daidzein, genistein (the last two are also constituents of soy).

Other constituents: flavonols (isorhamnetin, quercetin glycosides), coumestrol, phenolic acids (salicylic acid, p-coumaric acid), volatile oils.

General indications

Alterative, mild expectorant, mild antispasmodic, lymphatic.

Extracts

The isoflavone extract used in most trials has been Promensil® (Novogen Limited), standardised to contain 40mg of total of isoflavones: 4mg of genistein, 3.5mg of daidzein, 24.5mg of biochanin A, and 8mg of formononetin. An 80mg version is also sometimes used in trials.

Pharmacokinetics

Isoflavones are isolated from red clover via alcohol extraction: in 25% aqueous ethanolic extracts these constituents are present only in low quantities, usually as glycosides.

The isoflavones biochanin A and formononetin are hydrolysed by β-glucosidases in the jejunum and liver,[5] releasing genistein and daidzein, the main isoflavone constituents of soy. Metabolism and absorption (influenced by food and healthy gut flora) are highly variable, and the isoflavones have a half-life of 13–16 hours.[6]

There have been suggestions relating to *in vitro* studies that red clover isoflavones might have higher bioavailability compared with soy and that red clover clinical trials tend to show more efficacy for menopausal symptoms compared with those evaluating soy products.[7] However, other clinical trials have not shown a significant difference from placebo, particularly for relieving hot flushes,[8] and so it is probably safe to say it that red clover has a mild effect.

As noted, isoflavones bind to ER-β preferentially over ER-α. Red clover extract has also been found to bind with μ- and δ-opiate receptors, which have a role in the opioid system in regulating temperature, calming mood, and influencing hormonal levels and actions, and there is clinical evidence to support these effects, potentially suggesting a different mechanism for its effects in menopausal problems.[9]

Menopausal symptoms

A meta-analysis in 2017 with Promensil® (at a dosage providing 80mg of isoflavones, shown to be sufficient to raise plasma isoflavones to a level comparable with the plasma isoflavone content of populations consuming a soy-rich diet) found it effective for hot flushes, and to show effects on the Kupperman Index as a whole, indicating that red clover may have a clinically significant effect on menopausal symptoms in general and not just on hot flushes specifically.[10]

Subjective symptoms of vaginal atrophy (vaginal dryness) and objective symptoms (maturation value) showed significant improvement with the 80mg isoflavones dose of red clover, together with a reduction in symptomatic palpitations and a significant improvement in subjective scores of depression.[11] In another trial, supplementation with this dosage of red clover extract also resulted in a subjective improvement of scalp hair and skin status, as well as libido, mood, sleep, and tiredness in postmenopausal women.[12]

There are other somewhat contradictory results for red clover on menopausal symptoms and to complicate matters, research with Trifolium is often interpreted together with that on soy isoflavones and or isolated isoflavones, and a distinction is not always made. In meta-analysis, different red clover products with very different chemical profiles have been compared,[13] a typical problem with systematic reviews of herbal medicines. Different extraction methods using the same batch of *Trifolium pratense* have shown considerable differences in oestrogenic activity. The most effective extraction seems to be with ethanol content 70% or above and high pressure. But there is still enough evidence to indicate its use for hot flushes and other menopausal symptoms.

Increasing and protecting bone density

There is some clinical evidence favouring the use of red clover isoflavones for bone density after the menopause, with 57–85.5mg (Rimostil®) daily for 6 months increasing BMD of the proximal radius and ulna in healthy postmenopausal women,[14] and red clover-derived isoflavones (26mg biochanin A, 16mg formononetin, 1mg genistein, and 0.5mg daidzein for 1 year) reducing the loss of lumbar spine BMD and BMC in women age 49–65 years, indicating that isoflavones have a potentially protective effect on the lumbar spine in women.[15]

Skin

The phenolic compounds found in Trifolium could explain the traditional use of Trifolium for chronic skin conditions. Both *in vivo* and *in vitro* studies with phenolic compounds have demonstrated inhibition or reversal of the signs of ageing (wrinkles or hyperpigmentation), and inhibition or slowing down of the development of various skin-related diseases, including skin cancer, skin problems (acne), as well as demonstrating efficacy in healing chronic wounds and burns.[16]

Reduced risk of coronary vascular disease

Most trials have shown no effect, but in one clinical study, a red clover extract providing 80mg isoflavones daily reduced total cholesterol and LDL in postmenopausal women.[17] Results from another, small clinical study, suggested that isoflavone supplementation from red clover may favourably influence blood pressure and endothelial function in postmenopausal Type 2 diabetic women. Body mass index (BMI) did not change compared to pre-treatment.[18] A systematic review concluded that red clover reduces levels of triglycerides and increases high density lipoprotein cholesterol.[19] This effect is common to soy and flax seed, too.

Anti-proliferative effects

The isoflavones biochanin A and genistein inhibit cell proliferation *in vitro*, and genistein inhibits cell proliferation by inhibiting tyrosine kinases and DNA topoisomerases I and II.

Benign prostatic hyperplasia (BPH) and prostate cancer

Daily oral administration of 60mg of an isoflavone extract from red clover in patients with BPH showed a decrease in size and in total PSA levels but an increase in all three liver transaminases.[20] A trial for prostate adenocarcinoma patients using 160mg/day of red clover-derived dietary isoflavones, containing a mixture of genistein, daidzein, formononetin, and biochanin A, showed that apoptosis in low to moderate-grade tumours was significantly higher than in control.[21]

Contraindications and adverse effects

No significant adverse events have been reported in the literature, though the rise in liver transaminases in one study suggests some challenge to the liver. None of the controlled, clinical trials has reported adverse effects at doses up to 160mg of isoflavones per day. Coumestrol has been shown to exhibit both mutagenic and clastogenic (chromosome-breaking) properties in cultured human lymphoblastoid cells.[22]

As with soy, there has been debate about the oestrogenic effects in breast cancer and other oestrogenic related conditions, but clinical evidence likewise suggests this is not a problem. Meta-analysis of randomised, controlled clinical trials on soya and red clover (*Trifolium pratense*) isoflavones found no impact on mammographic breast density in postmenopausal women, nor was there any change in this measure in a trial taking Promensil® providing 40mg isoflavones daily for a year.[23-25]

Endometrial effects

In human research, purified isoflavones extracted from red clover (P-07) lacked an effect on endometrial proliferation, with no changes in thickness of lining in uterus in postmenopausal women.[26]

Dosage, preparations, usage

Trials using Trifolium used standardised extracts for isoflavone content, whereas the traditional 25% aqueous ethanolic extracts tend to be low in isoflavones, and infusions particularly so, which might explain the relative lack of traditional use for gynaecological problems. To have confidence that a liquid extract contains any significant amount of isoflavones, either look for verification or choose a 45% or 60% ethanolic extract.

Clinical trials

There is plenty of research support for using the Trifolium extract, Promensil® used in most clinical trials, where the most effective dosage tended to be 80mg isoflavones. That would correspond to an extract of the whole herb of 480mg or 20–40ml 1:2 per week provided the isoflavones have been efficiently extracted.[27]

Summary of actions, indications and research findings for Trifolium pratense

The main history of use of red clover has been for skin complaints, as a lymphatic and alterative (a designation given mostly to plants we would now call anti-inflammatory), for:

- Burns, ulcers
- Psoriasis
- Eczema
- Skin cancers

Red clover has also been much used as an expectorant, particularly for dry and spasmodic coughs. More recently, it has been researched (in the form of Promensil®) and used for hormonal problems particularly around the menopause:

- Hot flushes
- Libido, mood, sleep, and tiredness
- Potentially protective against osteoporosis
- Metabolic syndrome: decreases triglycerides and increases HDL levels
- May also help blood pressure postmenopausal Type 2 diabetic women
- Has shown efficacy in BPH and prostate cancer

Hops, Humulus lupulus, Cannabinaceae

Lupulus means a 'little wolf', as the plant climbs over other plants as a wolf does a sheep. Both the genus name and the common name from Anglo-Saxon hoppan (to climb or jump) and its earlier Indo-European roots.

This is another plant steeped in history, mentioned by Avicenna (980–1037) in al-Qanun fi'l-tibb. Ibn-Al Baitar (1188–1248)[28] praised its digestive and calming properties,[29] although the calming effect was a bit too much for Hildegard von Bingen (1098–1179), who wrote in Physica, 'it is not much use for a human being, since it causes his melancholy to increase, gives him a sad mind, and makes his intestines heavy', but also paying tribute to its best known use, 'its bitterness fends off decomposition of beverages and increases shelf life'. This was well known to German monks, who added hops for their preservative action when making beer. The antibacterial properties of hops have long been confirmed.

Over the centuries, many more herbalists, including Paracelsus (1493–1541), have recommended hops as a digestive aid, diuretic,

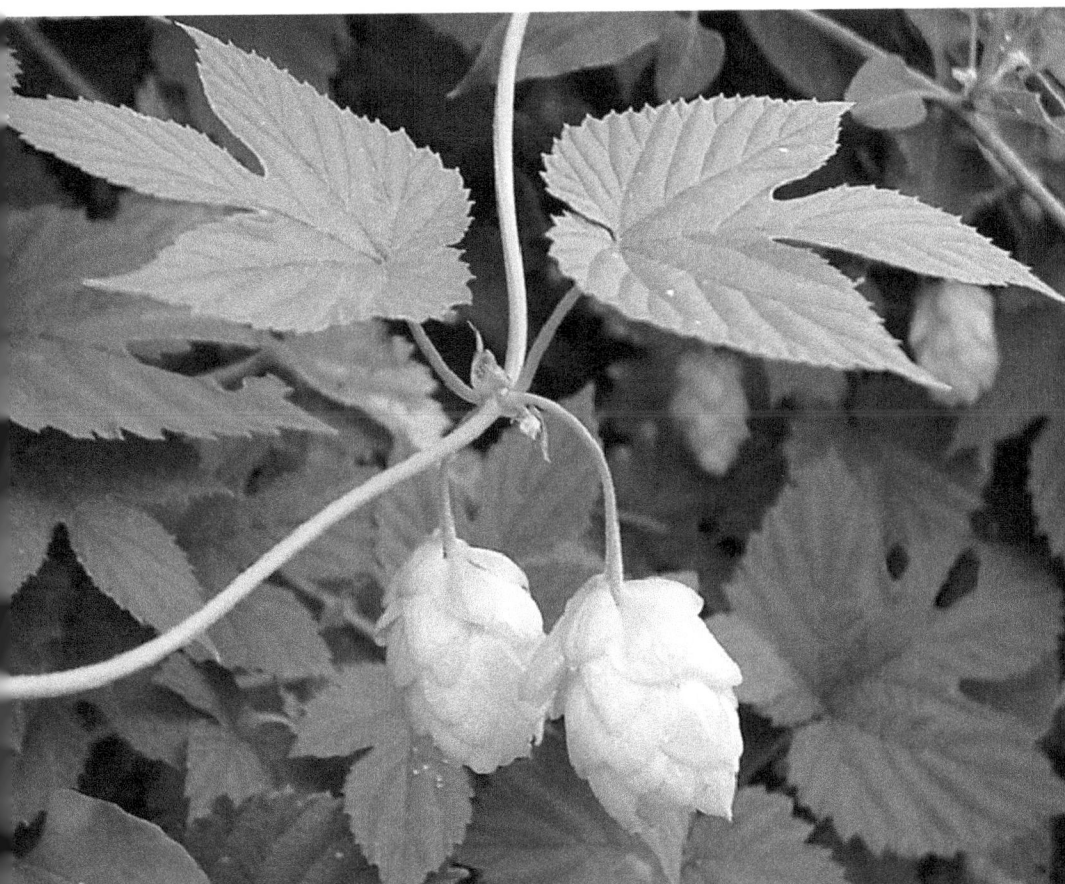

cholagogue, and bitter, and for its calming and appetite-stimulating effect, used both for anorexia due to gastritis and for sleeplessness (particularly sleep latency).[30]

King George III (1738–1820), whose nervous problems are legendary, used hop pillows to calm himself.[31] Several writings recommended the use of hop pillows, teas, or extracts for sleeping problems associated with nervous disturbances.[32] It was believed that hops acted through a strong and heavy odour, causing somnolence.

Native American, European and Eclectic herbalists also used hops as a sedative and bitter tonic, and for sleep disorders and digestive problems associated with nervous tension or stress. Native Americans and later the Eclectics used a fomentation, dipping a muslin bag filled with hops into hot water, wrung out and applied over painful acute local inflammations. This was applied to facial neuralgia, over an ulcerating tooth, used for earache in children.[33] Another historic use was against hair loss, washing the head with beer to increase hair growth.

In Ayurvedic medicine, hops were used for restlessness associated with nervous tension, for headache, and for indigestion and as a sedative, hypnotic, and antibacterial.[34] Hops have also been regularly mentioned for sexual neurosis, priapism, and as an anaphrodisiac. It is fascinating how many independent traditional uses, for nervous tension, poor appetite, sexual excitement and sleeplessness corroborate each other.

Hops gained interest in relation to gynaecological conditions when it was observed that women hop pickers regularly began menstruating 2 days after beginning to pick hops, and so research began into the oestrogenic properties of hops.

Constituents

Hop resins, polyphenols and essential oils are important for brewers. Isomerised products of hop resins give beer its bitterness, and its polyphenols promote the precipitation of proteins, while hop essential oils give the beer a distinctive hoppy flavour.

The main constituents form a very unusual combination:

- Resinous bitter principles: ρ iso-α- and β-acids. The bitter principles are known to break down rapidly during storage, and the α- and β-acids are particularly susceptible to oxidation. The iso-α acids (there is more than one isomer) are extracted and commercially used in brewing beer.

- Essential oil that yields sesquiterpenes (myrcene, linalool, humulene, caryophyllene, 2-methyl-3-butene-2-ol the latter increase after storage (soporific)).
- Flavonols: quercetin, kaempferol, and myricetin.
- Flavonoids: the chalcones, prenylnaringenins (6- and 8-prenylnaringenin), xanthohumol and isoxanthohumol.

General actions

Sedative, hypnotic, spasmolytic, aromatic bitter, oestrogenic.

Sedative and hypnotic action

There are stories of hop pickers getting drowsy,[35] and certainly a long and widespread use of hops to help with sleep. The compounds mainly responsible for its sedative action are the bitter resins and essential oils.

The crude extract has a high affinity to a wide range of receptors in the nervous system, including GABA (A and B), glutamate (AMPA, NMDA, kainite), glycine, CCK (A and B), and chloride ion channel receptors. The α-acids have proved to the be most potent sedative components *in vivo*.[36] The effect on GABA receptors is presumably the most important factor for the sedative action,[37] and perhaps the decreased gut motility is due to the effect on CCK receptors, which decrease contractions of the smooth muscle of the gut. A volatile degradation product of hop bitter acids, 2-methyl-3-buten-2-ol (dimethylvinyl carbinol), also has sedative properties and could be the reason for the effectiveness of hop pillows. This constituent increases during storage, and may be formed after ingestion as well.[38]

As always with herbs, there are always several (or many) modes of action, and sleep-inducing effects may also be centrally mediated through activation of melatonin receptors, which are responsible for circadian rhythms (*in vivo*).[39] Unlike the related *Cannabis sativa* (hemp or marijuana), hops do not contain cannabinoids, but caryophyllene present in both plants does bind to endocannabinoid receptors, and is another possible cause for the decrease in gut motility in hops.

Clinical trials for insomnia

Studies, always in combination (typically with *Valeriana officinalis*) when used internally, show a positive effect on both subjective and objective measures.

- Reductions in the sleep latency and wake time have been found, with sleep stage 1 reduced and slow-wave sleep increased; patients felt refreshed in the morning,[40] with improved quality of sleep[41] and improved quality of life,[42] similarly to taking benzodiazepine and bromazepam (Lexotanil).[43] EEG recordings indicated improved sleep stage patterns (slow-wave sleep and REM) in sleep-disturbed volunteers.[44] Sleep latency (the time required to fall asleep) was improved compared to using valerian on its own.[45]
- One study found that effects did not appear until after 28 days, suggesting that continued treatment over a month can be helpful in insomnia. However, another clinical trial showed that after a single dose the EEG-derived parameter 'sleep quantity' (calculated from the electrohypnogram) proved the valerian/hops combination superior to placebo, and concluded the combination can be used successfully using a single dose.[46] This does suggest that there are multiple modes of action, a purely sedative one and an effect on circadian rhythms. However, sleep is psychologically complex, so this is somewhat speculative.
- Hops reduce the stimulant effect of caffeine taken 60 minutes after oral administration:[47] typically a herbalist would suggest taking the herbs around 1 hour before bedtime.
- Hop baths on three successive days improved both objective and subjective sleep quality.[48]

Oestrogenic effects

Hop picking used to be a popular country summer holiday for poorer families from cities, a change of rhythm and a chance of sunshine, despite the long working days in the fields. Women who did this often began menstruating two days after beginning to pick hops, and that stimulated research into the oestrogenic properties of hops. The flavonoid chalcones, 8-prenylnaringenin and xanthohumol have been the main focus of attention. They have inherent oestrogenic activity but inhibit aromatase, thus decreasing endogenous oestrogen production, decrease breast cancer cell line proliferation and induce apoptosis *in vitro*.

8-prenylnaringenin, the most potent phytoestrogen, is metabolised from isoxanthohumol during the production of beer or, after ingestion, converted by the intestinal bacteria. It has a preference for ER-α, mimicking (though weakly) the action of 17β-oestradiol. It is slightly uterotrophic with an oestrogenic effect on mammary glands.

Xanthohumol is (both *in vivo* and *in vitro*) a 'broad-spectrum' cancer chemopreventive with antibacterial properties (there has been much research into its potential topical application for treating acne vulgaris).

Clinical evidence for using hops for menopausal symptoms

- One small clinical trial demonstrated that 8-prenylnaringenin is quickly and completely absorbed in the human intestine and that relevant plasma levels are achieved. This was inferred from a decrease of LH levels.[49]
- Daily intake of a hop extract reduced vasomotor symptoms and other menopausal symptoms. No dose-response relationship could be established, but a higher dose appeared less active,[50] a phenomenon that has also been found in studies of *Cimicifuga racemosa*. A study indicated reductions after 16 weeks for the Kupperman Index, visual analogue scale and Menopause Rating Scale.[51] Another trial showed a reduction in the number of hot flushes as well as decreased incidence of palpitations, insomnia, irritability and sweating.[52]
- Vaginal application of a gel with hops (also including hyaluronic acid, liposomes, and vitamin E) in an open, non-controlled study demonstrated a marked effect on vaginal dryness and associated symptoms. Dryness, itching, burning, dyspareunia, inflammation, and rashes all improved.[53]
- Hops have been shown to possess an oestradiol-like effect on osteogenic differentiation *in vitro* and *in vivo* studies with increased bone density (BMD),[54] and a cross-sectional study of 1697 healthy women (mean age 48.4 years) found increased BMD in women beer drinkers.[55]

Antibacterial, antiseptic, and tuberculocidal, antiviral, antifungal uses

Although it does not figure much in traditional use outside of brewing, hops have marked antibacterial action. The β-bitter acids have the strongest antibacterial effects and hop extracts containing them have high activity *in vitro* against Gram-positive bacteria, confirming their use as a preservative. But there quite a number of indications that hops could be much more widely used therapeutically:

- An *in vivo* study demonstrated the inhibitory effects of hops on *H. pylori* strains isolated from patients with gastritis. The researchers concluded that hops can be used as an adjunct or even an alternative to antibiotics in the treatment of *H. pylori* infections.[56]
- Suggestions have been made that brewery workers had lower incidence of tuberculosis.[57] *In vitro* results showed that different concentrations of hop ethanolic extracts (4 and 8mg/ml) had a marked inhibitory effect on rifampicin-sensitive and resistant isolates of *Mycobacterium tuberculosis*.[58]
- One study showed that hop compounds, especially xanthohumol, as alternatives for treatment of infections caused by select anaerobic bacteria, namely nosocomial diarrhoea caused by resistant strains.[59]
- Xanthohumol and the lupulones both showed strong inhibitory activities against all strains of acne-causing bacteria, and xanthohumol, humulones and lupulones all showed moderate to strong inhibition of anticollagenase.[60]
- Xanthohumol has also show antiviral activity against bovine viral diarrhoea virus, cytomegalovirus, herpes simplex virus Type 1 and 2 and human immunodeficiency virus 1, and indications of antifungal activity and the ability to inhibit replication of *Plasmodium falciparum*, the causative agent of malaria.[61]

Antioxidant, anti-inflammatory, antihyperlipidaemic, hypoglycaemic, antiobesity, anti-ageing

It may seem a bit much to lump all of these properties together but as we have seen, there is a great deal of overlap between these effects, and one might also refer to them as generally protective against tissue and cardiovascular damage.

- Systemic administration and *in vitro* research both demonstrate an anti-inflammatory effect of hop bitter acids on acute local inflammation.[62]
- ρ iso-α acids ameliorated joint damage *in vivo*,[63] and a 6-week, open-label trial of people with knee osteoarthritis taking 1,000mg of ρ iso-α acids produced a 54% reduction in WOMAC Global scores.[64]

- Xanthohumol, iso-α-acids and matured hop resin acids (*in vivo* and *in vitro*) have a beneficial effect on lipid metabolism, glucose tolerance, and body weight,[65] so hops offer great promise in diet-induced obesity and Type II diabetes. Diabetic subjects treated with isohumulones have shown reduced plasma glucose, triglyceride, and free fatty acid levels to a level similar to antidiabetic medication, with improved insulin sensitivity, increased liver fatty acid oxidation, together with a decrease in size and an increase in apoptosis of hypertrophic adipocytes. Patients also showed reduction in systolic blood pressure and in the levels of serum markers of liver disorder.[66]
- In a study using non-alcoholic beer, elderly nuns had reduced markers of cardiovascular risk and of inflammation. Researchers concluded that non-alcoholic beer or hops can contribute to a reduction in age-associated pathologies.[67]

Anti-cancer

- Xanthohumol has potential in cancer treatments. As an antioxidant it is more potent than vitamin C and vitamin E,[60] inducing apoptosis of cancer cells, having anti-proliferative effects (*in vitro*), modulating biotransformation of carcinogens, and inhibiting angiogenesis.[68]
- Further anti-cancer properties include protecting cells against DNA damage by mutagens by inhibiting their activation, inhibiting DNA synthesis and proliferation of cancer cells *in vitro*, inactivating oxygen radicals and inducing apoptosis. An *in vivo* study also indicates that xanthohumol protects against DNA damage and cancer induced by cooked food mutagens. The effects were observed with low doses of xanthohumol.[69] A clinical study also suggests that low doses of xanthohumol also protect humans against oxidative DNA damage.[70]
- The bitter acids have also been found to inhibit cell proliferation and angiogenesis, induce apoptosis and increase the expression of cytochrome P450 detoxification enzymes.

Hepatoprotective

Xanthohumol also inhibits several steps in the development of chronic liver disease, offering particular promise in obese patients with a predisposition to non-alcoholic fatty liver disease.[71] Based on these health-promoting properties, the production of a xanthohumol-enriched beer has been suggested.

Contraindications

Hops are traditionally contraindicated in depression, and the herb is not suitable for coldness, weakness or lethargy.

It has been said that because of activation of ER-α receptors the herb should be used cautiously over the long-term and best avoided by women with oestrogen receptor-positive breast cancer. However, as prenylflavonoids from hops have potential application in cancer prevention programmes and in prevention or treatment of peri- and post-menopausal hot flushes and osteoporosis, hops are actually useful in cancer prevention and possibly therapy. A hop extract, and particularly the compound 6-prenynaringenin, preferentially induce the non-toxic oestrogen 2-hydroxylation pathway in two different breast cell lines, hops appear to have a potentially protective role against breast cancer through oestrogen metabolism modulation.[72]

A clinical study of menopausal women to evaluate safety and pharmacokinetics confirms that short-term consumption of a chemically and biologically standardised preparation of spent hops is safe for women and that once-daily dosing might be appropriate.[73] Several *in vitro* studies suggest a protective effect for hops,[74] and an *in vivo* study indicates that hops do not have an oestrogenic effect on the uterus. There is also indirect epidemiological evidence of safety regarding breast cancer, too. Consumption of alcohol in adolescence and early adulthood predisposes to breast cancer, but no evidence has been found for a difference in risk between consumers of beer and other drinks.[75]

Summary of actions, indications and research findings for Humulus lupulus

Hop constituents, particularly the resinous and volatile constituents, bind to a wide range of receptors in the nervous system including GABA, glutamate, glycine, CCK and cannabinoid receptors, and this probably accounts for its sedative, hypnotic and spasmolytic effects.

Flavonoid chalcones, 8-prenylnaringenin and xanthohumol have a range of oestrogenic effects including aromatase inhibition, and xanthohumol and the bitter acids are antibacterial, anti-inflammatory (locally, and also beneficial for lipid metabolism and glucose tolerance), and cancer protective.

General indications

- Restlessness, anxiety.
- Neuralgia, headache.
- Nervous digestive problems: indigestion, dyspepsia, colon pain, spastic constipation, irritable bowel syndrome, mucous colitis, and other indications where bitters could be of use.
- Excessive sexual excitability.
- Sleeplessness (generally in combination with *Valeriana officinalis*): research indicates that it improves latency and quality of sleep.

Additional indications based on modern research

- Diabetes Type 2, obesity.
- Anticarcinogenic.
- Hepatoprotective.
- Menopausal problems (hot flushes, palpitations, insomnia, irritability and sweating).
- Improvement in bone density.
- Topically: ulcers, and as antibacterial.

Recommended dosage

1:2, 60% ethanolic extract, 1.5–3.0ml per day, 10–20ml per week.

Sage, Salvia officinalis

Introduction and history

The name Salvia (from Latin 'salvere', to preserve) may relate to its food storage properties or its ability to increase the fertility of women.[76] Sayings from the Middle Ages point at the high regard in which sage was held, even though nowadays it is much less venerated perhaps because of its culinary usage. An old French proverb points at its use in fevers and as a nervous tonic: 'sage helps the nerves and by its powerful might/palsy is cured and fever put to flight'; others are still more

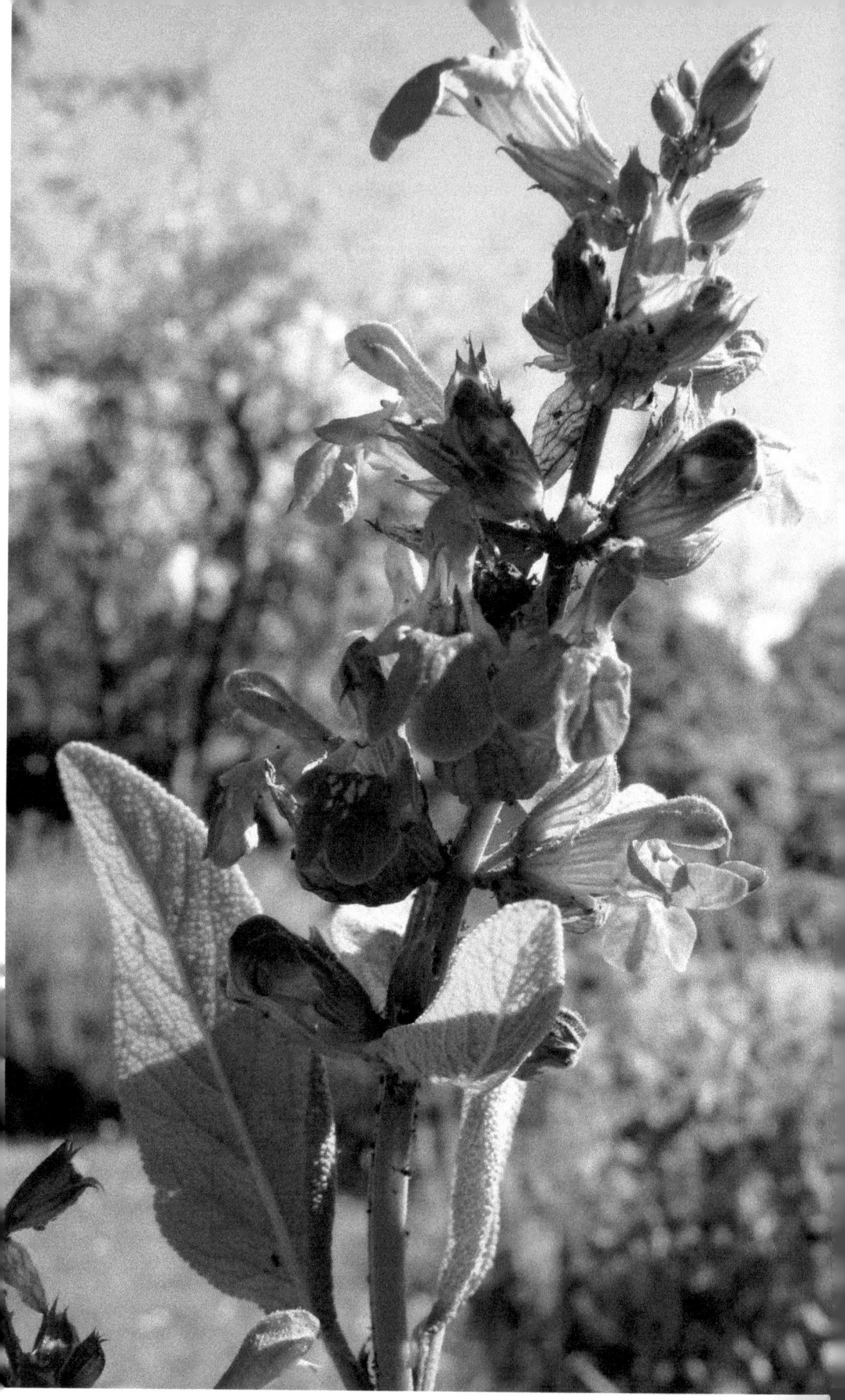

forthright 'Why should a man die while sage grows in his garden?' (*Cur moriatur homo cui salvia crescit in horto?*) and 'He that would live for aye/ Must eat Sage in May.'

Gerard says that 'Sage is singularly good for the head and brain, it quickeneth the senses and memory, strengtheneth the sinews, restoreth health to those that have the palsy, and taketh away shaky trembling of the members', and Culpeper and Hill both give tribute to its benefits for the brain, memory, and longevity. The current rediscovery of sage for cognitive and memory impairment, particularly in senile dementia, for nervous irritability and for hot flushes, clearly have a venerable history.

Sage's reputation makes it a strong candidate for inclusion among the adaptogens: it enhances abilities and is associated with strength and vitality into old age. Perhaps sage is a herb that can act as a pointer to the notion of supporting vitality within the western herbal tradition and to find analogues, based on the function of our general restorative herbs and immune tonics, to the Three Treasures of TCM (Jin, Qi, and Shen), and thus investigate the wealth of indigenous resources (nutritional as well as herbal) available to western herbalists in these terms.

Constituents

Phenolic acids:	Caffeic acid, 3-caffeoylquinic acid rosmarinic acid, salvianolic acids
Flavonoids:	Rosmarinic acid, luteolin-7-glucoside, apigenin, hispidulin, kaempferol, chlorogenic acid, ellagic acid and quercetin
Essential oils:	
Terpenoids:	α- and β-thujone (up to 30%), camphor, 1,8-cineole, α-humulene, borneol, pinene, limonene, β-caryophyllene
Diterpenes and triterpenes:	Carnosic acid, ursolic acid, carnosol
Polysaccharides:	Arabinogalactans, pectin

General indications

- Inflammations and infections of mouth and throat
- Excessive sweating

110   HERBAL MEDICINE IN TREATING GYNAECOLOGICAL CONDITIONS

- Menopausal hot flushes, night sweating
- Reducing and stopping lactation
- Febrile conditions
- Nervous debility, exhaustion
- Memory loss, Alzheimer's disease, dementia

Studies on Salvia officinalis

Cognitive and memory-enhancing effects, possible mechanisms

Salvia's antioxidant and anti-inflammatory actions offer long-term protection in the pathogenesis of dementia. Rosmarinic acid in particular has been shown to have neuroprotective, antioxidative, and anti-apoptotic effects against amyloid beta plaque toxicity in neuronal cells.[77]

A systematic review of clinical studies concluded that sage exerts beneficial effects by enhancing cognitive performance both in healthy subjects and patients with dementia or cognitive impairment.[78] In one such study, a hydroalcoholic extract improved cognitive functions in patients with mild to moderate Alzheimer's disease, and reduced agitation of patients.[79] Cholinergic activity has been identified for sage, acetylcholinesterase inhibitors being one of the main conventional drugs for treatment of Alzheimer's disease, used particularly for agitation and depression, and it is possible that this may be part of the explanation for this effect. Another might be, as discussed in the last chapter, that its oestrogenic activity causes increased activity in various neural circuits. There are indications that sage increases serotonergic activity in particular.[80] Dosage and preparations are likely to be important.

Other clinical studies for memory and cognition

- Aromas of essential oils of the Salvia species reproduce some but not all of the effects found following oral herb administration.[81,82]
- In young healthy adults, sage improved memory and cognition. With increasing dosage, the mood was elevated along with increased alertness, calmness, and contentedness. Both doses given (300, 600mg dried sage leaf) led to improved ratings of mood with the lower dose reducing anxiety and the higher dose increasing 'alertness', 'calmness' and 'contentedness' and improved mood and cognitive performance.[83]

- In healthy older volunteers (mean age around 73 years), sage improved cognitive function (167, 333, 666, and 1,332mg ethanolic extract). The 333-mg dose caused a highly significant enhancement of secondary memory. Interestingly, higher doses did not work nearly as well.[84]

Cognitive- and memory-enhancing effects *in vivo* and *in vitro*

- The ethanolic extract of *Salvia officinalis* potentiated memory retention, and it is thought that this is likely to be because of its interaction with muscarinic and nicotinic cholinergic systems involved in the memory retention process.[85] Cholinesterase-inhibiting properties have been shown *in vitro*.
- Sage and rosmarinic acid both improved cognition *in vivo* against diabetic memory impairment,[86] and the hydroalcoholic extract attenuates morphine-induced memory impairment.[87]

Menopause: hot flushes, metabolic syndrome, sweating, bone metabolism

Hot flushes

Clinical research in general supports traditional usage of sage in menopausal symptoms. In an open clinical trial there was a decrease in the intensity and total number of hot flushes and general improvement in the Menopause Rating Scale (MRS): somato-vegetative, psychological, and urogenital subscales decreased,[88] and another trial has shown similar general improvements along with reduced frequency, severity, and duration of hot flushes and night sweats in menopausal women.[89] No differences were found in oestradiol levels. One further study in which no significant differences between sage and placebo groups were found with respect to frequency, duration, and severity of hot flashes also found that a larger number of the patients taking sage noted an improvement in their overall clinical conditions.[90] Another study, using a combination product of Salvia and *Medicago sativa* (alfalfa)[91] showed a reduction in hot flushes and night sweating together with an increase in prolactin and thyroid stimulating hormone (TSH) in response to thyrotropin-releasing hormone (TRH) but no change in basal levels of oestradiol, LH, FSH, prolactin and TSH concluded this combination had central slight antidopaminergic action. It is thought that the flavonoids most likely play a role in the reduction of menopausal symptoms.

A pilot study also found *Salvia officinalis* effective in controlling hot flushes in prostate cancer patients treated with androgen deprivation therapy (oestrogen deficiency can also affect men as aromatase conversion of androgens is also needed for bone and skin metabolism).[92]

Perspiration-inhibiting effect studies

Several open studies were carried out mainly in the 1930s on patients or healthy volunteers, showing a definite ability to restrain sweating. A larger study from 1989 (unpublished) on patients with idiopathic hyperhidrosis found that excessive sweating induced by pilocarpine (a parasympathomimetic alkaloid) was inhibited by an extract of fresh sage. In a similar open study, patients were given dried aqueous extract of sage, (equivalent to 2.6g) or infusion of sage (4.5g herb daily) and a reduction of sweat was achieved in both groups.[93]

Metabolic effects on glycaemic control and lipid profile

As discussed in Chapter 7, the menopause involves a number of biochemical and hormonal changes in the body, one of which is a tendency towards metabolic syndrome, hence Type 2 diabetes, with less glycaemic control and more low-density lipoproteins in the blood. There is *in vivo* evidence to indicate that sage decreases blood glucose in normal and diabetic conditions,[94] reduces serum triglycerides and total cholesterol, and low-density lipoproteins (LDL) levels in diet-induced obesity, and that it also decreases body weight and abdominal fat mass.[95]

A number of trials of sage have been run with hyperlipidaemic Type 2 diabetic[96] and other hyperlipidaemic patients[97,98] in which the extract lowered:

- Fasting glucose in patients with hyperlipidaemia and diabetes.
- HbA1c (glycated haemoglobin2: gives clinicians an overall picture of average blood sugar levels over weeks/months).
- Total cholesterol, triglyceride and LDL-C, very low-density lipoproteins (VLDL).

The extract also increased HDL-C compared to baseline at endpoint. The beneficial properties of *S. officinalis* tea consumption on serum lipid profile have been also reported on non-diabetic healthy volunteers.

Bone resorption inhibition activity in vivo, *and* in vitro

Dried leaves have been shown to strongly inhibit bone resorption, an effect confirmed for the essential oils and monoterpenes borneol, thymol, and camphor *in vivo* using osteoclast resorption pit assay (a tool to study osteoclast and osteoblast differentiation and function).[99]

Acute pharyngitis

Topical application of sage liquid extract as a throat spray reduced throat pain in acute pharyngitis (randomised, double-blind, placebo-controlled study).[100]

Other actions based on *in vivo* and *in vitro* research

Anti-tumour activity

Sage infusion and methanolic extracts have shown anti-proliferative, antimigratory and antiangiogenic effects on several cancerous cell lines *in vitro* and similar effects *in vivo*,[101] with chemopreventive effects of sage infusion, on colon cancer *in vivo*.[102] Individual constituents contributing to this are diterpenes, ursolic acid, flavonoids (rosmarinic acid) and monoterpene compounds such as thujone, camphor, limonene, and 1,8-cineole.

Antioxidant

Carnosol, rosmarinic acid, and carnosic acid, caffeic acid all contribute to sage's powerful antioxidant properties *in vivo* and *in vitro*.[103,104]

Anti-inflammatory and antinociceptive properties

Sage leaf aqueous and butanol extracts have analgesic and anti-inflammatory effects *in vivo*[105] and help to control neuropathic pain in chemotherapy-induced peripheral neuropathy[106] with the flavonoids and terpenes in particular identified as the active substances. This analgesic effect and may explain sage's antinociceptive effect in patients with pharyngitis.[107]

Antimicrobial

The whole extract either as an ethanolic extract or an infusion, as well as the essential oils, oleanolic and ursolic acid, showed antimicrobial activity with bactericidal and bacteriostatic effects against both Gram-positive and Gram-negative bacteria.

- Antimicrobial effects are attributed to (terpenes and terpenoids) camphor, thujone, and 1,8-cineole.[108]
- The triterpenoids oleanolic acid and ursolic acid, and carnasol (a diterpenoid), have inhibitory action on growth of multidrug-resistant bacteria.[109]
- Antifungal properties have been identified with the phenolic fraction.[110]
- The antiviral activity of *S. officinalis* is most probably is mediated by safficinolide and sage one, two diterpenoids which are found in its aerial parts.[111]

Summary of traditional and modern use

Traditional indications

- Inflammation of mouth, tongue, throat—topically
- Flatulent dyspepsia, debilitated digestion, bilious and kidney disorders
- Excessive perspiration, hot flushes of menopause
- Nervous exhaustion, debility of the nervous system, joint pain, tension headache. Improve memory, stimulate senses, improve clarity of thought
- Galactorrhoea, to cease lactation (orally and topically)
- Excessive salivation, dysmenorrhoea, diarrhoea

Actions

- Antimicrobial: thujone, thymol, eugenol, rosmarinic acid, phenolic acids
- Antioxidant
- Astringent (high tannin content)
- Antispasmodic
- Carminative: volatile oil
- Antihidrotic

- Anxiolytic: the leaves contain compounds which interact with the GABA/benzodiazepine receptor
- Anticholinesterase: inhibits acetylcholinesterase activity
- Tonic to the nervous system, thujone being potentially restorative and calming: large doses, however, could lead to nervous excitability
- Inhibit milk production: Traditionally for reducing milk production, women will use one dose every 12 hours for 3 days to keep their supply down

Indications

- Memory loss, Alzheimer's disease, dementia
- Menopausal hot flushes, night sweating
- Possible use for osteopaenia
- Nervous debility, exhaustion
- Inflammations and infections of mouth and throat
- Excessive sweating
- Reducing and stopping lactation
- Febrile conditions

Dosage[112]

- 2.0–4.5ml of 1:2 per day
- 15–30ml 1:2 per week
- 1–3ml 1:2 would contain the quantities of essential oil used in the clinical trial (per day)
- 1–4g infusion three times a day

Contraindications

- Pregnancy (due to content of thujone, although this is a theoretical concern).
- Lactation (unless to stop or retard milk flow).
- Do not exceed dosage recommended, and not long-term, although one may use low thujone varieties of sage. Intake of thujone is avoided if use infusion, and polyphenols are still extracted to a very high degree. Up to 6 cups of average food sage tea or up to 3 cups of average medicinal sage may be ingested daily.[113]

CHAPTER FOUR

Key herbs containing steroidal saponins

Dioscorea villosa, *Wild yam, colic root, rheumatism root*

The progesterone myth

As many practitioners will know, over the years it has repeatedly been said that wild yam is a source of natural progesterone, or that the body will convert diosgenin into progesterone. The truth is that saponins from yam species were used as a raw material for the production of corticosteroids and sex hormones including progesterone for some years, but not using biochemical pathways that exist in the human body. Yams are not a source of progesterone or other sex hormones, and wild yam cream does not contain progesterone. Progesterone produced from diosgenin is sometimes added to creams that are then labelled 'natural progesterone', and they do contain progesterone but there is nothing particularly natural about it—it is simply progesterone cream, and as such, a form of HRT. However, if there is no mention of progesterone at all then it probably contains none, nor does there seem to be any obvious traditional use of external application of wild yam.

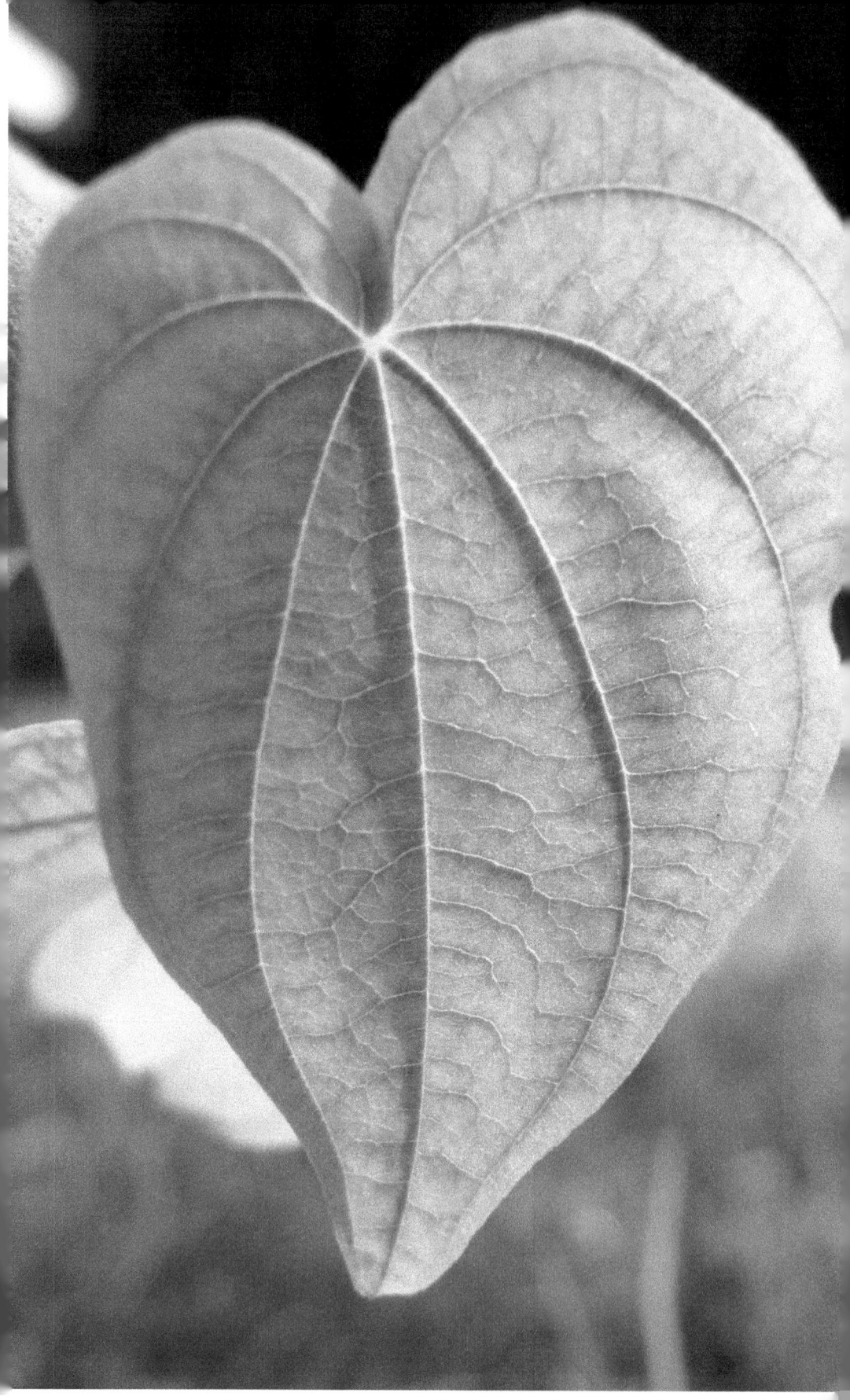

Historical use

American Indians have used *D. villosa* for pains associated with rheumatism and arthritis, colic and intestinal cramps, to relieve labour pains, for nausea and spasms during pregnancy, as well as for the treatment of bilious colic. It was one of the Eclectics' favourite herbs for spasmolytic activity and a specific in bilious colic. According to Prof. J. King: 'it gives prompt and permanent relief in the most severe cases in bilious colic, and in all forms of colic and other painful abdominal neuroses, and all forms of gastrointestinal irritation'.[1]

Ellingwood in 1908 describes being called to see a woman, pregnant for about 4 months, with possible threatened abortion, having 'labour pains':

> I gave her the following prescription: Morphine, 1/4 grain; sp. hyoscyamus, 10 drops, in a dram of hot water, and ordered her to be given one dram of sp. viburnum in hot water every hour until contractions and pains had ceased. When I saw her the following morning the pains were slightly lessened, but they still came on in frequent intervals. I then ordered the viburnum discontinued and gave her sp. Dioscorea, one dram, in four ounces of water, in teaspoonful doses every hour, whereupon the pains had ceased entirely.
>
> This case was interesting to me, as there were strong evidences that this woman was going to have an abortion. The influence of the Dioscorea in this case, was to antagonise the tendency to muscular spasm, and to control the contractions. This may be an old remedy, but it is new to me in this condition, and I am confident it exercised an important influence in preventing the abortion in this case.[2]

Modern times

Although wild yam has been used for centuries for relieving rheumatism and arthritis, colic and intestinal cramps, labour pains, and nausea and spasms during pregnancy, it is now generally thought of as one of the oestrogenic herbs because of the presence of diosgenin, the aglycone of dioscin, used industrially to produce progesterone and cortisone.

In the 1930s, animal glands were used, but in the 1950s American chemists identified that saponins from yam could be chemically modified to produce glucosteroids and sex hormones. This modification only happens in the lab, but nevertheless it has been claimed that Dioscorea is progestogenic. Wild yam root picking became important in Mexico. At one time wild yam provided about 90% of the world's raw material for steroid drug synthesis.

Yam is clearly a very useful herb for spasmodic conditions of the digestive and the female reproductive system, and for inflammatory conditions.

Constituents

- Steroidal saponins—protodioscin and several other glycosides of diosgenin (spirostanols and furanostanols, varying with the time of harvest)
- Flavonoids. Two flavan-3-ol glycosides have been isolated from *D. villosa*[3]
- Phytosterols (sitosterol, stigmasterol, taraxerol)
- Alkaloid (dioscorine)
- Tannins

Glycosides such as dioscin are broken down in the large intestine by microbial activity to form the aglycone diosgenin. This breakdown needs a healthy gut flora.

Pharmacology

There is not a great deal of research on hormonal effects of wild yam, perhaps because the common misunderstanding about progesterone-mimicking effects made such research less respectable. It is relatively clear that wild yam has some oestrogenic effects on the body, probably mediated by the hyphothalamo-pituitary axis due to feedback effects.

In postmenopausal women, it has been proposed that steroidal saponins bind to vacant receptors in the hypothalamus (in a low oestrogen situation) and so decrease the symptoms of oestrogen withdrawal, and also increase the production of oestrogen precursors from the adrenal cortex. Even though the amount of diosgenin absorbed in the body is likely to be small, even trace amounts of hormone-like substances can have a significant oestrogen-like effect on the hypothalamus.

Before the menopause, diosgenin competes with endogenous oestrogens. As the its oestrogenic components have a weaker effect on hypothalamic receptors than endogenous oestrogens, the total oestrogenic effect on the hypothalamus is reduced. The body responds as though the oestrogen levels are lower than they really are and stimulates the pituitary to make more FSH, hence oestrogen production increases.

Tribestan® and the actions of diosgenin

Most recent research on the oestrogenic effect of dioscin has used *Tribulus terrestris* leaves rather than Dioscorea. Traditionally, Tribulus fruit has been mostly used in Ayurveda for the urinary system, and in the reproductive system for spermatorrhoea, impotence and uterine disorders after parturition.[4] Research on the leaf has taken place mostly in Bulgaria using Tribestan®, a concentrated extract of Tribulus (leaf, some stem) standardised to 45% furostanol saponins as protodioscin. Tribestan is quite widely used in Europe for menopausal symptoms, to relieve hot flushes, insomnia and depression.*

The research indicates that Tribulus leaf normalises production of LH in men and FSH in women, maintaining normal testosterone and oestrogen levels respectively, and so in women Tribulus leaf could help with normal ovulation.[5]

Clinical trials using Tribestan®

- A 5-day treatment of eight healthy women (aged 28–45) increased serum FSH concentration, which returned to pre-treatment levels on cessation of treatment.[6]
- LH was more strongly influenced in males, indirectly stimulating testosterone secretion. Stimulation of growth hormone and aldosterone led to suggestion of mild activation of anabolic processes. None of the hormones exceeded normal levels.[7]
- Female Infertility: a clinical study evaluated *Tribulus terrestris* (Tribestan®) and pharmaceuticals for ovulation induction in women with

---

*The location of harvesting is important: the leaf from Bulgaria tends to be high in protodioscin and Tribulus from the Mediterranean region has high contents of furostanol saponins. The furostanol glycosides (including protodioscin and prototribestin) readily convert into spirostanol saponins due to exposure to enzymes in the plant during harvesting and processing.

oligo/anovular infertility. During the three-month follow-up, ovulation rates were highest with epimestrol (74%), followed by *Tribulus terrestris* (60%), clomiphene (47%) and cyclofenil (24%).[8] Treatment with Tribulus and ovulation stimulant on days 5 to 14 was better than treatment with either single agent. Tribulus extract every day on the other hand resulted in no improvement in ovulation parameters, led to longer menstrual cycles, menorrhagia, increased libido, and general nervousness with insomnia.
- An open study on menopausal women showed a beneficial effect on hot flushes, sweating, insomnia and depression. There were no changes in LH, prolactin, oestradiol, progesterone and testosterone, although FSH tended to be lower. Libido was enhanced in 70%.
- In a small study in 2014, Iranian women had improvement in the desire, arousal, lubrication, satisfaction and pain domains of the FSFI (Female Sexual Function Index), particularly the satisfaction domain.[9] A recent (2018) study found Tribulus to be effective for the treatment of premenopausal women with hypoactive sexual desire in reducing the symptoms (improvements in desire, sexual arousal/lubrication, pain, orgasm, and satisfaction) with increased levels of free and bioavailable testosterone.[10]

Clinical studies of yam related to menopause

In a clinical study using yam (*Dioscorea alata*, a related species to *Dioscorea villosa* and also containing diosgenin), postmenopausal women took 390g of yam for 30 days. The results showed that the plant:

- Increased serum concentrations of oestrone, sex hormone binding globulin (SHBG), and oestradiol
- Did not change serum concentrations of dehydroepiandrosterone sulphate, androstenedione, testosterone, FSH or LH
- Decreased free androgen levels (perhaps related to the increase in SHBG)
- Decreased urinary concentration of 16 α-hydroxyoestrone
- Decreased total cholesterol concentration

The authors concluded that these effects might reduce the risk of breast cancer and cardiovascular diseases in postmenopausal women.[11] *In vitro* studies also indicate that wild yam extract can downregulate ERα expression in human breast cancer cells.[12]

- Predictably, a clinical study with topical wild yam cream in women suffering from menopausal symptoms appears to have little effect.[13]

Clinical studies on Dioscorea and diosgenin for cholesterol metabolism

As mentioned above when discussing sage, one of the main features of the menopause is a tendency to metabolic syndrome, i.e. hyperlipidaemia and insulin resistance, increasing the risk of cardiovascular disease and late-onset diabetes. Diosgenin has been shown both *in vitro* and *in vivo* to interfere with absorption of dietary and endogenous cholesterol and to enhance cholesterol secretion into bile,[14] so both mechanisms suggest a cholesterol-reducing effect.

- Diosgenin inhibits atherosclerosis *in vivo*.[15]
- On a yam-rich diet (not *Dioscorea villosa*, but diosgenin-rich nonetheless), plasma cholesterol concentration decreased significantly in postmenopausal women.[16] (*Dioscorea villosa* does have much higher concentration of diosgenin but is not usually eaten).
- A Dioscorea-modified pill (spp. not stated is reported to have had a positive effect in patients with vascular cognitive impairment but no dementia (VCIND) measured using a mini-mental state examination and clinical dementia rating scale).[17]
- A small study in people aged 65–82 years taking *Dioscorea villosa* (dosage undefined) showed:
  ○ No change in serum dehydroepiandrosterone sulphate.
  ○ No changes in total cholesterol or LDL-cholesterol.
  ○ Reduction of serum lipid peroxidation and serum triglycerides, and increased HDL-cholesterol levels. The authors concluded that Dioscorea acts as an antioxidant to modify serum lipid levels.[18]

Other effects found from *in vivo* and *in vitro* studies

- Anti-inflammatory and anti-nociceptive effects of *Dioscorea villosa* and diosgenin[19] support traditional usage.
- Diosgenin reduced subacute intestinal inflammation associated with indomethacin.[20]
- Diosgenin administration prevented some cholestatic effects of oestrogen[21] (interesting in relation to the traditional use of *Dioscorea villosa* for bilious colic).
- Hypoglycaemic, antioxidant, and anti-proliferative activities.[22]
- A protective effect of *Dioscorea villosa* against alveolar bone loss.[23]

Summary of actions, indications and research findings for *Dioscorea villosa*

Actions

- Spasmolytic
- Cholagogue
- Hypolipidaemic
- Anti-inflammatory
- Antirheumatic
- Oestrogenic

Therapeutic indications

- Gastrointestinal spasm, spasmodic griping pain in stomach and bowels or irritation including intestinal colic, bilious colic, cholecystitis
- Dysmenorrhoea
- Morning sickness, false labour pains, threatened miscarriage and for ineffective, hypertonic uterine contractions during labour
- Inflammatory conditions, arthritis, rheumatoid arthritis
- May assist in the reduction of blood lipids
- May regulate ovulation and enhancement of fertility, modulating perimenopausal symptoms (oral use only!!), although there is no tradition of use in these conditions
- Maintaining bone density after the menopause

Preparations

- Decoction of dried root: 2–4g three times daily
- Tincture 1:2 or 1:3, 45%: 2–6ml three times daily
- Fluid extract 1:1, 45%: 2–4ml/three times daily[24]

Suggested combinations

Dysmenorrhoea and ovarian cramping: *Cimicifuga racemosa, Viburnum prunifolium, Valeriana officinalis, Anenome pulsatilla*
Threatened miscarriage: *Viburnum prunifolium*
Menopause: *Panax ginseng, Cimicifuga racemosa, Verbena officinalis*
Intestinal colic: *Matricaria chamomilla*

Adverse reactions

As with all saponin-containing herbs, oral use may cause irritation of the gastric mucous membranes and reflux. To minimise this side effect wild yam should be taken with food.

Chamaelirium luteum

Should it be used, and can it be substituted?

Chamaelirium is on the United Plant Savers 'At Risk' list.[25] As of 2010, at least 90% of plants sold are thought to have been collected from the wild.[26] So it is discussed here not necessarily with a view to using it in practice, unless it is known for certain to have been sustainably produced, but rather by understanding its actions to have a standard to refer to when using substitutes.

There are good substitutes, but *Aletris farinosa* is not seen as one by most herbalists. Its substitution for Chamaelirium arose from a misunderstanding: Chamaelirium and Aletris were commonly confused during the nineteenth and early twentieth centuries, and the Materia Medica of the time generally mention this adulteration. All seem to suggest, as Felter did in 1922, that Aletris is probably nothing more than a gentle stomachic and tonic, employed to promote the appetite and aid digestion[27,28] and that any further therapeutic reputation was due to its adulteration with Chamaelirium. Most of the actions of Chamaelirium may be found by using, perhaps in combination, *Achillea millefolium*, *Alchemilla vulgaris*, *Dioscorea villosa*, *Rubus idaeus*, *Tribulus terrestris*, or *Asparagus racemosus*.

Constituents

- Steroidal saponins:
  - Chemical investigation has led to the isolation of 15 steroidal glycosides, 12 of them unique to Chamaelirium. Some have displayed significant anti-proliferative activity.[29,30]
- Bitter principle

Pharmacology

There has been speculation that the steroidal saponins in Chamaelirium have similar effects to those in Tribulus, with an action on the hypothalamic-pituitary-ovary axis leading to increase of FSH, stimulating ovulation. But despite the wide use of this herb, little information is available.

Traditional use

Native Americans used *Chamaelirium luteum* as a tonic, diuretic, emetic, sialagogue, emmenagogue, vermifuge, antiscorbutic, for 'female conditions' and to prevent miscarriages, a range of uses that seem to indicate a generally stimulatory, activating profile. It might be that there are both systemic effects from the sapogenins, and reflex actions from stimulating and toning the mucous membranes of the digestive tract. The Eclectics used it in digestive disorders such as indigestion, dyspepsia, colic, loss of appetite, and as a tonic for the sexual organs. It was seen as a uterine tonic, specifically for when the tissues were very relaxed, leading to the feeling that the contents of the pelvis were falling out of place, and causing pain in the back and down the thighs and back of legs. They describe Chamaelirium as toning the uterus and thereby preventing miscarriage and the tendency to abort, and useful also in leucorrhoea, amenorrhoea, dysmenorrhoea, atonic forms of prolapse, passive haemorrhage and menorrhagia.

The plant was also used as a nervous tonic in irritability and depression, especially if associated with uterine troubles. It has been suggested that it was useful for the relief of vomiting during pregnancy.

Chamaelirium was also used as a tonic to the urinary tract, and was said to have some benefit in diabetes insipidus.[31] Small doses were employed.

The Eclectics cautioned against its use in sensitive patients and in irritable uterine conditions.[32]

Summary of actions and indications

Actions

- Reproductive tonic, uterine tonic, improving their function and nutrition, pelvic warming
- Emmenagogue
- Hormone modulator with amphoteric effect on hormonal secretion by the ovary
- Sialagogue
- Bitter tonic
- Vermifuge
- Emetic in large doses but in small doses also used as antiemetic in pregnancy

Therapeutic indications

- Typical picture: fullness, heaviness, congestion in the pelvic area with lumbar pains, down the thighs, and back of legs
- Uterine prolapse
- Strengthens the uterus: prevents miscarriages and tendency to abort
- Endometriosis
- Amenorrhea, dysmenorrhoea (with bearing down feeling), irregular menstruation
- Restlessness, general weakness, fatigue
- Dysfunctional uterine bleeding
- Menopausal symptoms
- Ovarian cysts
- Anorexia, anaemia, infertility
- Antiemetic and anti-nausea in pregnancy

Combinations

- Used with *Dioscorea villosa* L., *Viburnum opulus* L. for threatened miscarriage

Preparations and dosage; 1–2g as infusion or decoction

- Fluid Extract 1:1 45%, 1–2ml three times daily
- Tincture 1:5 45%, 2–5ml, three times daily (BHP 1983)
- Large doses may cause gastrointestinal irritation, with nausea and vomiting

Alternatives to Chamaelirium

Alternative remedies covering the digestive uses of Chamaelirium are not hard to find. The main reason for the popularity of Chamaelirium with practitioners has been its versatility as a general tonic for the female reproductive system. Some of these actions overlap with those of other saponin-rich herbs: Dioscorea, particularly in pregnancy, in alleviating nausea and the risk of miscarriage, and Tribulus, as a general reproductive tonic.

Neither of those herbs has a specific action as a uterine *tonic*, both being associated more with an anti-inflammatory, antispasmodic and generally oestrogenic profile. So, for Chamaelirium's specifically uterine profile, herbs such as raspberry leaves as a tonic for the last trimester of pregnancy and particularly as an aid to trouble-free delivery (partum preparator), and more generally *Achillea millefolium* and *Alchemilla vulgaris* suggest themselves. These will be briefly discussed here but are presented in more depth in the companion volume to this book, which discusses herbs with specific functions for gynaecological complaints, and treatment of a wide range of gynaecological problems, where this book addresses more specifically the hormonal basis of treatment and herbs with a more generalised physiological effect.

Achillea millefolium

Yarrow is not a saponin-rich herb—its main constituents are volatile compounds (volatile oils, proazulene), sesquiterpene lactones (bitter and often stimulating), and flavonoids. It shares some of the digestive tonic actions of Chamaelirium, probably due to its aromatic and bitter aspects, and is both drying/styptic and a circulatory stimulant, helping perfusion of tissues as it relaxes blood vessel walls. Culpeper regards it as specific for the 'bloody flux'.[33] Yarrow has something of an amphoteric effect on the uterus. Through its action as a circulatory stimulant it has tonic, emmenagogic and trophorestorative properties, but it is also useful in cases of excessive uterine bleeding. According to Scudder, it acts directly on the reproductive organs of the female in atonic amenorrhoea and menorrhagia.[34]

Alchemilla vulgaris

Lady's mantle has broadly similar indications to yarrow, being used since antiquity for menorrhagia, for, as an emmenagogue, and also as a powerfully wound healing herb, both internally and externally, not only being anti-inflammatory, antioxidant but also encouraging tissue healing and inhibiting elastase, thus preserving the skin's elasticity. Like many western herbs, this is one that is probably undervalued for being too familiar. Lady's mantle was seen as particularly useful, like raspberry leaves, to promote contraction during labour, and to restrain bleeding associated with the birth, and the name may also convey, apart from the appearance of the leaves, something of the respect given for its protective properties. Its astringent properties were also useful for vomiting, excessive discharge of fluid from the body, diarrhoea, and leucorrhoea. In a clinical trial for menorrhagia in 341 teenage girls in Romania using FE 50–60gtt 3–5 times per day, the volume of flow reduced when used 10–15 days before period, the cycle shortened, and premenstrual administration prevented menorrhagia from recurring.[35]

Asparagus racemosus

In Ayurvedic medicine, Shatavari is regarded as the main rejuvenating tonic for women, and a counterpart to *Withania somnifera* in men. It grows widely at low altitudes throughout India and is a member of the Liliaceae. The dried roots are used. As a result of excess harvesting and destruction of habitat, the species is now threatened in its native habitat, However, though not frost-resistant, Shatavari can be cultivated sustainably in temperate climates.

Ancient classical Ayurvedic literature recommended Shatavari in cases of threatened abortion, and saw it as a bitter-sweet, emollient, cooling, nervine tonic. In terms of treating female problems, it is used as a galactagogue and aphrodisiac. It also has carminative, stomachic and antiseptic properties, and an ulcer-healing effect probably via strengthening the mucosal resistance or cytoprotection. Shatavari is used in South-East Asia for promoting appetite and providing nourishment to children. A decoction of the young root with the bark removed was traditionally used by Aboriginal Australians as a wash for scabies, infected or ulcerating skin lesions and chicken pox.

Shatavari is often said to mean 'a hundred husbands', referring to its power as a female tonic and aphrodisiac, but this is perhaps fanciful, and it seems more likely that it means 'a hundred roots', referring to the plant's rhizomes. Despite its long and venerable history as a tonic, there is relatively little clinical research on Shatavari, and most studies are *in vitro* and *in vivo*.

Constituents

- Steroidal saponins, saponins of the furanostanol-type, such as Shatavarins I–IV
- Alkaloids, including the non-hepatotoxic pyrrolizidine alkaloid asparagamine A
- Other constituents include mucilage, isoflavones, and sterols (sitosterol)

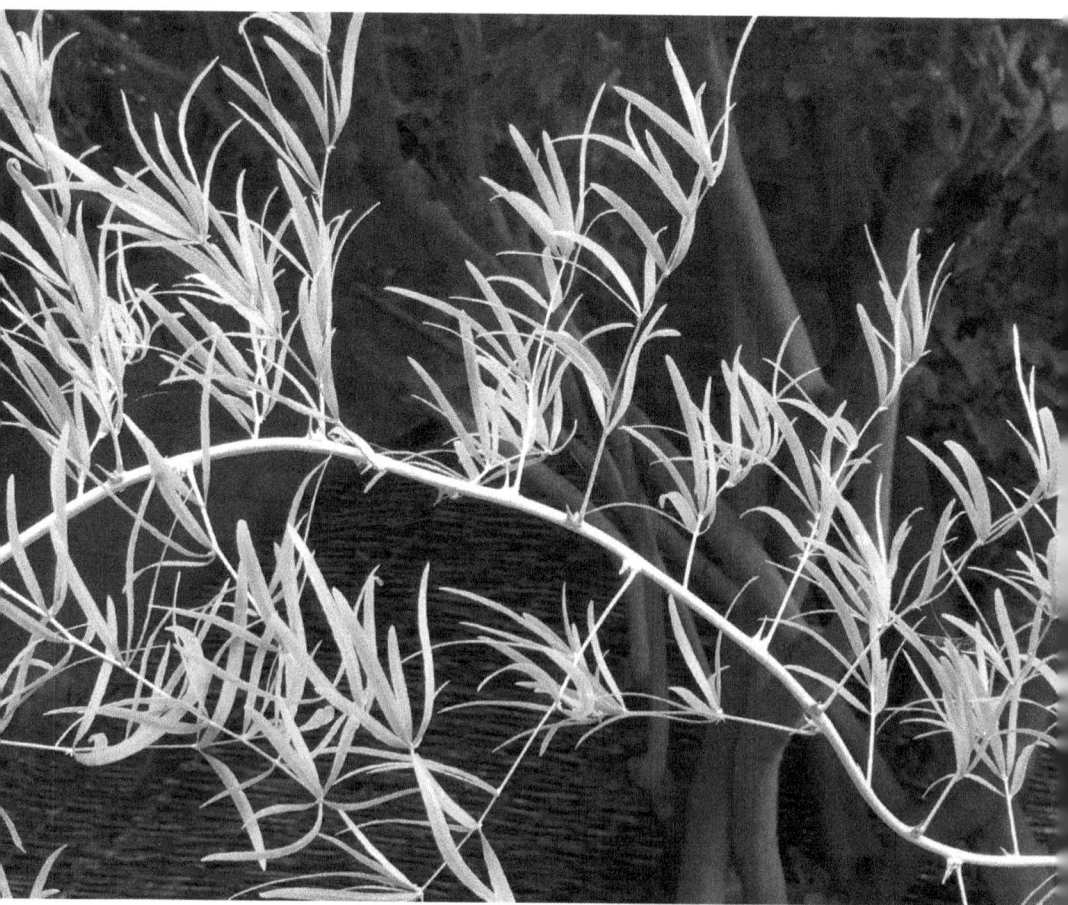

Steroidal saponins

It is speculated that as with other herbs rich in steroidal saponins such as Tribulus, the effect is on the Hypothalamus-Pituitary-Ovary axis, in the case of delayed menses increasing serum FSH[36] and initiating ovulation. It is speculated that:

- In a low oestrogen environment the steroidal compounds bind to vacant receptors in the hypothalamus and so decrease the symptoms of oestrogen withdrawal.
- In postmenopausal women, sapogenins may act directly or indirectly via hypothalamus and/or pituitary gland to increase the production of oestrogen precursors from the adrenal cortex.
- Pre-menopause: Because the oestrogenic substances are very weak compared to the normal oestrogens that bind to the hypothalamic receptors, the body responds as though the oestrogen levels are lower than they really are by increasing FSH, hence oestrogen production increases.
- *In vivo* research also suggests the possibility of a direct oestrogenic[37] effect, and it is thought that it may act directly on the mammary gland or via the pituitary and adrenal glands.
- In women who have a long follicular phase, stimulation of ovulation results in the earlier formation of the corpus luteum, which will increase the progesterone to oestrogen ratio for a longer part of the cycle, so the net result is increased oestrogen in the follicular phase, but a shorter period of oestrogen excess.

Clinical studies

Galactagogue effect

No increase was observed in prolactin levels in women complaining of secondary lactational failure;[38] however, serum prolactin was found to increase in a clinical trial in lactating mothers,[39] with infants up to 6-months-old and deficient lactation. The mothers were selected because the infant was crying just after feeding, there was a painful sensation in the breasts during the time of feeding, and mothers were exhibiting loss of appetite or the manifestation of an anxiety disorder.

Secondary outcomes were better weight of both mother and infant, subjective satisfaction of mothers regarding the state of lactation, and wellbeing and happiness of babies (subjective rating by mother). It is interesting to wonder how much of the improvement resulted from a direct change in hormone levels (given the lack of change in prolactin levels in secondary lactational failure), and how much from other properties (tonic, appetite stimulant, carminative and nervine).

Animal trials: several *in vivo* studies have shown an increase in milk yield, and in guinea pigs an increased growth of mammary glands, alveolar tissue and acini.[40]

Digestive system

Antiulcer activity

- *Clinical study:* Shatavari powder relieved symptoms of patients with duodenal ulcer.[41] It has no antisecretory or antacid properties, and heals duodenal ulcers without inhibiting acid secretion, so Shatavari may have a cytoprotective action.
- *In vivo*: The methanolic extract of fresh roots of *A. racemosus* has shown an ulcer protective effect of against acute gastric ulcers and an increase of mucosal defensive factors like mucus secretion, cellular mucus, life span of cells, antioxidant effect.[42]

Promotion of gastric emptying

- This was shown in healthy volunteers,[43] indicating a possible use in dyspepsia

It is perhaps best to regard Shatavari as an overall tonic, with oestrogenic effects but also with antioxidant, anti-inflammatory effects and widespread trophorestorative effects particularly on the female reproductive system, nervous system, liver and stomach.

A full list of in vivo effects found for *A. racemosus* includes:

- Antitussive[44]
- Preventing post-operative adhesions[45] (associated with increase in the activity of macrophages)
- Uterine spasmolytic,[46] antioxytocin (Shatavarin 1, competitive block of oxytocin induced contraction pregnant uterus[47])
- Hepatoprotective (reduced levels of alanine transaminase, aspartate transaminase and alkaline phosphate),[48] prevents hepatocarcinogenesis[49]

- Antineoplastic,[50] immunomodulatory,[51] antioxidant[52]
- Antidepressant[53] and stimulant[54,55]
- Enhances memory and protects against amnesia[56]
- Aphrodisiac, anti-stress,[57] oestrogenic[58]
- Diuretic, antiurolithiatic
- Anti-inflammatory, hypoglycaemic,[59] analgesic, antidiarrhoeal[60]

In vitro research shows:

- Antibacterial activity, antiprotozoal activity, molluscicidal activity[61]

Summary of actions and indications for Asparagus racemosus

Actions

- Tonic action on the female reproductive system
- Sexual tonic/aphrodisiac
- Adaptogen (often combined with *Withania somnifera* and *Ocimum sanctum*)
- Galactogogue
- Spasmolytic
- Demulcent for dry and inflamed membranes of lungs, stomach, kidney, sexual organs, and therefore possible for vaginal dryness
- Promotes appetite and providing nourishment to children

Therapeutic indications

- Irregular menstruation
- Menopausal problems
- Promoting conception: sexual debility and infertility (both sexes)
- Insufficient lactation
- Threatened miscarriage
- Leucorrhoea
- General debility, fatigue, infections, body ache
- Promoting appetite in children

Dosage

- Up to 2–3g of powder per day.
- Lower doses are used by infusion or decoction.

- The recommended adult dosage of 1:2 45% liquid extract is 30 to 60ml per week.

Combinations

- Shatavari combines well with other tonic herbs, such as *Withania somnifera*.
- As with all saponin-containing herbs, oral use may cause irritation of the gastric mucosa and reflux. To minimise this, Shatavari should be taken with food.

CHAPTER FIVE

Actaea racemosa (widely known as *Cimicifuga racemosa*) and *Vitex agnus-castus*

Common myths concerning black cohosh

A great deal of what is popularly said of black cohosh is wrong. Firstly, it is not really a phyto-oestrogenic plant. Secondly, there is no evidence that it promotes breast cancer; rather the reverse. And thirdly, its reputation for causing liver damage seems to have little basis either in theory or fact, although that is not true of some plants that have been misleading labelled as black cohosh. Even though many herbalists know all of these things, what will perhaps surprise many is how small a dose is generally effective: most clinical trials use doses that are equivalent to rather less than 5ml of a 1.5 tincture per week.

Popularity

In 1997, over ten million monthly units of *Cimicifuga racemosa* extract were sold in Germany, the United States, and Australia for peri- and postmenopausal complaints. One major reason was that despite initial optimism, HRT failed to become the treatment of choice for many menopausal women, partly because of increased risk of stroke, heart

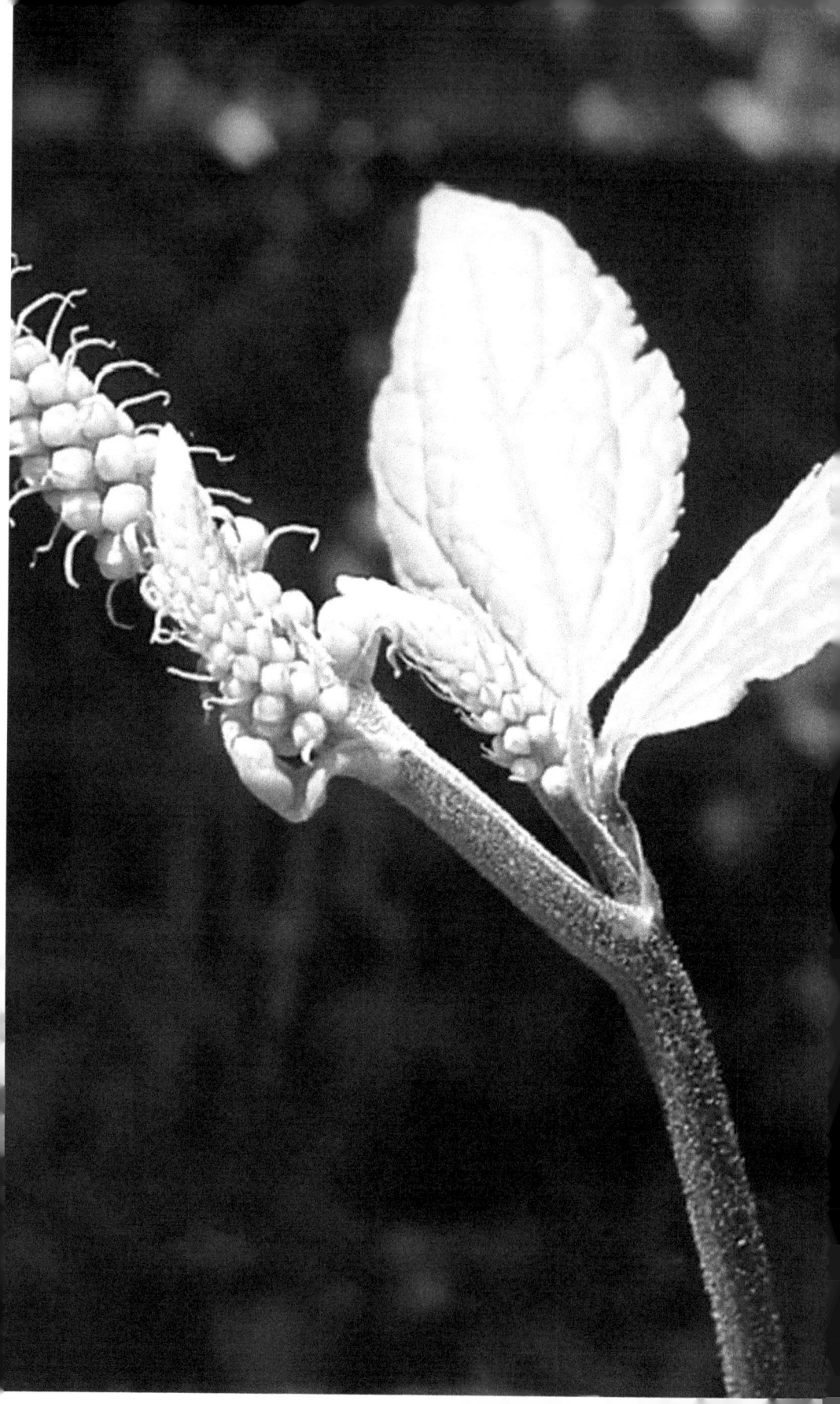

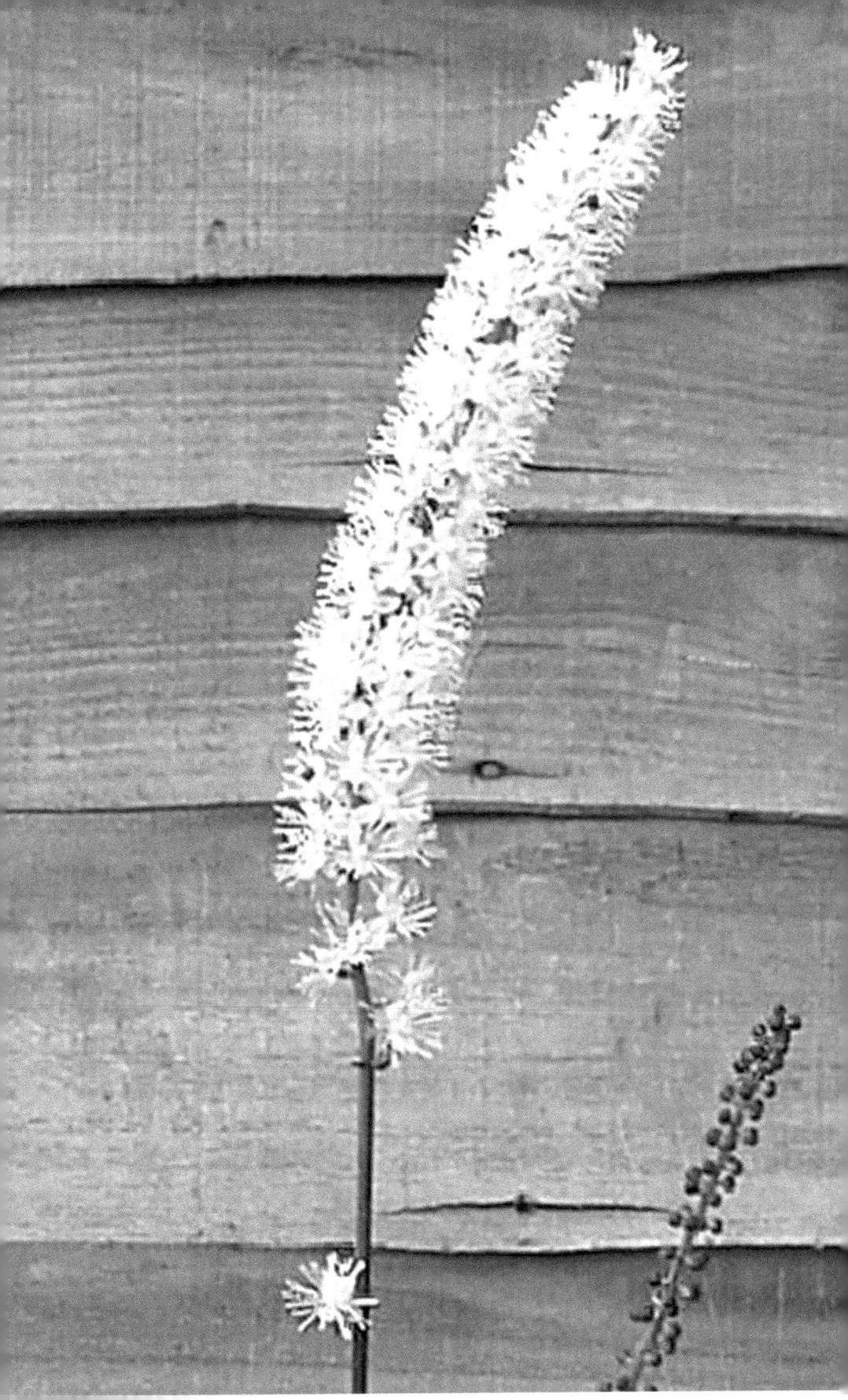

diseases, and breast cancer, hence the popularity of a herbal product promising many of the benefits but with greater safety.

The use of black cohosh for gynaecological complaints came to Germany in the nineteenth century. Since the 1950s, German gynaecologists have increasingly used it for intermittent bleeding, disturbances in the menstrual cycle, PMS, and climacteric complaints (especially hot flushes and psychic complaints). When HRT was first developed its uptake was low as it was plagued by side effects, and black cohosh proved itself a suitable alternative to hormonal therapy. By 1962, 14 clinical studies of black cohosh for perimenopausal symptoms, involving 1,500 patients, had been performed, and of course there have been many more since, but there are questions of quality and particularly of bias as most have been carried out by the manufacturer of the main available product, Remifemin®.

First people use

Black cohosh is native to the deciduous forests of Eastern North America. The botanical genus has oscillated between *Actaea* and *Cimicifuga* since it was first classified, but for the majority of that time it has been *Cimicifuga*. The root was widely used by a number of native American tribes particularly for pain management and inflammation. Its medical uses were first recorded by Barton, in 1801, who called it 'squawroot', and wrote: 'Our Indians set a high value on it'. Rheumatic limbs were placed over the steam, or used as footbath, and steamed sweat bath, and a decoction was also taken internally. It was also used as an analgesic for other types of pain including dysmenorrhoea, childbirth, and also as an emmenagogue and for slow parturition.

The Eclectic physicians

Known variously in the in United States Pharmacopoeia as Cimicifuga, black cohosh and black Snakeroot, it was also known among the Eclectics as Macrotys, as the genus was so designated in Eaton's *Manual of Botany*.[1] Macrotys occupied a central place in the Eclectic Materia Medica for rheumatic and gynaecological complaints, and it features prominently in various versions of *The Eclectic Dispensatory of the United States of America*.[2] John King, co-author of its first edition, is likely to have been a strong influence in establishing it, as both a leading lights of Eclectic medicine and a specialist in obstetrics and gynaecology.

The range of uses of Macrotys was broadly similar to that of native Americans. These uses can be summed up as:

- Relaxing muscle tension particularly in rheumatic complaints
- Relieving neuralgia, particularly rheumatic neuralgia
- Febrile conditions accompanied by distress
- Regularizing the menstrual cycle particularly around menarche
- As a partum praeparator taken in the weeks before childbirth
- Nervous coughs

Macrotys was seen as a general ovarian and uterine tonic, promoting regular contractions of the uterine muscle. It was regarded as especially efficacious in chronic ovaritis, endometritis, menstrual derangement, amenorrhoea, dysmenorrhoea, menorrhagia, frigidity, sterility, threatened abortion, uterine subinvolution, and for stimulating labour.

Among physiomedicalists, too, black cohosh had a considerable reputation. In his *Physiomedical Dispensatory*, Cook claimed that it had both soothing and stimulating qualities, whereby it could reduce pain and spasm locally by soothing tissues, while also being used as an expectorant.[3]

For dysmenorrhoea, Scudder[4] indicated it 'in cases of tardy, slow, irregular, scanty, or protracted menstruation' while it was also employed in some cases of amenorrhea (Webster 1893).[5]

Constituents

- Triterpene glycosides, xylosides, actein, cimicifugoside, 27-deoxy-actein. These are complex molecules and the main actions of *Cimicifuga* are ascribed to them.
- Alkaloids and dopamine derivatives.
- The isoflavone formononetin in the aerial parts of the plant (however, we use the root, so this is irrelevant).
- Phenolic constituents: caffeic acid and derivatives, Isoferulic and salicylic acid.
- Other constituents: tannins, resins, fatty acids.

Mode of action[6]

Oestrogenicity used to be measured by the effect of a drug or herb on uterine tissue, but as the understanding of oestrogen α and β receptors has grown, it was realised that it means something more complex.

In Cimicifuga's case, however, even this refinement does not give the picture fully because its effect on menopausal symptoms appears not to depend on oestrogen receptors, as the herb does not seem to interact directly with them.

There is some clinical as well as *in vivo* evidence that *Cimicifuga racemosa* is osteoprotective; an *in vitro* study has shown that black cohosh induces osteoprotegerin (OPG, a bone marker). As this effect is inhibited by oestrogen receptor antagonists, an oestrogenic effect is implied.[7] However, there does not appear to be any direct oestrogenic effect on endometrial or breast tissue.[8]

Effect on pituitary hormones

There is a correlation between raised LH levels and hot flushes in postmenopausal women. In *in vivo* and some human studies, Cimicifuga has inhibited luteinizing hormone (LH), which might explain a beneficial effect.[9] Cimicifuga in combination with clomiphene actually increased LH in PCOS patients.[10] However, most trials of *Cimicifuga racemosa* by itself in postmenopausal women showed no effect on LH;[11] but what *has* been shown is significant inhibition of prolactin release from cultured pituitary cells indicating the presence of dopaminergic compounds.[12]

Neurotransmitter activity

Dopaminergic activity leads to lower prolactin levels, and high prolactin levels have been associated with a decline in oestrogen levels and premature reduction in bone density. This action would be similar to *Vitex agnus-castus*. Dopaminergic activity could also explain the reduction in hot flushes. Dopaminergic agonists also cause decrease in proliferation of MCF-7 cells (breast cancer cell line) and so rather than black cohosh being contraindicated in breast cancer because of oestrogenic activity, which as we have seen is not the case, it is actually useful because of its dopaminergic effect and the consequent inhibition of prolactin. Before the menopause, this would tend to increase the level of progesterone in the luteal phase of the menstrual cycle.

Recent research suggests a wider range of neurotransmitter-mimetic effects. As well as dopaminergic activity, noradrenergic, serotonergic and GABAergic effects have been demonstrated.[13] Cimicifuga contains actein-like triterpenes with GABAergic activity and a serotonin analogue,[14] which would also have an effect on menopausal symptoms such as hot flushes, mood swings, anxiety, insomnia. Oestrogens affect brain neurotransmitter levels and receptor density,[15] and so black cohosh having activity at the same receptors would compensate for lower levels of oestrogens.

A further synergistic effect seems to happen in the endogenous opioid system, disturbance of which is associated with hot flushes. It appears from a pilot study that in postmenopausal women black cohosh has an impact on the same regions and neurotransmitter systems.[16]

The importance of using the whole plant

All in all, it is most likely Cimicifuga acts via multiple mechanisms in different tissues, including indirect oestrogenic (or anti-oestrogenic) effects, influence on serotonergic, dopaminergic and other neurotransmitter pathways, and antioxidative and anti-inflammatory activity. The efficacy of methanolic extracts of the root is dependent upon at least three different fractions with a synergistic action.

Clinical trials

Pharmacokinetics

In a Phase 1 clinical trial of healthy menopausal women given oral doses, the triterpenes were found to be readily absorbed into the bloodstream, with a half-life of around 2 hours, and excreted via the bile and faeces.[17]

Osteoprotective effects

A clinical trial showed that *Cimicifuga racemosa* and conjugated oestrogen have comparable effects on serum markers of bone metabolism. The action is different, however. Bone-specific alkaline phosphatase, a marker for bone formation, increased under Cimicifuga, which stimulated osteoblast activity but decreased with conjugated oestrogens, which inhibited osteoclast activity.[18]

Increased muscle tone in urinary bladder

Improvement in muscle tone in the bladder indicates a possible effect on urinary incontinence.

No changes in endometrium

Cimicifuga did not lead to changes in the endometrium, and this may be the most important difference with HRT, that the herb may be prescribed without the worry over triggering uterine cancer.[18]

Lowering pH in vagina

Cimicifuga increased the number of superficial cells, responsible for lowering pH in the vagina, in a vaginal smear. Lower pH levels prevent ascending infection.[18] Cimicifuga also led to an increase of lubrication in sexual activity.[18]

Helpful in infertility alongside clomiphene

One trial demonstrated improved pregnancy rates in women with unexplained infertiliy treated with clomiphene together with black cohosh compared with clomiphene alone. The regime was *Cimicifuga racemosa* 120mg/day given from days 1 to 12 of the cycle, clomiphene (used to stimulate ovulation) from days 3 to 7 and human chorionic gonadotrophin injection (HCG) when ovulation appeared close. Those that also took black cohosh group had:

- Higher pregnancy rates
- Thicker endometrium measured on the day of the HCG injection
- Higher serum progesterone concentrations in the luteal phase (days 21 to 23), indicating better ovulation

Clomiphene is thought to have anti-oestrogenic effects on the follicle and on the endometrium, which could explain its failure in certain women. It was suggested by the researchers that Cimicifuga blocks that anti-oestrogenic effect and aids follicular development, as there was an increase in endometrial thickness and a (non-significant) increase in oestradiol for the black cohosh group.[19]

A similar trial for women with PCOS, i.e. receiving *Cimicifuga racemosa* alongside clomiphene, compared to clomiphene alone, also significantly improved pregnancy rates and also showed improvements in the cycle and in progesterone levels.[20,21]

Reduces menopausal symptoms in perimenopausal women

Many clinical trials have been done on Cimicifuga's effect on menopausal symptoms. In particular, it seems effective for patients suffering from moderate menopausal symptoms as opposed to mild symptoms, and particularly in early menopausal symptoms.[22]

Menopausal symptoms following breast cancer

In a trial where Cimicifuga was used for over 12 months following treatment for breast cancer, there significant reduction in the more severe symptoms particularly in younger patients.[23] In a short trial of only 2 months with some patients using tamoxifen, many of them older women, there was significant reduction in sweating, and in combination therapy with tamoxifen, Cimicifuga helped with reduction of hot flushes and improved quality of life.[24] *In vitro* research also suggests that Cimicifuga enhances the anti-cancer effect of tamoxifen in oestrogen-sensitive breast cancer tissue.[25]

Helpful in women with fibroids

A 12-week trial using Remifemin® offered the conclusion that it is a valid herbal medicinal product in patients with uterine myomas, providing adequate relief from menopausal symptoms and inhibiting growth of the myomas in contrast to tibolone.[26]

In vivo *and* in vitro *research*

Anti-proliferative effects

- Inhibition of proliferation of both oestrogen-positive and oestrogen-negative human breast cancer cells
- Slowing the growth of oestrogen-dependent tumours
- Promoting apoptosis of breast cancer cells and androgen-dependent and -independent prostate carcinoma cells[27]

As Cimicifuga does not bind to the known oestrogen α or β receptors, anti-tumour activity may be mediated via another mechanism. Several possible modes of action have been suggested.

- Cimicifuga compounds potently inhibit growth of human prostate cells *in vitro*, which may be mediated via aryl hydrocarbon receptor (AhR) activation, leading to inhibition of tumour growth. AhR receptor activation may explain why Cimicifuga also has anti-proliferative action on ER-negative breast cancer cells.*
- Dopaminergic anti-proliferative action.
- An as yet unknown third subtype of oestrogen receptor.
- Antioxidant and anti-inflammatory effects.

Effect on hepatic and lipid metabolism

Cimicifuga increases leptin sensitivity (increasing the sense of satiety after eating) *in vivo* and had a favourable effect on hepatic and lipid metabolism, with reduced fat deposition and protection against atherosclerosis.[28]

Summary of actions and indications for Cimicifuga racemosa

Actions

- Neuroendocrine effect: dopaminergic and serotonergic receptor binding
- Nervine
- Oestrogen modulation/oestrogen-like effect
- Correction of progesterone depletion due to high prolactin levels
- Uterine and ovarian tonic
- Anti-inflammatory, antioxidant, anti-proliferative in hormone-dependent cancers
- Analgesic
- Spasmolytic

Specific indications

- Effective especially in perimenopausal women with more severe symptoms (hot flushes, mild depression, and other symptoms associated with cyclical or climacteric changes such as myalgia). Helpful in breast cancer patients when taking tamoxifen. Looks promising

---

*AhR is widely expressed in breast tissue and tumours, and is a target of some aromatic xeno-oestrogens, hence its name.

on the effect of bone metabolism and may have a role to play in osteoporosis.
- Helpful in fertility treatment, for those taking clomiphene, and other conditions requiring reduction in LH Levels (ovarian failure, infertility, miscarriage, cyst formation, PCOS).
- Premenstrual syndrome, amenorrhoea, dysmenorrhoea, menorrhagia, ovarian pain, endometriosis.
- Arthritis, neuralgia, myalgia, sciatica.
- Respiratory conditions; whooping cough, asthma.
- Tinnitus.[29]

Safety

Black cohosh has an extremely good safety record. Theoretical concerns have been raised about promotion of hormone-dependent cancers and as discussed, this is based on misunderstanding of the mode of action of the herb, which actually has anti-proliferative effects.

The other concern has been hepatotoxicity, and there are genuine safety cases that have implicated products purporting to contain black cohosh. In the many clinical trials using authenticated *Cimicifuga racemosa*, serious liver disease has not occurred. A critical review in 2010 found (69 cases) that the assessed data raises serious doubts on the initial claims of causality for Cimicifuga as the evidence was of poor quality, especially when spontaneous reports are considered. There were major inconsistencies for the same patient regarding reported data.

Analysis of all cases disclosed confounding variables:[30]

- *poor case data quality*
- *uncertainty of BC product, quality, and identification*
- *undisclosed indication*
- *insufficient adverse event definition*
- *lack of temporal association and rechallenge*
- *missing/inadequate evaluation of alcohol use*
- *comedication, comorbidity, reexposure test, and alternative diagnoses were not excluded*

Data so far does not support the concept of hepatotoxicity due to black cohosh.

A study investigating the potential mechanisms of hepatotoxicity: on 100 healthy postmenopausal women for 12 months found no significant changes in hepatic artery blood flow, portal vein blood flow or total hepatic blood flow, or in any liver function tests. They concluded that daily administration of 40mg/day CR for a period of 12 months in postmenopausal women did not adversely affect the liver.[31]

Mis-identification of herbs

Between 2005 and 2009, Health Canada received six reports of liver adverse reactions suspected of being caused by black cohosh. Analysis of three products associated with these revealed that they did not contain black cohosh, but found the presence of other related species.

A review followed of the authenticity of all licensed products containing black cohosh which resulted in withdrawal of products that did not contain authentic black cohosh, including products reported in four of the adverse reaction cases.[32]

Side effects

A meta-analysis of nine trials[33] (more than 1,400 participants) concluded that reported side effects were no different between black cohosh and placebo groups.

- GIT disturbances (most common)
- Frontal headache with a dull, full or bursting feeling
- High doses: nausea, vomiting, vertigo, headache, hypotension, impaired vision, impaired circulation
- Rare case reports of idiosyncratic hepatic reactions have been reported
- Mutagenicity, teratogenicity and carcinogenicity tests are negative

Dosage

It has been suggested that too high a dose makes black cohosh ineffective. In a clinical trial comparing the effects of a daily dosage of 40mg against 127mg, similar results in safety and efficacy was observed in both dosages.[34]

In clinical trials of many herbs, an extract standardised for one particular fraction or constituent is used and may be more concentrated than a liquid extract, but Remifemin® is not standardised and so is roughly equivalent to a 1:1 liquid extract. The dose in clinical trials is between around 50mg and 120mg per day, with 80mg per day being typical. When that is converted into a tincture or liquid extract equivalent dosage, this is actually a very small dose. For a 1:10 60% tincture, this equates to 6ml per week.

Below is a conversion of a daily dosage of 80mg to typical dosages when used in tinctures:

0.6ml	of a	1:1	per week
1.2ml	of a	1:2	per week
1.8ml	of a	1:3	per week
2.4ml	of a	1:4	per week
3.0ml	of a	1:5	per week
6.0ml	of a	1:10	per week

To extract the triterpene glycosides a tincture needs at least 60% ethanol, although this need not apply to the final ethanol content depending on the manufacturing method.

Vitex agnus-castus

Vitex myths

Vitex is one of those herbs that seems, like quite a few others in this book, to have become progressively more misunderstood as theories of its hormonal actions emerged. The key with some of these herbs, particularly ones whose history of use is so rich, is to look closely at how they have been used in the past. It is not really possible to maintain that centuries of practice that have led to modern formulations and pharmaceuticals were somehow accidental. There were certainly myths, too, but consistent patterns are revealing, for example strewing Vitex to deter amorous males, and the puzzle of it being used both as a galactagogue and as an aid to weaning. Both of these are likely to do with dosage: at high concentrations, Vitex inhibits prolactin release and reduces milk output. At low concentrations, it increases it, and so it is at these low concentrations that it might have an anaphrodisiac effect in both sexes and be a galactagogue in women.

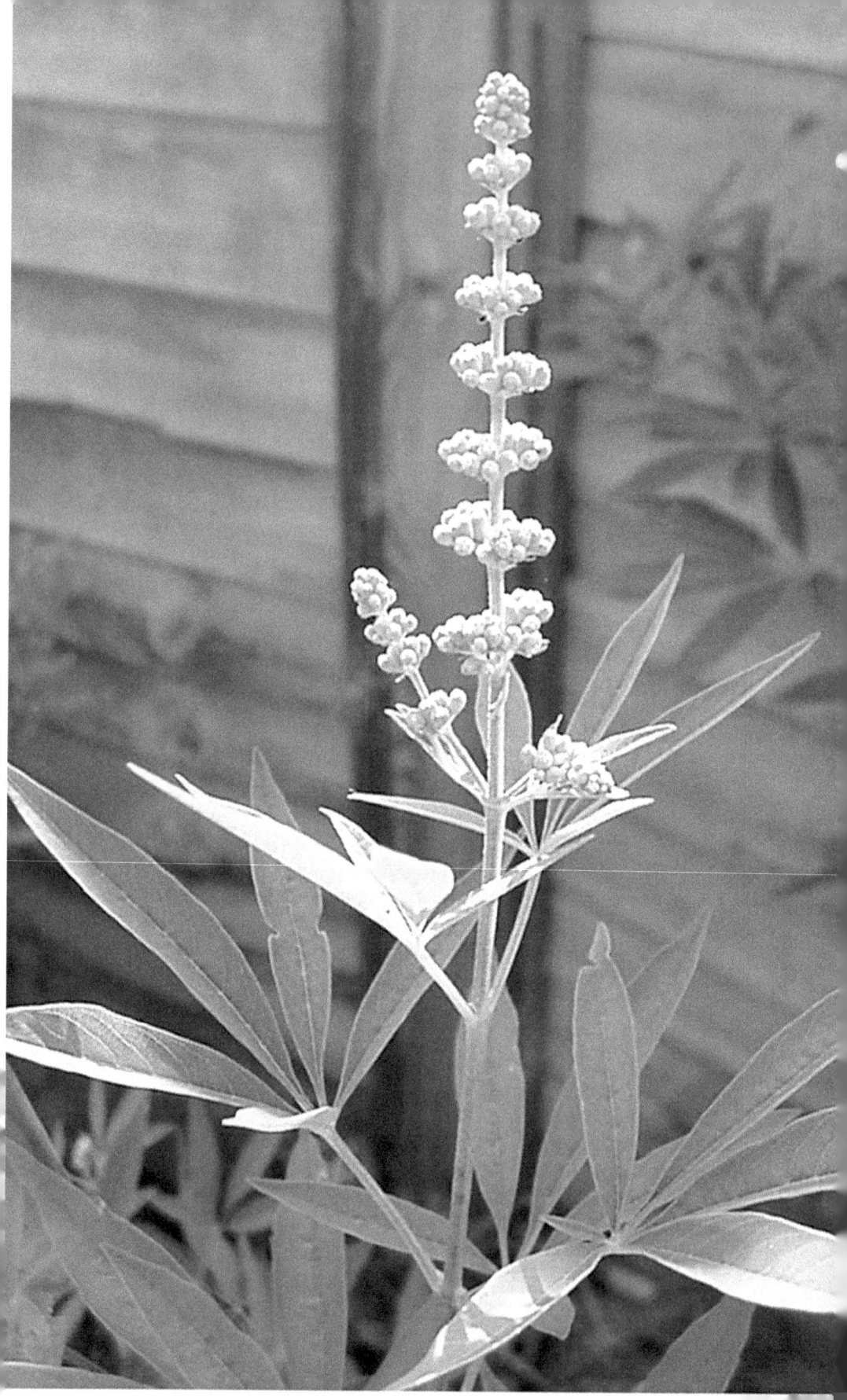

The second myth around Vitex is when it should be taken. The taking of drop doses early in the morning arose only in the 1950s in one research trial, and it is likely to be more effective either taken through the day, like most preparations, or in an evening dose, depending on the indication.

Other theories are that it is contraindicated in PCOS, is contraindicated for depression in PMS and directly promotes progesterone production. The first two of these have little merit, and the last is an oversimplification. But then Vitex is a complex herb and needs careful study and careful use.

Traditions

Antiquity

Vitex has been used medicinally for more than 2,500 years. It was an important plant for much of this time, as it is for modern herbalists, and accordingly it is worth looking at in some detail. The fruits were prescribed in ancient Egypt, Greece, Iran, and Rome for treating gynaecological and other sexual health problems.

Various names point to the reputation of Vitex to curb sexual appetite, among them chaste tree and monk's pepper tree, pointing to its ability to curb male sexual appetite. In medieval Europe, chasteberry was popular among celibate clergymen as it was thought to reduce unwanted sexual libido.[35] Vitex flowers at the time of the Thesmophoria, an ancient Greek festival held in honour of Demeter, the Greek goddess of agriculture, fertility, and marriage. During this festival, women who remained chaste during the festival covered their beds with its leaves. The Romans, following the Greek traditions of linking the plant with chastity, called it agnus (lamb) castus (chaste) – the 'lamb' reference may have been added in Christian times. The Vestal Virgins carried twigs as symbol of chastity.

Two other names, Indian spice and wild pepper, refer to the fruits' use as a pepper substitute: they have a pungent scent and flavour similar to black pepper.

Most traditions suggest use of herbal wine as an effective way of taking Vitex, and this was how the ancient Greeks and Romans prepared it; both Hippocrates and Dioscorides recommended this form, just as today we would mainly use it in the form of a tincture.

According to Hippocrates, ca. 400 BCE, 'If blood flows from the womb, let the woman drink dark wine in which the leaves of the chaste tree have been steeped'. Once again, this has a parallel with the present-day herbalist, who often would use significant amounts of Vitex in the case of heavy bleeding, especially flooding. Hippocrates also recommended it for treating injuries, inflammations, enlargement of the spleen, and to help the uterus to expel the afterbirth.

Dioscorides (around 50 CE), a Greek physician attached to the Roman military, follows similar principles to Hippocrates, and also suggests, along the lines of the Greek tradition, that Vitex is able to curb sexual appetites, with women placing the foul-smelling branches and leaves upon their bed to deter men. He also said it was good for stimulating mother's milk, and that it goes to the head and brings sleep. This is certainly close to some of the modern research findings presented later in this chapter, in the section 'Melotonin release'. Dioscorides further recommends mixing it with *Mentha pulegium* (pennyroyal) for headaches, with menstrual difficulties (which Gerard quotes directly many centuries later), again closely akin to modern practice, although pennyroyal is now used less than other emmenagogues.

From the Middle Ages to the Enlightenment

In the Middle Ages from the Middle East to Southern Spain during the 'Islamic Golden Age' many scholars introduced new plants to the system of medicine inherited from the Greeks, and extended the uses of the old ones. There was keen appreciation of medical theory and the actions of medicinal plants, so the characterization of their medical uses rewards close attention. In Traditional Persian Medicine,[36] *Vitex agnus-castus* (alongside *Foeniculum vulgare*, *Anethum graveolens*, *Pimpinella anisum*, and *Nigella sativa*) was found to be among the most effective galactagogues. Likewise, in Iranian traditional medicine its leaves and fruits were used for increasing milk.[37]

Many writers over the centuries have confirmed its use of encouraging milk production, and breast feeding decreases post-partum fertility ('lactation amenorrhoea': increased prolactin and consequent reduction in oestrogen levels suppress the periods). Once again seemingly contradictory information indicates opposite actions at high and low dosages.

From 1600 onwards, Vitex was widely used as a common folk-remedy for female hormonal imbalances as well as for stimulating the milk flow. Gerard and other Renaissance herbalists recommended Vitex for inflammation of the uterus and as an emmenagogue: 'The decoction of the herbe and seed is good against pain and inflammations about the matrix, if women be caused to sit and bathe their privy parts therein; the seed being drunke with Pennyroiall bringeth downe the menses, as it doth also both in a fume and in a pessary...'

Contradictory information about whether Vitex cools or stimulates passions recurs in the literature of Enlightenment times. James, in his *Pharmacopeia Universalis* (1747), regarded Vitex as only repressive to the passions in people who were excessively hot, because of its drying nature, which might act to dry up excess 'seed', but that because of its hot nature, it could actually be a stimulant of sexual desire where the person was 'cold'.

The dose dependency of Vitex's effects may be either because some constituents themselves are stimulatory or inhibitory at different doses, or because different constituents with contrasting effects have their influence at different dosages. In any case, probably because it did not convincingly fit any available medical theory, the English began to lose interest from the 1700s to the twentieth century. A French medical herbal book of the late 1800s, describes the use of Vitex to cool the passions, but offers doubts that it had that effect and rather considered that it had 'a very stimulating property'. The Eclectic medical works only mention it in passing, saying that it cools passions, or has stimulating properties, but without mentioning for which sex. Chasteberry was, however, still used as an emmenagogue and to stimulate lactation.[38]

Research between 1930 and 1950

In 1938, a German researcher, Gerhard Madaus, using a series of animal experiment to determine which part of the plant had the greatest biological activity. Madaus found that extracts of the leaves, fruits, and bark retarded oestrus (heat) in female rats, without evidence of adverse effects on reproductive performance. The fruits had the greatest activity.

During the Second World War, *Vitex agnus-castus* was used in Germany as galactagogue, and clinical confirmation of the effectiveness of chaste tree fruit preparations in stimulating milk production in German women under stress from Allied bombing was published in several papers (1941, 1942, and 1943). In the 1950s, animal studies further confirmed an experimental lactation-stimulating action. The first clinical work confirming Vitex's galactagogue activity (using Agnolyt) was published in 1953.[39]

Constituents

Diterpenes (clerodadienols, vitexilactone, rotundifuran, and 6-beta,7 beta-diacetoxy-13-hydroxy-labda-8,14-dien)
Flavonoids (casticin, isovitexin, apigenin, kaempferol, quercetagetin, orientin)
Iridoid glycosides (aucubin and agnuside)
Essential oils (cineole, limonene, sabinene, pinene)

Pharmacology

A study published in 1954 on women with amenorrhoea describes a dramatic improvement in menstrual regularity among patients with cystic hyperplasia of the endometrium.[40] This suggested progestogenic activity, a view supported by research in the 1960s and which still finds its way into present day textbooks.[41] It was proposed that the mechanism was that *Vitex agnus-castus* stimulates LH secretion. This has now been disproven: present day studies indicate that Vitex does not directly affect levels of follicle-stimulating hormone (FSH) or luteinizing hormone (LH).[42]

Dopaminergic activity and the clerodadienols

The major dopaminergic compounds are the clerodadienols, a subgroup of the diterpenes in the plant. These are very stable and resistant to almost any treatment. The clerodadienols are highly lipophilic compounds that easily pass the blood-brain barrier and can access brain dopaminergic systems and their postsynaptic receptors.

Research indicates that Vitex causes a decrease of prolactin secretion as a result of dopamine receptor agonism. Dopaminergic activity inhibits prolactin secretion from the anterior pituitary gland. This could well explain Vitex's effectiveness in PMS and menstrual problems, as increased prolactin levels are associated with premenstrual mastalgia, corpus luteal insufficiency and infertility, and reduced aromatase activity. So the progesterone theory is not entirely wrong, but it is an oversimplification. As increased prolactin inhibits corpus luteal development, leading to reduction of the secretion of progesterone in the luteal phase of the menstrual cycle, chasteberry's inhibition of prolactin excess can *indirectly* increase progesterone by correcting luteal phase deficiency.

It has been suggested that these diterpenes may also be a beneficial adjunct in the treatment movement disorders; Parkinson's disease, Periodic Limb Movement disorder and restless leg syndrome, Huntington disease and Essential Tremor.

Studies with effect on prolactin

Clinical trials have indicated that after 3 months of treatment with Vitex for hyperprolactinaemia, the supraphysiological release of prolactin due to stress, and prolactin pulsing associated with LH pulses were normalised. Thus, LH pulses resulted in increased progesterone and oestradiol levels.

In an *in vivo* study assessing the effect of Vitex on lactating animals and their offspring, a decrease in milk consumption in the offspring was observed, and a high rate of mortality resulted compared with untreated animals. Normal milk consumption patterns resumed in the offspring when the dams were no longer given the extracts.[43] This contradicts earlier studies in the 1950s and indicates a possible dose-dependent effect of Vitex on prolactin levels, with an increase in prolactin at low doses and a decrease in prolactin when higher doses of Vitex are given.

In a clinical study on healthy males, using a mother tincture (1:10) at doses of 120mg, 240mg, and 480 per day for 2 weeks, lower doses indeed caused a rise in prolactin (120mg, 2–3gtt of FE or 5gtt of 1:2), whereas higher doses led to a much-reduced secretion (480mg, 10gtt of FE or 20gtt of 1:2).[44] In men, prolactin inhibits the secretion of testosterone, so low doses should indeed decrease sexual appetite. So, the dose-dependent effect on prolactin would certainly seem to be the clue to the contradictory writings in relation to Vitex being a galactagogue (lower doses), or an antigalactagogue (higher doses), decreasing sexual desire (lower doses), and increasing (or normalizing) it (higher doses).

Casticin and other flavonoids

Casticin is found in a number of medicinal plants other than *Vitex agnus-castus*, among them other *Vitex* spp., *Artemisia annua* (in which it has been shown to enhance the antimalarial effect), *Artemisia abrotanum*, and *Achillea millefolium*.

- Studies have also affirmed the anti-inflammatory properties of casticin, with several molecular mechanisms identified and have suggested a wide range of other actions and properties:
  - anti-asthmatic, tracheospasmolytic, lung injury protection.
  - analgesic, rheumatoid arthritis amelioration.
  - antihyperprolactinaemic, oestrogenic.
  - Opioidergic.
  - liver fibrosis attenuation.
  - anti-angiogenic, antiglioma, and activities.[45]
  - immunomodulatory properties, anti-cancer properties, enhances apoptosis.[46]
- *In vitro*, casticin is effective against many cancer cell lines via different molecular mechanisms.
- *In vitro*, casticin and other constituents have been shown to have anti-inflammatory activity and lipoxygenase inhibition.[47]
- Casticin has neuroprotective effects, following middle cerebral artery occlusion *in vivo*.[48]
- Casticin and other flavonoids have been recognised to have the main role in the antioxidant effect of the plant.

Oestrogenic activity

In vitro studies have demonstrated oestrogen receptor binding for some constituents of *Vitex agnus-castus*, namely apigenin and linoleic acid. These constituents are commonly found in many seed oils, and apigenin is also found in many herbs including chamomile. Most of these plants are not considered to be 'oestrogenic' and, as Vitex is not a rich source of either apigenin or linoleic acid, these substances are unlikely to exert any direct oestrogenic effect.[49]

Some clinical trials have demonstrated an increase in both progesterone and oestrogen when treating latent hyperprolactinaemia, however. Again, this is likely to be due to correction of deficient corpus luteal function associated with that condition, and resulting in low levels of both progesterone and oestrogen.[50] Therefore, if you are improving corpus luteal function you would expect to increase oestrogen as well as progesterone. Even at higher doses, Vitex is unlikely to increase oestrogen beyond normal levels in such circumstances because it appears to simply normalise corpus luteal function as its dopaminergic activity decreases prolactin release from the pituitary.

Melatonin release

Dioscorides said of Vitex that it 'brings sleep'. Some clinical studies confirm this use, and show a dose-dependent increase of melatonin secretion (between 0.6 to 2.4g/day of dried berries, in divided doses taken three times daily), especially during the night. Melatonin output was approximately 60% higher in those taking Vitex and began approximately 1 hour after the light was turned off. It was concluded that the promotion of sleepiness observed by some patients taking Vitex during the trial might be a result of the stimulation of endogenous melatonin secretion.[51]

This could be of interest in insomnia in older people, as this is thought partly to be related to reduced melatonin levels, and interestingly also it has been shown that melatonin was able to delay the endocrine changes that occur during the course of menopause. This makes it an intriguing herb for use in the menopause, not necessarily for its hormonal effects but the effect on melatonin.

Opioid receptors

Vitex has shown affinity to opiate receptors[52] – both μ and δ receptors,[53] perhaps due to casticin – and that might play a part in the plant's efficacy in PMS.

In vivo *reduction in LH and testosterone, leptin*

- Intraperitoneal injections of Vitex *in vivo* decreased LH and testosterone levels. The authors concluded that these results indicate one could use Vitex for pathological cases with increased LH and testosterone levels.[54] Obviously, we do not use it this way, but it does indicate possible use in treatment of PCOS, where some have thought Vitex contraindicated because of the belief that it *increases* LH.
- Leptin (the 'satiety hormone' made by adipose cells, which helps to regulate energy balance by inhibiting hunger) was found to be reduced in animal studies.[55]

Other in vivo *and* in vitro *studies*

- Vitex has been shown to have effects as a prophylaxis for osteopaenia.[56] After 3 months, a slight, statistically not significant, osteoporosis-protecting effect has been seen.

- Improvement in learning and memory (interesting in the light of the neuroprotective effect of casticin).[57]
- Effective in preventing non-alcoholic fatty liver disease and oxidative stress, both of which are frequent causes of abnormal liver functions in the postmenopausal period.[58]
- May have beneficial effects on ageing and age-related kidney disease.[59]
- Hypoglycaemic, with pancreatic protective effects in naturally aged and ageing-model mice.[60]
- Reduction or prevention of epileptic activity *in vivo*, decreasing ADD and S5D (length of convulsion) in a dose-dependent manner.[61]
- Pharmacological studies confirm that *V. agnus-castus* exhibits antibacterial activity, and the methanolic extract has antifungal activity against *Candida albicans*.
- Insect repellent activity.

Clinical trials

Clinical studies have demonstrated that *Vitex agnus-castus* is beneficial in the treatment of premenstrual syndrome, abnormal menstrual cycle, amenorrhea, mastodynia, and hyperprolactinaemia (all related to increased level of prolactin).[62]

A systematic review of many clinical trials confirmed that Vitex is effective in the treatment of premenstrual syndrome, premenstrual dysphoric disorder, and latent hyperprolactinaemia.[63,64]

PMS

- General reduction of PMS symptoms,[65–67] including depressive symptoms, anxiety, craving, and hyperhydration, irritability, mood changes, anger, headache, insomnia, and breast fullness. Vitex taken over three cycles gave symptomatic relief, but duration of symptoms was not changed. It was equally effective for women taking OCP. Once treatment stopped symptoms gradually retuned to baseline within three further cycles.[68] Differences become even more significant after 3 months of treatment. So the full benefits require at least three menstrual cycles to become established.
- PMS in perimenopausal women: A combination of Hypericum (5,400mg) and Vitex (1,000mg/day) was not useful for typical menopausal symptoms, but beneficial for late-perimenopausal women, for

whom it caused a marked reduction in PMS-like symptoms.[69] In another clinical study, late-perimenopausal women took *V. agnus-castus* dry with reductions in anxiety, depression, cravings, and hydration.
- Migraine related to cycle: reduction in frequency and duration (days with headache) of monthly attacks,[70] and reduction of PMS symptoms.
- Premenstrual dysphoric disorder (PMDD): patients responded well to fluoxetine and Vitex in combination. Fluoxetine was more effective for psychological symptoms (depression and irritability) while Vitex diminished the physical symptoms (breast tenderness, cramps, food cravings, swelling).[71,72] A systematic review confirmed that Vitex for treatment of PMS/PMDD is a safe and efficacious,[73] despite many people thinking it is contraindicated for depression in PMS.

Hyperprolactinaemia and cyclic mastalgia

- Effective as treatment of cyclical mastalgia,[74] comparable to flurbiprofen (nonsteroidal anti-inflammatory drugs). Both medications significantly reduced the complaints.[75]
- A clinical trial reported it reduced prolactin secretion, normalizing a shortened luteal phase, increasing mid-luteal progesterone and 17β-oestradiol level.
- The intensity of mastalgia in patients treated with Vitex decreased after one or two treatment cycles and remained reduced after the third cycle. *Fructus agni-casti* performs similarly to bromocriptine with respect to lowering serum prolactin and reducing breast pain but with better patient compliance and lower cost.[76]

Intrauterine device induced bleeding, and menorrhagia

Vitex (dosage not stated) taken three times a day during menstruation (day 1 until day 8) for 4 months was compared with mefenamic acid for IUD-induced bleeding. In the mefenamic acid group, bleeding was decreased significantly more than the Vitex group in the first 3 months but during the 4th month, the mean difference was not statistically significant.[77]

In a trial in Iran, mefenamic acid or Vitex (dosage not stated) were given in patients complaining of menorrhagia. Both caused reduction of menstrual blood loss and increase in Hb content (oral iron was given to those with low Hb), with no statistically significant difference between them. In comparison with mefenamic acid, Vitex caused much fewer complications.[78]

Severe dysmenorrhoea

The effectiveness of Fructus agni-casti (Agnucaston® tablet 4mg once a day) was similar to that of ethinyl oestradiol/drospirenone in patients with primary dysmenorrhoea.[79]

Acne vulgaris

An open study male and female, with different forms of acne found that after 6 weeks of treatment with Vitex extract and a topical disinfectant; 70% of the cases experienced total resolution, with the highest success rate reported for acne vulgaris, follicularis and excoriated acne (in some people, picking at acne goes to an extreme point when the skin tissues get damaged seriously). The group that was not treated took 30–50% longer to achieve similar results.[80]

Survey among herbalists (paper NIMH): 80% of herbalists used it for acne.[81]

Menstrual cycle irregularities and fertility

A regime of 20mg of the plant extract (Ze 440) taken for three consequent menstrual periods (observational study) resulted in remission or improvement of menstrual cycle irregularity and specific symptoms such as polymenorrhoea, oligomenorrhoea, and amenorrhoea, dysmenorrhoea, intermenstrual bleeding, hypermenorrhoea, menometrorrhagia, ovulation bleeding, and premenstrual or postmenstrual bleeding. Among the women taking part who had a desire to have children, 23% became pregnant during treatment with the Vitex extract: 91% of the physicians and 92% of the patients were 'satisfied' or 'very satisfied' with the achieved treatment outcomes.[82]

Another study including women with hyperprolactinaemia demonstrated improved menstrual cyclicity by an increased average number of luteal days from 3.4 days (±5.0) to 10.5 days (for 3 months).[50] In another study of women with menstrual irregularity and infertility, menstrual cyclicity was significantly improved among those taking a

Vitex-based preparation, Mastodynon®: in women with amenorrhoea or luteal insufficiency, pregnancy occurred in the Mastodynon® group more than twice as often as in the placebo group.[83]

Study of the effects of FertilityBlend®[84]

FertilityBlend®, a mixture of Vitex, green tea, L-arginine, vitamins (including folate) and minerals, was taken by women of 24–42 years who had tried unsuccessfully to conceive for 6–36 months. As it is a mixture, it is not strictly possible to attribute the results solely to Vitex, but it is the only herbal medicine in the mixture and so the results appear to be indicative at least. The findings were:

- A trend towards increased mean mid-luteal progesterone. The average number of days with luteal phase basal temperatures over 98°F increased, and both short and long cycles were normalised.
- After 3 months, 26% of women in the treatment group became pregnant compared to 10% (4 out of 40) in the placebo group. Three of the remaining women in the treatment group conceived after 6 months on FertilityBlend® (32%).
- Women with luteal phase defects due to latent hyperprolactinaemia had reduced prolactin release after 3 months, with luteal phases normalised and deficits in luteal phase progesterone synthesis eliminated.
- 17 beta-oestradiol rose in the luteal phase.

The tested preparation is thought to be an efficient medication in the treatment of luteal phase defects due to latent hyperprolactinaemia.

Restless leg syndrome

Restless leg syndrome has been associated with dopamine deficiency and so dopamine agonists can be used in treatment. As a way of researching plant-based treatment that could avoid potential side effects of pharmaceutical dopamine agonists, patients with restless leg syndrome (RLS) received tablets containing extract of the fruit of chaste tree (*Vitex agnus-castus*, equivalent to 360mg/day of dried herb) over 1–29 months, on the basis of the herb's own dopaminergic effects.[85] Some of them were also taking drugs (L-dopa or pramipexol, a dopamine agonist). There was a positive effect in those taking Vitex alone as well as for those that were on medication, and the group on medication were able to reduce their dosage of the drugs or cease the use of drugs.

Effects on fracture healing

In a double-blind, randomised, placebo-controlled trial, women with long bone fracture demonstrated that co-administration of magnesium and *V. agnus-castus* (4mg dried fruit extract of *V. agnus-castus*) could enhance the fracture healing,[86] significantly improving the osteocalcin level. The serum concentration of vascular endothelial growth factor was increased in the Vitex-only group. The overall results suggesting that administration of *Vitex agnus-castus* plus magnesium may promote fracture healing and given that 30% of postmenopausal women suffer from bone fractures at some point, this study may indicate a useful role for Vitex here, too.

Main actions

- Prolactin inhibitor (unusually high amounts are suspected to be responsible for impotence and loss of libido)
- Dopamine agonist
- Indirectly progestogenic
- Galactagogue (dose-dependent, i.e. small doses only)
- Increases melatonin

Indications

The PMS symptoms that respond best are:

- Mastalgia
- Fluid retention
- Irritability
- Depressed mood
- Anger, mood changes
- Headache, migraines related to the cycle
- Premenstrual aggravations (such as mouth ulcers, orofacial herpes, epilepsy)

Menstruation problems

- Irregular menstruation and related infertility
- Secondary amenorrhoea
- Metrorrhagia (from functional causes)
- Oligomenorrhoea
- Polymenorrhoea, especially when marked by progesterone deficiency (cystic hyperplasia of the endometrium) and latent hyperprolactinaemia

Hyperprolactinaemia

- breast cysts
- fibrocystic breast disease
- benign prostatic hyperplasia
- erectile dysfunction or infertility in men
- galactorrhoea

Several autoimmune diseases have been linked to higher levels of prolactin in the blood, systemic lupus erythematosus (SLE), rheumatoid arthritis (RA), Sjögren's syndrome, and juvenile arthritis. For SLE, serum prolactin concentrations have been correlated with both clinical activity and remission.

Other indications

- Insufficient lactation (very low doses only, certainly less than 150mg/day)
- Infertility due to decreased progesterone levels or hyperprolactinaemia
- Acne (in both sexes)
- Perimenopausal PMS-like syndromes
- Poor sleep maintenance, insomnia
- Restless leg syndrome
- Uterine fibroids, endometriosis, follicular ovarian cysts
- Possibly osteoporosis

When to take Vitex

Many herbalists use Vitex in the morning and suggest that use as a single morning dose is most effective as the body is more hormonally active or receptive in the morning. However, that regimen is based on the first trials in the 1950s, and does not reflect the traditional use nor the more recent research done on prolactin levels. If the aim is to block prolactin sleep time peaks, some say that it needs to be used at night as it does in the treatment of prolactin-associated infertility. If there is significant hyperprolactinaemia, use throughout the day.

Dosage

A study examining the clinical effects of three different doses of the Vitex extract in patients suffering from PMS found improvement in a 20mg group that was significantly higher than both placebo and an 8mg treatment group. The higher dose of 30mg was no better than the 20mg. The study used a dry extract (6–12:1), extraction solvent: 60% ethanol m/m.

The dose of 20mg per day corresponds to 180mg crude material a day, or 0.18ml of FE, approximating to 1ml of 1:5 (20gtt) – a weekly dose 1.4ml FE or 7ml of 1:5.[87] The German Commission E recommended 30–40mg/day of extract of dried fruit which is standardised based on 0.6% casticin, and this would mean a weekly dose 2–3ml FE or 10–15ml of 1:5 tincture.

Clinical trials have used a variety of doses:

- Fluid extract: 1–2.5ml of extract daily.
- Dried fruit: 1.5–3mg daily as decoction.
- Dried extracts in pill or capsule form: 2–500mg twice daily.

The key to finding the right dose is to take into account the clinical indications, use typical dosages (not too low if one is trying to reduce prolactin secretions) and adjust over several months. Higher doses are indicated for short-term treatment in the case of excessive uterine bleeding and restless leg syndrome.

As a slow-acting herb, it needs to be taken for 3–6 months in cases of amenorrhoea. Weiss suggests that Vitex needs to be taken for a year before regular menstruation is re-established.[88] Infertile women with amenorrhea can remain on *V. agnus-castus* for 12–18 months unless pregnancy occurs during treatment.

Indications and dosage

Contraindications

Use cautiously in pregnancy and only in the first trimester, when the pregnancy depends on the corpus luteum for progesterone production. Higher doses (greater than 250mg/day) should be avoided during lactation.

There are no drug interactions recognised or reported by systematic reviews.[89] No herb-drug interactions have been reported, but caution is advised for its concomitant use with dopamine agonists or antagonists.

Side effects

Chasteberry is well tolerated; reported adverse effects are minor: most commonly gastrointestinal disturbances (particularly nausea) and skin conditions (acne, pruritus, and rashes).

Occasionally reported: headache, fatigue and hormone-related symptoms, such as menstrual cycle changes, mastalgia, and weight gain.

Concerns have been expressed that chaste tree use might mask a prolactinoma.

Case report: After three endocrinologically normal cycles while undergoing unstimulated *in vitro* fertilization treatment, a woman took Vitex (no dosage given) at the beginning of a fourth IVF treatment cycle. In this fourth cycle, her serum gonadotrophin and ovarian hormone measurements were disordered. She had symptoms (no symptoms given) suggestive of mild ovarian hyperstimulation syndrome in the luteal phase. Two subsequent cycles were endocrinologically normal.[90] This has not been reported anywhere else, in systematic reviews or clinical trials.

CHAPTER SIX

Paeonia lactiflora and *Glycyrrhiza glabra*

Traditional use

The combination of peony and liquorice in equal or near-equal parts has been quite intensively used in Chinese medicine and perhaps even more so in Kanpo, the Japanese 'barefoot' medical tradition derived from it, to relieve spasms. Both the Chinese name, 'Shao-Yao-Gan-Cao-Tang' and the Japanese derivation, 'Shakuyaku-kanzo-to' or the formula code TJ 68 are used in research papers investigating its use for muscle cramps. It seems to be both very well tolerated and very effective, far more so than either plant used individually, so an example of genuine synergy. In recent years, the combination, as PGD (Peony-Glycyrrhiza Decoction), has been investigated more for its hormonal effects, particularly for PCOS and hyperprolactinaemia, and there is no doubt that it helps to regulate the menstrual cycle and correct excess testosterone production in the ovaries.

The species of liquorice most widely used in Chinese medicine is *Glycyrrhiza uralensis*, but two other species, *G. inflata* and *G. glabra*, the latter native to Europe commonly used in western herbal medicine are used interchangeably. All three species contain glycyrrhizin, although they each contain different polysaccharides, which are currently of pharmacological interest, and so some therapeutic differences between the three species may soon emerge.

Peony and liquorice have been used as medicines in Europe for at least 2,000 years. *Paeonia officinalis*, or common peony, was cultivated for that purpose in classical antiquity and is mentioned as both a treatment of epilepsy and as an emmenagogue by Hippocrates and Dioscorides. Paeonia actually takes its name from Paeon, physician to the gods and a pupil of Aesculapius. However, common peony, native to South-East Europe, has different properties to *Paeonia lactiflora*, the species used in Chinese medicine, which we are discussing in this chapter. Common peony has much less studied by pharmacologists, and it does not contain paeoniflorin, the constituent generally seen as most pharmacologically active.

Paeonia lactiflora

Despite what might be expected from the name lactiflora, i.e. milky, the flowers can be white, red, or pink. The Chinese name 'bai shao' refers to white, too, but denoting rather the colour of the root after its bark is stripped and it is processed. In Chinese medicine 'bai shao yao' is said to nourish the blood, nourish and balance the liver, reduce acute pains, soothe the liver and be astringent to yin. The root is also thought to remove stagnant blood. The former use of *Paeonia officinalis* root as an emmenagogue is interesting as *Paeonia lactiflora* also has effects on the endocrine and nervous systems, and the high reputation and cultivation of *P. officinalis* in earlier times may indicate a possibility of useful further investigation.

Constituents

The monoterpene paeoniflorin is the major active component and has received the most research attention.

Other constituents are flavonoids, proanthocyanidins, tannins, terpenoids, triterpenoids, and polysaccharides.

Preclinical studies suggest a range of actions including:[1]

- Spasmolytic
- Improving memory, anti-epileptic activity

- Hepatoprotective, anti-atherosclerotic—associated with lipid peroxidation inhibition
- Inhibiting hydrochloric acid secretion, appetite suppressant and stimulating metabolism
- Antimutagenic, immunomodulating
- Antioxidant, protects endothelium from negative effects of hyperlipidaemia; anticoagulant, fibrinolytic, inhibits platelet aggregation

Clinical studies using total glycosides of peony (TGP)—water/ethanol extract

Studies confirm anti-inflammatory, hepatoprotective and immunoregulatory activities:

- Enhancing orthodox treatment in rheumatoid arthritis. The combination of methotrexate and leflunomide used in active rheumatoid arthritis is associated with liver toxicity. In a clinical trial, peony reduced the incidence and severity of liver damage while enhancing the effects of these drugs.[2]

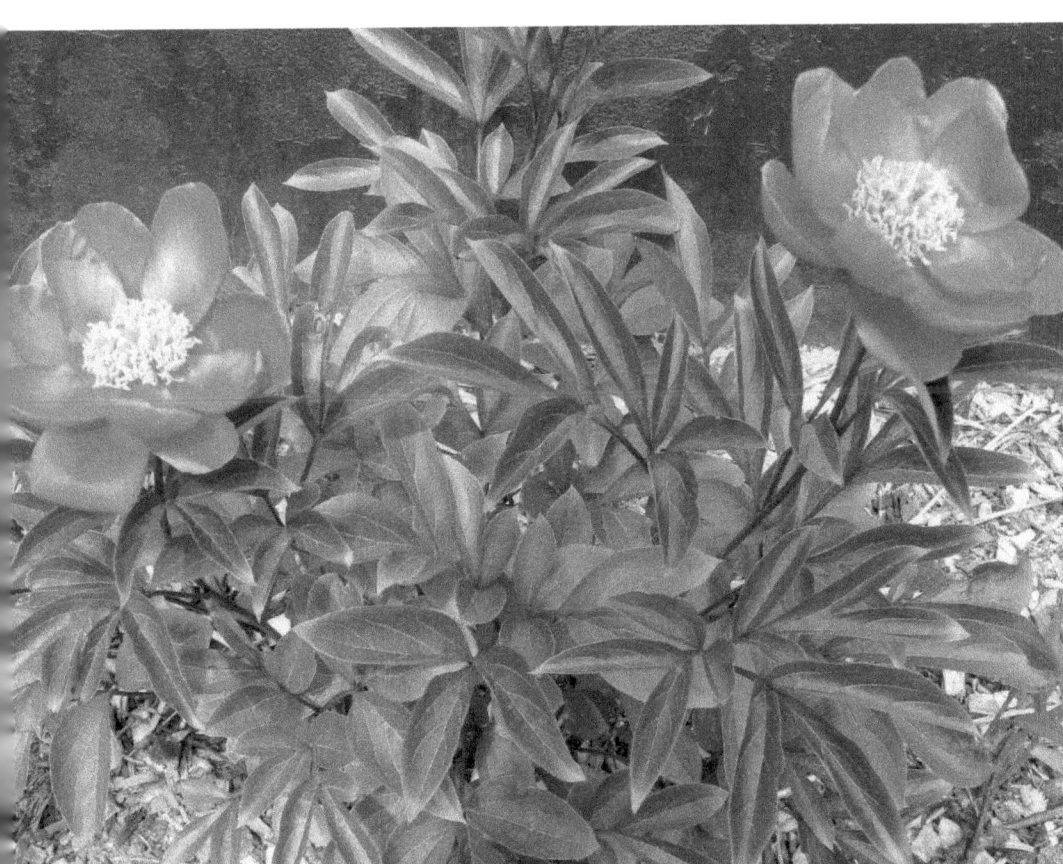

- In a retrospective study of Sjögren's syndrome (no systemic involvement), with patients receiving the extract for over 2 years, saliva secretion was increased, and serum gamma-globulin decreased from the 6th month. Schirmer's test (for sufficiency of tear secretion) improved after 12 months, the initiating time being 6–12 months.[3] A review found that combination with an immunosuppressant showed greater efficacy compared to immunosuppressant alone in improving exocrine function (saliva flow test and Schirmer's test), as well as inflammatory indices ESR and CRP, and immunoglobulins (IgM and IgG).[4]
- Albuminuria and inflammatory markers diminished in Type 2 diabetes mellitus patients with diabetic kidney disease.[5]
- A clinical trial in chronic cor pulmonale with pulmonary hypertension also found peony to be of benefit, but in this trial, it was given intravenously so extrapolation is uncertain.[6]

Liquorice

Liquorice 'root' actually consists of rhizomes, which form an extensive network anchoring the plant in relatively loose, sandy soils in its native coastal and estuarine regions. It is widespread and so familiar across most of the world, and so widely used medicinally and for so long that there is little point in giving another exhaustive presentation on this plant when we are mainly interested in particular contexts. Discussion of uses in, for example, ulceration (whether internal or external) or for sore throat and coughs, will be very limited, the main focus being here on its more general physiological, and particularly endocrine, effects.

Medicinally, the rhizome has been used over thousands of years (the name Glycyrrhiza very clearly 'sweet root' is certainly accurate) in Egyptian, Chinese, and Indian civilizations. In Greece and Rome, it was taken as a general tonic and for respiratory complaints. Theophrastus (371–287 BCE) administered it in honey to treat asthma. In the first century, Pliny the Elder advised its use in the form of a lozenge to clear the voice and postpone hunger and thirst, and as powder to sprinkle on mouth ulcers and films on the eyes.

Ancient Hindus believed that liquorice increased sexual vigour, ironically as we think it reduces testosterone levels. This indication is,

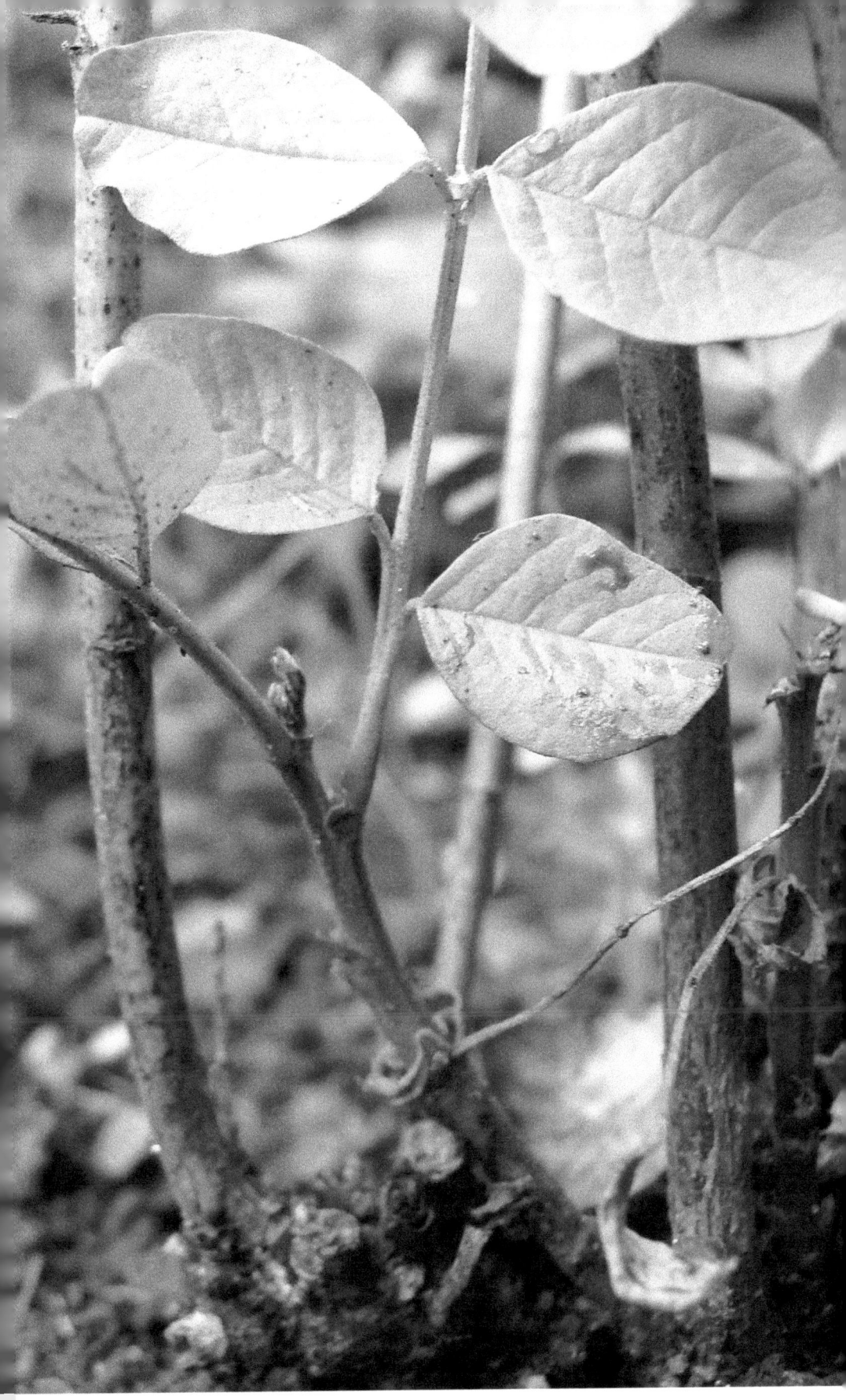

however, compatible with the plant's characterization as a general tonic, and the Ancient Chinese thought that liquorice root gave them strength and endurance.

In more recent centuries, Glycyrrhiza has been a staple for herbalists, including Nicholas Culpeper, who wrote that it 'serves as an emollient, demulcent, attenuant, expectorant, detergent' and that the root 'abates thirst in dropsies'.

Of course, it is very familiar in the form of confectionery, though it is typically only a minor ingredient in liquorice sweets, where it is combined with aniseed or similar extracts of umbelliferous plants. That is probably a good thing because it makes it harder to consume the amounts that might lead to water retention and high blood pressure. By far the majority of liquorice in commerce is actually used to sweeten the flavour of tobacco in cigarettes.

Constituents

Triterpenoid saponins: glycyrrhizin (also known as glycyrrhizic acid or glycyrhizinic acid—GZA—which is 50–170 times sweeter than sugar); glycyrrhetinic acid (GA, the aglycone of glycyrrhizin).

Flavonoids: isoflavonoids, chalcones, liquiritin.[7]

Actions

Glycyrrhiza has been extensively researched and demonstrates a wide range of actions:

- Antibacterial, inhibits oral bacterial adherence, antiviral, antifungal, antimalarial
- Anti-inflammatory, antioxidant, immunostimulatory, anti-mutagenic
- Anti-allergenic expectorant, antitussive, decongestant
- Stimulates gastric and tracheal mucus secretion (thus demulcent and expectorant)
- Antiulcer, wound healer
- Antispasmodic
- Anti-hepatotoxic and anti-hyperglycaemic
- Memory enhancing

Effect on the endocrine system

In vivo studies have shown that Glycyrrhiza reduces testosterone (free and total) and increases oestradiol. These effects occurred primarily in the ovary through enhanced aromatization of testosterone to 17-beta-oestradiol and increased ovulation rates, and not through changes to FSH or LH levels. It was thought that it interferes with 17 beta-hydroxysteroid dehydrogenase (which catalyses the conversion of androstenedione to testosterone).[8] *In vivo* studies have also shown an influence of *Glycyrrhiza uralensis* on the morphological features of polycystic ovaries.

Clinical trials related to sex hormones

A drop in serum testosterone and increase in 17-hydroxyprogesterone has been observed in men,[9] as well as a moderate decrease in the serum concentrations of dehydroepiandrostenedione sulphate (DHEAS, a metabolite of DHEA, hormonally neutral but neurotrophic). Decreased plasma testosterone has also been recorded in healthy women (22–26 years old) during the luteal phase of the menstrual cycle, returning to pre-treatment levels after discontinuation.

Drops in renin activity and aldosterone levels have been noted during therapy, while blood pressure and cortisol remained unchanged.[10] Gender may influence the action of liquorice, with aldosterone inhibition being greater in men, but its mineralocorticoid effects, raising blood pressure in people with essential hypertension, are not sex dependent.[11] Parathyroid hormone, 25-hydroxycholecalciferol and urinary calcium have been observed to increase, with authors suggesting that effect of liquorice on calcium metabolism is probably influenced by several components of the root, which show aldosterone-like, oestrogen-like and anti-androgen activity.[12]

Authors have also suggested that liquorice could be considered an adjuvant therapy of hirsutism and polycystic ovarian syndrome. Adding liquorice to spironolactone provided a synergistic effect on androgen excess in PCOS patients, with metrorrhagia lower in patients receiving the combination. The addition of liquorice also reduced both the side effects related to the diuretic activity of spironolactone (hypotension related to volume depletion) and the activation of the renin-aldosterone system.[13]

In another clinical study liquorice reduced body fat mass without any change in body mass index,[14] and it has also been observed to decrease the frequency and severity of hot flushes.[15]

Combination product, equal parts Paeonia and Glycyrrhiza

Spasmolytic effect of the combination

In vivo, ex vivo and *in vitro* research all confirm the spasmolytic effect of Paeonia and Glycyrrhiza and it appears to be the result of an interesting synergy whereby peony extracts interfere with acetylcholine *release* into the neuromuscular junctions while liquorice extracts interfere with acetylcholine's *activity* there.[16] One study found that concentrations of paeoniflorin and glycyrrhizin that were individually too low to inhibit muscle contraction were very active when applied simultaneously *in vivo*.[17] However, this study needs to be interpreted cautiously as glycyrrhizin is not absorbed but its aglycone, glycyrrhetinic acid (GA). Other studies do, however, suggest that GA is responsible for the inhibitory effect of Paeonia and Glycyrrhiza on myometrial contraction.[18,19]

In vitro results suggest that the combination may exert its action against dysmenorrhoea through preventing prostaglandin production: the effect on oxytocin- and prostaglandin F2α-induced contractions is different to the effect on KCl-induced contractions.[20]

Clinical trials with combination equal amounts of Paeonia and Glycyrrhiza

Relieves muscle cramps and muscle pain

- Hepatic cirrhosis: muscle cramps were relieved, along with the typical severe side effects of muscle weakness and central nervous system (CNS) depression that tend to occur as side effects of treatment[21]
- Muscle cramps also relieved in patients with diabetes mellitus,[22] undergoing dialysis[23,24] alcoholism,[25] cerebrovascular disease[26] or lumbar spinal stenosis[27]
- The combination also relieves muscle pain related to the cancer drug, paclitaxel (Taxol®), and carboplatin therapy[28]
- Reduces dysmenorrhoea in women with uterine fibroids,[29] inhibits contraction of uterine smooth muscles in pregnant women[19]

Inhibits prolactin

In vivo and *in vitro* studies show that PGD affects modulation of dopaminergic system, reducing prolactin levels and consequently normalizing progesterone levels by removing corpus luteum suppression by prolactin.[30] The dopaminergic inhibition of prolactin is the same mechanism of action as with *Vitex agnus-castus*, and Cimicifuga also exhibits a dopaminergic effect among other nervous system actions.

Clinical trial on prolactin levels

Clinical studies have demonstrated the effectiveness of PGD in alleviating antipsychotic-induced hyperprolactinaemia[31,32] resulting from the inhibition of dopaminergic activity that normally suppresses prolactin release. It is therefore beneficial for people on antipsychotic medication suffering from oligomenorrhoea or amenorrhoea. It also reduces abnormal involuntary movements (EPSEs, or extra-pyramidal side effects) more effectively than bromocriptine, without the side effects of exacerbating psychosis and changing other hormones,[33] and reduces sexual dysfunction in men caused by risperidone-induced hyperprolactinaemia.[34] In cases of anovulation, it aided menstrual resumption,[35,36] and progesterone and oestradiol increased.[37]

Reduces testosterone levels

Amenorrhea, oligomenorrhoea, irregular menstrual cycles, luteal insufficiency, and infertility are frequently associated with hyperandrogenism associated with excessive testosterone production in the ovary, for which the paeoniflorin and glycyrrhetic acid and glycyrrhizin in combination have shown a clear benefit. *In vivo* studies suggest that paeoniflorin, glycyrrhetic acid, and glycyrrhizin affect the conversion between delta 4-androstenedione and testosterone to inhibit testosterone synthesis, and stimulate the aromatase activity to promote oestradiol synthesis by the direct action on the ovary.[38]

Other preclinical studies have shown that the combination influences testosterone production by the ovaries but not by the adrenal glands. There was a dose-dependent decrease in testosterone production in ovaries, and delta 4-androstenedione production by ovaries was increased: the ratio of testosterone to delta 4-A was lowered.[39]

Clinical studies on PCOS Patients

As a treatment for PCOS, Paeonia and Glycyrrhiza combination is a common recommendation. The follow-up book to this one will look in more detail at PCOS, which is only briefly discussed here and at the end of this one.

In one trial, the oestradiol/testosterone ratio increased within 24 weeks of treatment: after 12 weeks, testosterone was only lower in the patients who became pregnant. It was concluded that the combination was effective for decreasing free testosterone levels and achieving pregnancy in patients with PCOS, by increasing the activity of aromatase in the ovary, thus promoting the conversion of testosterone to oestradiol, and thus lowering serum testosterone. The combination has also been shown to have an effect on catecholamines, and this was thought responsible for also improving lowering the LH/FSH ratio in the trial.[40] A further small trial also showed lowered serum testosterone levels, along with the induction of regular ovulation and pregnancy in oligomenorrhoeic and hyperandrogenic patients.[41]

The efficacy of Paeonia and Glycyrrhiza combination in PCOS seems to vary according to the type of polycystic ovary syndrome treated.[42] A small trial on infertile Japanese with polycystic ovary contrasted the effects on patients with general cystic and peripheral cystic patterns. Overall, plasma testosterone was decreased and (25%) became pregnant, but the plasma testosterone concentration in the case of the general cystic pattern was significantly higher than that in the women with a peripheral cystic pattern, and the pregnancy rate in those with the general cystic pattern was lower.

A further small trial in women with acne vulgaris, with the combination taken for 12 weeks, showed decreased serum free testosterone compared to baseline values, and a concomitant reduction in the number of comedomes.[43]

Summary of the actions and indications of Paeonia and Glycyrrhiza

- Normalizing ovarian function by reducing prolactin levels and increasing the activity of aromatase, which promotes oestradiol syntheses from testosterone
- Normalizing LH/FSH ratio
- Spasmolytic
- Anti-inflammatory

Clinical indications

- Androgen excess
- PCOS
- Hyperprolactinaemia (thus similar to Vitex)
- PMS, PCOS, ovulatory failure, infertility, endometriosis, adenomyosis, uterine fibroids, mastalgia, menopausal symptoms
- Dysmenorrhoea
- Uterine overactivity in pregnancy
- Other indications: nephritis or kidney problems related to type two diabetes
- Muscle cramps (as in cramps due to hepatic cirrhosis, diabetes, undergoing dialysis, alcoholics, cerebrovascular disease)

Dosage

Paeonia officinalis:
4.5–8.5ml/day of 1:2, 45% (Chinese Pharmacopoeia dosage: 6–12g dried root), 15/30ml per week of 1:1 45%
Glycyrrhiza glabra:
2–5ml 1:1 25% per day, 15–35ml per week but the higher end of that range should not be prescribed long-term.

Japanese clinical trials with a Paeonia and liquorice combination used an extract equivalent to 4–6g/day of dried Paeonia root and 4–6g of *Glycyrrhiza glabra* per day. However, aqueous ethanol is a more effective solvent than water for many of the constituents, and thus one could potentially use less. All the trials used equal parts of each herb.

Adverse effects

Liquorice can cause pseudoaldosteronism (aldosterone levels are actually suppressed; the symptoms are oedema and weight gain with hypokalaemia and hypertension). Liquorice-induced inhibition of aldosterone secretion differs between the genders (it is higher in men) and is not influenced by blood pressure. Risk factors are patient age (>60 years) and dosing period (>30 days) as well as co-administration of drugs inducing hypokalaemia.[44]

Peony's efficacy is probably reduced with antibiotics, as the gut flora is responsible for cleaving the aglycones of peony glycosides and thereby activating these constituents. Damage to the gut flora by antibiotics might interfere with this process.[45]

Table 6.1: Effects of herbs on hormonally-related functions

	Effects of Phyto-Oestro-Genic Herbs	Mastalgia	Reduces Hot Flushes	Menstrual Migraines	Decreases LH	Increases Bone Density	Res Cholesterol, LDL triglycerides	Increase HDL	Indication for Mood	Effect on Memory	Glucose Control	Insomnia
Soya			C	E	C	C	C	C	C Depression, and anxiety			
Trifolium pratense			C	E		C	C	C	C Depression			
Flaxseeds			C	E		E	C Lowers BP				C	
Humulus lupulus			C	T Headaches	C	C			Anxiety, Irritability		C	C
Salvia off.			C			E	C	C	C Depression Calming	C	C	
Asparagus racemosus			E				?		T nerve tonic	E	E	
Tribulus terrestris			C						Depression			
Dioscorea villosa			E?			E	E	E				
Chamaelirium luteum			E						T Irritability & depression			
Cimicifuga racemosa			C	T	? Increases & reduces	C	C		C Anxiety & depression			X
Glycyrrhiza glabra and Paeonia lactiflora	C					E			E			

PAEONIA LACTIFLORA AND GLYCYRRHIZA GLABRA 177

General Tonic	Tonifies Reproductive System	Lubricates	Effect on Bladder	Helpful in Breast Cancer	Demulcent Mucous Membranes/	Helpful of Atrophy Vaginal	Sexual Debility	Palpitations	Energy	General Wellbeing	Prolapse	PMS	Menstrual Irregularities	Fertility	Increases SHBG	Galactagogue	Threatened Miscarriage
		C		C										C			
				E?		C		C									
		C		C	T					C		C				C	
				E?		C gel	T Opposite	T									
T			C	E						C	C					T Opposite	
T	T		X	E	T	E	T	T	T	T				E		C	T
		C				C								C			
														E	E		T
T	T		T							T		T	T				T
	C	C	C	C	C	C		X				E	T	C alongside clomiphene			
												E	E	E			

(Continued)

Table 6.1: Continued

Effects of Phyto-Oestro-Genic Herbs	Mastalgia	Reduces Hot Flushes	Menstrual Migraines	Decreases LH	Increases Bone Density	Res Cholesterol, LDL triglycerides	Increase HDL	Indication for Mood	Effect on Memory	Glucose Control	Insomnia
Vitex agnus-castus	C	C For early vaso-motor symptoms	C		E			C PMS-related, depression, anxiety, irritability, anger			E Restless legs; C PMS
Panax ginseng		C				C		C Nervous tension, depression, anxiety			C
Foeniculum vulgare		C						PMS-related-stress, depression			
Valeriana officinalis		C									
Trigonella foenum-graecum		C									
Pimpinella anisum		C									

Key: C: confirmed by clinical trials; E: extrapolated from *in vivo* and *in vitro* research; T: theoretical based on known pharmacological actions.

General Tonic	Tonifies Reproductive System	Lubricates	Effect on Bladder	Helpful in Breast Cancer	Demulcent Mucous Membranes/	Helpful of Atrophy Vaginal	Sexual Debility	Palpitations	Energy	General Wellbeing	Prolapse	PMS	Menstrual Irregularities	Fertility	Increases SHBG	Galactagogue	Threatened Miscarriage
												C		C		C	
							C	C	C	C	T						
		C Cream									C						
											C						

CHAPTER SEVEN

Herbs, HRT, and the menopause

As with much to do with herbs and hormones, there is a widespread myth attached to herbal medicine and the menopause, namely that you in effect get HRT without the side effects by doing things the natural way. The 'forever young' image implies there is something wrong with getting older. That idea has nothing to do with nature. But the thing is half true, all the same. The menopause is a transition to a different phase of life, and can be made more comfortable, and the new phase much healthier, with proper attention to diet, and with the help of herbs. But that is not hormone replacement.

The main characteristics of the menopause

The menopause is most easily thought of as signalling the end of the monthly periods and the sudden decline in oestrogen levels. It is also obviously known as a time of change that is partly welcomed and partly dreaded. The reduction in oestrogen leads to a wide range of symptoms such as hot flushes and night sweats, cognitive instability, sleep disturbances, and vaginal atrophy, together with increased risk of some cancers, metabolic syndrome, cardiovascular disease, and osteoporosis. It is not unique to the middle years, though, as these events also happen during lactation, and through extreme calorie restriction, exercise or medical causes.

Some evolutionary biologists argue that after 50, one is on the evolutionary scrapheap—evolutionary pressure is to maximise the bearing and nurturing of children as soon as the capability is there at the expense of being able to do so in later years. After the childbearing years, one is not passing on useful genes, particularly as in much of human history the years after the menopause have been generally not so many. That seems a rather bleak view and is somewhat overstated. Death rates in societies living close to nature do not accelerate quickly between 50 and 65. But the 'bleakness' is also linked with our society's obsession with looking and feeling young. To escape from that is actually a kind of liberation!

There is certainly a major change of physiology taking place, and two ways to characterise it. The first is to say that the menopause resembles the time of lactation, where high levels of prolactin suppress reproductive hormones and the menstrual cycle, where raised blood glucose and triglycerides may enrich breast milk and where flushing may help to keep an infant warm (In a pilot study on postmenopausal women, the cognitive performance of women who reported having hot flushes during their menopausal years was better than in women who did not experience them, so here there is perhaps an adaptive value to them).[1] Lactating mothers lose significant bone density during while breast feeding lasts, in providing the calcium that the baby needs.[2] Another way to look at it is that female physiology begins to resemble that of men: less oestrogen, a tendency to fat deposition in the viscera rather than more peripherally, and similar cardiovascular changes and markers.[3] This might make it clear that health and lifestyle advice, too, should be similar in some ways for both sexes in later years to improve cardiovascular fitness as well as bone health.

One question that is sometimes asked is whether problems experienced in the menopause are somehow due to living an artificial lifestyle, partly because of not accepting the change, partly because of diet and lifestyle, particularly xeno-oestrogens. Should one be thinking of this as primarily a matter of adjustment? Well, diet and lifestyle have a very great role in ameliorating the transition, but we cannot fully emulate the lives of our Palaeolithic ancestors, when changes in metabolism of fats and sugars would generally have made far less difference than in a time of nutritional excess and a sedentary lifestyle. But even with a proper programme of exercise and diet the challenges are also very real in many cases. Not only is there a major physiological change, but with the increasing tendency to have children later, and for adolescents to stay home into adulthood, more women than ever are combining the roles of mother and provider during this time (making the notion of liberation somewhat illusory!) and the addition of a changing hormonal picture does not lighten the pressure. Theorizing about the evolution and traditional lifestyles can be helpful in giving a bigger picture and for contextualizing some of the changes, but of course the main thing is to have an ally who is also expert in the detail—at least to the extent that expertise is possible in such a complex and partially known field.

Timing and incidence of natural and artificial menopause

The menopause is defined as starting after a year without menstrual periods, at an average age of 48 to 52 years, after a phase of usually 4–5 years called the perimenopause, although in one in every hundred women, it occurs prematurely. In two-thirds of these women, there is no cause. In the remaining third, premature menopause is caused by:

- Metabolic/systemic disease
- Infections
- Lack of blood supply to the ovaries
- Smoking
- Radiation and or chemotherapy (in 30% menses return within 1 year)
- Tamoxifen and certain drugs that suppress menses used, e.g. in endometriosis
- Oophorectomy: Bilateral oophorectomy triggers the most dramatic form of menopause, with an increased risk of osteoporosis, cardiovascular disease, and vulval atrophy indicating that the ovaries do play an important role after the menopause

The main events in the physiology of the perimenopause

The perimenopause generally begins at somewhere between 41 and 51 years of age, with irregular ovulation (as there are few ovarian eggs left—the 1–2 million at birth are now just a few thousand). Physiological characteristics of this phase include:

- The length of the follicular phase shortens: there is an increased incidence of anovulatory cycles (hence heavy bleeding), and lower levels of progesterone.
- Hormonal tests will show an FSH increase, which can be the first sign. Seen in follicular phase when oestradiol levels lower. The cycle can still be regular and measurements of FSH may be normal as the test detects only a certain number of the over 60 FSH peptides. FSH typically increases 10- to 20-fold for about 1–3 years after last menstrual period.
- During the perimenopause, the chances of conceiving are lower, though not negligible, and this is quite a common time for an unplanned pregnancy to happen.
- Lower levels of oestrogens are found 6 months to a year before the true menopause, and progesterone declines before this. Lower progesterone levels lead to abnormal menstruation (excessive blood loss, absent period, persistent, and more frequent menstruation), which can be distressing. It is important in the case of irregular bleeding to exclude pathological causes, e.g. endometrial carcinoma, whose incidence increases at this time.
- Approaching the menopause, oestrogen levels rise very high (up to twice the level of a normal cycle) then fall rapidly. Follicular production drops from 700 to 30pg/ml within 2–3 days.
- PMS tends to get worse around perimenopause. The symptoms may be due to relative change in relationship of oestrogen to progesterone.

The main events in physiology of the postmenopause[4]

Oestrogen is too low for the uterine lining to build up, and menses are absent, as there is no longer any production of the most powerful oestrogen, oestradiol, in the follicles. FSH levels and to an extent LH levels become very high due to the loss of negative feedback.

The skin becomes less elastic, blood vessels also become stiffer and the arterial intima can thicken, leading to increased risk of cardiovascular disease. Bone resorption begins, and the epithelium of the vagina and vulva becomes drier and thinner, with loss of elasticity and shortening of the vagina, often causing dyspareunia. Oestrogen also affects the nervous system and central neurotransmitters: lower levels affect mood, sexual desire, memory and cognition, and temperature regulation.

Postmenopausal women derive almost all their oestrogen (oestrone more than oestradiol, in contrast to the reproductive years) from the aromatization of androgens androstenedione and testosterone produced in the adrenals and the ovaries under the influence of LH and FSH. The conversion takes place predominantly in fat, muscle, skin and brain. Over time, the adrenals become the most important source for the hormones. Surprisingly, though, women with bilateral oophorectomy have reduced formation of those hormones by the adrenals, so even more severe oestrogen depletion.

SHBG decreases due to the relative increase in testosterone (and is also reduced in hypothyroidism, obesity and hyperprolactinaemia), making the sex hormones more bioavailable so there is some measure at least of compensation.

Many of the physiological and psychological symptoms of the menopause are not directly due to hormones but secondary effects of oestrogen depletion on neurotransmitter systems, particularly serotonergic, adrenergic and dopaminergic pathways. The lower level of serotonin has an effect on thermoregulation in hypothalamus, causing hot flushes and night sweats.[5] SSRIs (serotonin reuptake inhibitors) have been found to reduce hot flushes by 60–70%. A reduction in oestrogen is thus also linked to depression and a sensation of warmth, but also to an associated increase in heart rate and anxiety, as the level of adrenaline is raised in response to low oestrogen.

Adrenaline can also cause downregulation of triiodothyronine (T3) receptors. When adrenaline is continuously elevated, the body tries to balance by lowering oestrogen and thyroid hormone, so this, coupled with tissue desensitization to T3, can exacerbate low oestrogen levels and also lead to functional hypothyroidism. Both oestrogen deficiency and hypothyroidism can cause a loss of energy, depression and bone demineralization.

Changes during the premenopausal and postmenopausal period as well as during pregnancy have also been associated with incidence of autoimmune diseases and cancers of the uterus, ovaries and breast. The mechanisms are not well understood, but involve cross-talk between oestrogen-signalling pathways and dopamine, epidermal growth factor, insulin, IGF-1 (insulin-like growth factor), cyclic AMP and other substances. It is not so much that this is a dangerous time of life as that a physiological transformation is taking place and needs an adjustment and not attempt to ignore it or to reset the physiology to that of the reproductive years. However, at least the attempt to establish HRT as a standard treatment led to insights into the menopause and its physiology through one of the biggest health studies ever performed, the Women's Health Initiative Study.

Women's health initiative study

This large-scale clinical trial of 161,808 menopausal women in the US tested combined hormones or oestrogen alone for cardiovascular outcomes and bone density; dietary modification (low-fat and high fruit, vegetable, and grain diet) for cardiovascular and breast cancer risks; and calcium/vitamin D for osteoporosis. It was halted prematurely in 1998 after 5.2 years (the planned duration was for 8.5 years), due to increased risk of invasive breast cancer, coronary heart disease, stroke, pulmonary embolism, and clots from hormonal therapy, and particularly combined hormonal therapy. The summary findings from this and associated studies on HRT were:

- HRT use reduced risk of colorectal cancer and fractures.
- Research that continued with oestrogen only did not find increase of heart disease but there was still an increase in strokes and clots.
- HRT increased death due to heart disease in the first year of use, compared to placebo.[6]
- One trial using only oestrogen for 10 or more years found that women were at greater risk of developing ovarian cancer, the risk increasing with length of use.[7]

As a result of the trial, many more women began looking for natural alternatives to HRT,[8] and that meant a significant focus both among women in many countries, among herbal medicine suppliers, and among researchers to find out what herbs are helpful in the menopause, and this has been a major driver for new research and new understandings of the roles of phyto-oestrogens in particular.

Why does HRT not work well?

We already saw that the simple one substance-one receptor idea is wrong—oestrogen receptors, as we know, come in two main types, alpha and beta. Oestrogen also affects receptors for some neurotransmitters, which contributes to its effects on mood and awareness. It gets much more complex. The steroid hormones being cholesterol-based, pass through cell membranes and have effects on cell nuclei through nuclear receptors, which are a type of transcription factor (i.e. switches that activate sections of DNA). But steroid receptors, and particularly the sex steroid receptors, can receive multiple inputs, i.e. are not only affected by their primary hormone. These steroid receptors include oestrogen receptors ER α and β, androgen receptors, glucocorticoid receptors, progesterone receptors and mineralocorticoid receptors. Furthermore, actions at one receptor can influence the expression (i.e. the density) and activity of others.[9]

An example of this is how progesterone upregulates activity of oestrogen at oestrogen receptors, the probable reason that breast cancer was seen more commonly in the WHI study (see next section) in women who were also taking progestogens, alongside an increased incidence of breast cancer in women with insulin resistance and diabetes.[10] Progesterone can induce or prevent breast cancer, probably depending on time of life and general hormonal background: on the preventive side, progesterone induces apoptosis and cell differentiation, but it also promotes growth driven by peptide growth factors (epidermal growth factor, insulin, IGF-1) and cAMP (as also do FSH and LH levels[11]). These factors—mostly also mentioned above in reference to oestrogen receptor cross-talk—tend to promote breast cancer and also stimulate ERα even in the absence of oestrogens.

There is no simple, clear picture that says 'use oestrogenic herbs, and they will be gentler than HRT and so you have the benefits without the risks'. As we will discuss later in the book, the menstrual cycle is a rhythm of nature, orchestrated by the nervous and endocrine systems as a whole. The menopause has to be respected and not masked, and embraced as a time of transition to something and not a change from something. It is rather a matter of making that transition as bearable as possible and helping women to prepare for a different rhythm.

As usual, there are three phases of treatment:

1. Initial relief of symptoms and alleviation of acute triggers
2. Nutritional, physiological and occupational support while the body adjusts and finds a new balance, withdrawal of pharmaceutical therapies as far as possible
3. Transition to minimal long-term maintenance (herbs and supplements)

Phase 1: manage symptoms, remove triggers

The integrity of the gut epithelium and efficient metabolism by the liver are crucial not only for the metabolism and excretion of hormones, but also to reduce the inflammatory load on the body. Many herbs will also need healthy digestion to be absorbed. So this has to be established at the beginning of herbal treatment.

Oestrogen metabolism and lifestyle advice

Mostly, women in and around the menopause will come to a herbalist because of some particular discomfort, be that physical or psychological (although it might also be prevention, e.g. of osteoporosis). As discussed, lifestyle and diet may be partly responsible for these. A low inflammatory diet and gut health may help not only with physical discomfort and blood sugar and lipid profile, but also with depression and irritability. So removing triggers is very important if it relieves distressing symptoms, but also in establishing the baseline for further treatment need for nutritional and herbal support. In other words, if tiredness and low mood are related to poor diet and digestive function and a lack of exercise, treating these symptomatically is potentially masking a problem and making it unclear what the real health needs are.

Having said that, a general anti-inflammatory strategy, while it is a very good basis for health, is unlikely by itself to deal effectively with all of the symptoms, and for the patient's comfort, peace of mind and confidence in coming for long enough for lasting improvement to take place, effective treatment of the more distressing symptoms should begin as soon as possible.

There is no clear cut-off point distinguishing initial from continuing treatment, but a rough guide would be that initial treatment is the first 1–2 months, followed by a transition over the following 2 months to the phase of treatment that is supportive and corrective of neuroendocrine health. That phase might last a few months or a year or more, depending on the previous history of health, after which a gentle withdrawal of herbal medicines to zero or to a minimal level of maintenance should follow.

It might be clear that a supportive rather than symptomatic outlook is important at the outset, however, for example when there are long-term problems that have just got worse in the perimenopause.

Diet and lifestyle

A happy medium is a good principle to follow when establishing a diet and exercise plan. Low body weight leads to greater reduction in bone density and vaginal dryness. Even before the perimenopause, being 15–20% below the ideal weight can cause oestrogen levels to fall below leading to an erratic cycle or absent menses with reduced fertility and bone density, and vaginal dryness. Over-exercising leads to decreased activity of 3 beta-dehydrogenase vital for the production of oestradiol in ovary, also leading to reduction of circulating oestrogens.

- Healthy exercising will help with metabolism, thyroid function, and bone density: ideally, a mixture of aerobic (for cardiovascular benefits) and strength exercise (for metabolism and bone density). Over exertion is potentially harmful to the joints and bones and it is important to build up gradually and keep a diary.
- Increase the intake of foods such as soya, flaxseed, legumes and nuts.
- Work on healthy bacterial flora to make phytoestrogens bioavailable:
  - Excess beta-glucuronidase is linked to an increased cancer risk, especially of oestrogen-linked cancer.
  - Probiotics and probiotic foods: lacto-ferments, root vegetables, beans and pulses will help to establish normal intestinal flora. Herbs that encourage healthy gut flora include garlic, *Berberis vulgaris*, *Artemisia absinthium*, slippery elm, and bitters in general.
  - Lots of vegetables and fruit not only for bowel health but to begin the process of nutritional support and for anti-inflammatory effects.
- Moderation: excess fibre leads to lower levels of oestrogen.
- Smoking causes endocrine disruption, pro-inflammatory biochemistry, increased FSH,[12] and an earlier menopause and increased incidence of osteoporosis.

Symptomatic herbal treatment: an overview of herbs

A 2017 review of herbal treatment of menopausal symptoms[13] showed that the following herbs were effective (in different ways) in the treatment of acute menopausal syndrome:

• *Cimicifuga racemosa*	• *Foeniculum vulgare*
• *Ginkgo biloba*	• *Glycine max*
• *Glycyrrhiza glabra*	• *Humulus lupulus*
• *Hypericum perforatum*	• *Medicago sativa*
• *Melissa officinalis*	• *Nigella sativa*
• *Oenothera biennis*	• *Panax ginseng*
• *Passiflora incarnata*	• *Pimpinella anisum*
• *Salvia officinalis*	• *Trifolium pratense*
• *Trigonella foenum-graecum*	• *Valeriana officinalis*
• *Vitex agnus-castus*	• *Zizyphus spinosa*

Quite a few of these herbs are useful for longer-term treatment, too, so there will be a bit of repetition between this section, initial intervention, and the next, of nutritional and herbal support in continuing treatment.

Treatment for specific symptoms

As mentioned, there are short-term and long-term strategies, but it is not a rigid distinction. For example, hot flushes and night sweats are likely to benefit from early treatment but may then clear up once dietary measures have their full effect, so herbal treatment would tend to be early. Depression and lack of energy obviously need both initial and persistent support, progressing from compensation and relief to support and tonifying and so are more long-term in scope.

The categorization is more important to the general strategy rather than to individual herbs. A rule of thumb applied to this plan is whether the strategy is still significantly helpful beyond 3 months.

Early on, it is important to establish confidence in treatment but make clear that it is groundwork and symptomatic intervention will be likely to lead to habituation if continued and will need adjustment, and it is important to realise that therapy will take time.

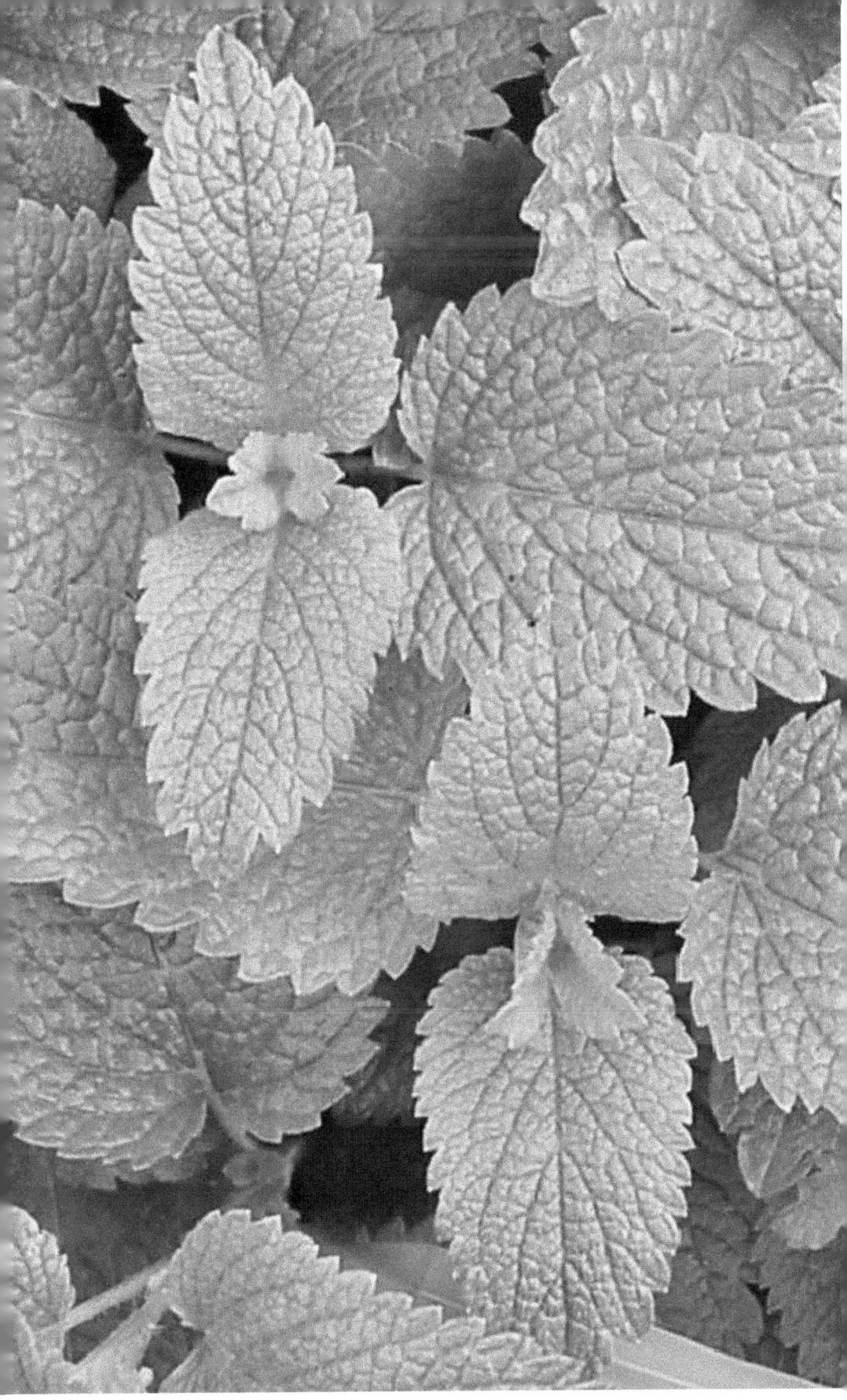

Hot flushes and night sweats

Salvia officinalis *and* Medicago sativa *(alfalfa)*

Of 30 menopausal women, hot flushes and night sweating disappeared in 20, four showed good improvement and the other six some reduction in symptoms. There was a significant increase in prolactin and TSH (thyroid stimulating hormone) response to TRH and the mixture was thought to have to have a slight antidopaminergic action.[14]

Foeniculum vulgare

A trial examining the effect of on menopausal symptoms in postmenopausal women showed a significant decrease in the mean Menopause Rating Scale scores after 4, 8, and 10 weeks.[15]

Humulus lupulus

Hops extract standardised to 100 or 250μg 8-PN (8-prenylnaringenin, the most potent oestrogenic constituent) showed significant effects on hot flushes after 6 weeks at the lower dose, but no effect was observed at higher doses. The lower dose was not significantly better than placebo after 12 weeks,[16] suggesting the possibility of habituation, and though it is hard to generalise, perhaps indicates it is useful as an initial intervention rather than a continued one. In a smaller study, Humulus extract showed weak efficacy over placebo when taken after placebo treatment until week 16;[17] another trial showed a general reduction in menopausal symptoms and a dramatic reduction in hot flushes.[18]

Trifolium pratense

A standardised extract of red clover isoflavones (Promensil) at 80mg/day was shown to be effective for treating hot flushes in menopausal women in a meta-analysis,[19] though this has not been a universal finding.

Glycine max *(Soy)*

There have been mixed results in trials with soy products in relation to hot flushes, perhaps due to differences in gut flora. Most clinical trials used products containing 50–100mg/day of isoflavones.[20]

Linum usitatissimum

Clinical trials have shown some beneficial effects on vasomotor symptoms.[21]

Valeriana officinalis

Exhibits serotonergic activity: valerenic acid has been identified as a potential partial agonist of the 5-HT5A receptor.[22] A clinical trial using 255mg valerian capsules three times daily showed a reduction in hot flush frequency and intensity.[23] A clinical trial with 60 postmenopausal women aged 45–55 years showed efficacy in the treatment of menopausal hot flushes.[24]

Cimicifuga racemosa

(See the chapter on Cimicifuga as it is not directly oestrogenic, and possibly also has an effect via serotonergic pathways).

A meta-analysis of clinical trials concluded that of the six trials that demonstrated a significant improvement, observed reduction of hot flashes in women, while other clinical trials have reported no significant difference from placebo for relief of hot flushes.[25] The bottom line with Cimicifuga is that low doses work as well as higher ones, but the effect on hot flushes is probably mild and that indicates a need to prescribe it along with other herbs, hardly a new idea to herbalists!

Astragalus membranaceus *and* Angelica sinensis *(Dang Gui Buxue Tang)*

A 1:5 combination of *Angelica sinensis, Astragalus membranaceus* (Dang Gui Buxue Tang/DBT) prescribed for acute menopausal symptoms proved superior to placebo in the treatment of mild hot flushes, but had no effect on moderate to severe hot flushes.[26] A multiple-dose escalation trial was performed in 60 postmenopausal women experiencing severe hot flushes and night sweats. The highest dose preparations at 6.0g/day significantly improved physical and psychological scores and significantly reduced vasomotor symptoms without affecting hormones or lipid profiles.[27]

Glycyrrhiza glabra

There have been very few clinical studies evaluating liquorice for the treatment of menopausal symptoms. One trial, with 90 women receiving liquorice (species not stated), showed a reduction in hot flushes. A clinical study comparing HRT with liquorice (1,140mg/day) to evaluate the effects of liquorice on hot flush symptoms in menopausal women found that liquorice was more effective than HRT in improving hot flush duration.[28] Another trial looked at *Glycyrrhiza glabra* in conjunction with an exercise programme and found improvement in terms of vasomotor, psychosocial, physical, and sexual health and quality of life with use of *Glycyrrhiza glabra* and exercise programmes in controlling the symptoms of menopause.[29]

Pimpinella anisum

In a clinical trial, 330mg three times a day was effective for frequency and severity of hot flushes in postmenopausal women.[30]

Trigonella foenum-graecum

Small group of postmenopausal women; 6g fenugreek seed powder decrease number of hot flashes and vasomotor symptoms, but the effect was smaller than that of HRT.[31]

Vitex agnus-castus

In postmenopausal women with hot flushes, shown to be effective treatment for the early vasomotor symptoms of postmenopausal women.[32]

Panax ginseng

Some clinical studies have indicated that it may be moderately effective in relieving postmenopausal symptoms while in others flushes, night sweats, nervous tension, headaches and palpitations dropped very quickly during treatment, with improvements in depression, insomnia and sexual problems, a sense of wellbeing, increased energy, and a positive effect on mood and anxiety.[33] It is thought that beneficial effects of ginseng on night sweats, hot flushes, energy and mood in the menopause are not mediated by hormone replacement-like effects, as physiological parameters such as FSH and oestradiol levels, endometrial thickness, maturity index and vaginal pH were not affected by the treatment.

The benefits of ginseng might be due to a short-term general stimulant effect, so that the herb is best used to bridge a gap rather than as a restorative.

Zizyphus spinosa

(Commonly used for abnormal sweating)

Night sweats, especially when accompanied by anxiety, irritability, palpitation, and insomnia. Actions are antihydrotic, hypnotic, sedative, hypotensive.

Vaginal dryness and vulvar atrophy

There is clinical evidence of the benefit of phytoestrogen-rich diet (phenolic phytoestrogens),[34] and the use of *Cimicifuga racemosa*, and fennel (5%) vaginal cream, application 5g per day, on vaginal atrophy in postmenopausal women. With fennel, the number of superficial cells increased, the number of intermediate and parabasal cells decreased and the vaginal pH decreased.[35]

Other useful measures include:

- Vitamin E in aloe gel
- Calendula pessaries
- Herbs containing steroidal saponins (*Dioscorea villosa, Asparagus racemosus, Tribulus terrestris, Chamaelirium luteum*)
- Omega 3 supplements
- Pelvic floor exercises[36]

Thrush and vaginal infections (bacterial vaginosis)

Decreased oestrogen secretion leads to thinning of vaginal walls, changes in blood composition and an imbalance in vaginal microflora with depletion of lactobacilli. This can lead to increased vaginal colonization by *Gardnerella vaginalis* and *Candida albicans*. The susceptibility should change as treatment progresses, but active symptomatic treatment is very welcome from the start. Probiotics positively alter the vaginal microflora and prevent vaginal infections.[37] Clinical trials of probiotic supplementation using vaginal *Lactobacillus rhamnosus* BMX54 indicate that it hinders bacterial growth especially after antibiotic therapy and is therefore strongly indicated as prophylactic treatment, in particular in high-risk patients.[38] In candida vaginal infection, clinical trials using probiotic capsules (*L. rhamnosus* GR-1 and *L. reuteri* RC-14) taken orally by postmenopausal women restored the normal vaginal flora.[39]

Herbal treatment

Clinical trials of herbal treatments have also shown good efficacy for *Calendula officinalis*,[40] thyme, Propolis, *Myrtus communis*, and garlic vaginal cream, which was as effective as clotrimazole cream.[41] Other preparations used in clinical practice include pessaries of tea tree EO, Thymus linalool EO, Lavandula EO and a wash made with Propolis, *Commiphora molmol* and Calendula 90%, diluted with water.

A general strategy can include the following:

- Restore mucous membranes and pH with *Cimicifuga racemosa, Hydrastis canadensis* (internal use)
- Immune support (*Echinacea angustifolia, E. purpurea*)
- Increase pelvic circulation: uterine tonics/emmenagogues (*Achillea millefolium Angelica sinensis, Artemisia vulga*ris)
- Diet: rich in vegetables, and fruit, low on sugar, and including lacto-fermented foods e.g. sauerkraut

Recurrent urinary tract infections

These are often caused by residual urine retention after voiding, changes in vaginal and bladder tone, pH and microflora, loss of lactobacilli and increased colonization by *E. coli*. Studies indicate that those with recurrent UTI have preponderance of uropathogens on the introitus and in vagina.

Vaccinium macrocarpon, cranberry: clinical trials suggest that cranberry is more effective at preventing rather than treating UTIs: the mechanism is generally thought to involve inhibition by some of the proanthocyanidins in cranberry juice of adhesion of *E. coli* that firmly attach to uroepithelial cells. Intake of fermented milk products and fresh berry juices has also been linked with decreased risk of recurring UTI. Lactobacilli producing hydrogen peroxide have been found in a healthy bladder, keeping the bladder in its preferred acidic state, and inhibiting pathogenic bacteria from adhering to vaginal and uterine wall, so it looks as though the mode of action is similar to that of cranberries, which is good to know, as not everyone likes to drink cranberry juice every morning.

Arctostaphylos uva-ursi (bearberry): The antimicrobial compound could be arbutin, which is hydrolysed in the gut to produce glucose and hydroquinone that can be further oxidised to para-quinone. Alkaline urine is required for this to work, so bicarbonate of soda is recommended alongside this.

Hormonal herbs: *Cimicifuga racemosa* (influences pH, bladder tone, and mucosa), *Chamaelirium luteum* (tonic for the pelvic area).

Toning the bladder: *Equisetum arvense*

Preventing bacteria adhering to the bladder: *Glycyrrhiza glabra*, Cranberry

Antibacterial, antiseptic: *Hydrastis canadensis, Arctostaphylus uva-ursi, Thymus vulgaris*

Demulcent: *Agropyron repens, Zea mays, Althea officinalis* radix.

Immune support: *Echinacea* spp., *Astragalus membranaceus, Baptisia tinctoria,*

Diet: sugar free, lots of vegetables to make the urine alkaline. A systematic review and metanalysis found that probiotic strains of Lactobacillus are effective in preventing recurrent urinary tract infections in adult women.[42]

Insomnia

Postmenopausal women taking HRT have been shown to have significantly improved sleep quality and reduced night-time restlessness and waking, and still better for combined progesterone with oestrogen, but not just progesterone. Night-time hypoglycaemia can cause a drop in glucose levels causes release of chemicals that stimulate the brain so eating complex carbohydrates with protein can help to maintain sleep. Sleep apnoea needs to be considered.

Important herbs for insomnia in the menopause

Valeriana officinalis (when anxiety plays a role).
- *Valeriana officinalis* and *Melissa officinalis*: a trial (160mg/day valerian) led to a reduction in sleep disorders.[43]
- *Hypericum perforatum (mood can have negative effect on sleeping)*. See below, *Continuing treatment.*

- *Vitex agnus-castus* (at night as it increases melatonin).[44] Melatonin has been shown to synchronise the circadian rhythms, and improve the onset, duration and quality of sleep,[45] and is effective in patients with long-term insomnia who are withdrawing from benzodiazepines.

Other herbs used for insomnia in clinical practice

Many other herbs address both the nervous and endocrine picture

- *Humulus lupulus* (oestrogenic effects)
- *Salvia officinalis*
- *Lactuca virosa*
- *Cimicifuga racemosa*
- *Panax ginseng* (sometimes people are too tired to sleep well).

Uterine prolapse

- Pelvic floor exercises
- Uterine tonics: traditional evidence.
  - *Angelica sinensis*
  - *Leonurus cardiaca*
  - *Capsella bursa-pastoris*
  - *Chamaelirium luteum*
- *Astragalus membranaceus*
- *Panax ginseng*

Phase 2: continuing treatment, physiological support for transition

Once symptoms are under control and an action plan has started to take effect, it is possible to start working with the terrain, so to speak. That means compensating for dysbalance, tonifying organs that have been under stress and restoring function within a new hormonal and nervous pattern.

HRT withdrawal and herbal support

As discussed, HRT is not a good answer for any length of time. Withdrawal is best worked out with the help of their GP, the reduction being gradual enough to minimise rebound effects.

Usually it is best to start herbal treatment before reducing HRT. After 4 weeks of being on both, the herbs and HRT, reduce the HRT dosage. Once the symptoms are under control lower HRT dosage again: this process can take 3–6 months.

Nutrition

A month or two into treatment is obviously a good point to review the dietary measures agreed: are they easy to stick to, do they seem to help? It takes a few weeks for gut flora to adjust, and this may need to be explained.

The most important general point about the diet at this point is that it deals effectively with free radicals, or as they are more accurately now categorised, reactive oxygen species (ROS). This is particularly important because of the raised risk of some cancers and because of the shift to low-density lipoproteins in the blood and the tendency to insulin resistance. Recalling that female and male physiology begin to resemble each other more in the menopause, this may be something of benefit to couples, too. The critical factor in the ageing process is not a healthy or a misspent youth, generally, but the lifestyle adopted from 50 onwards. Both exercise and diet help the cells regenerate for longer, something that can be observed in terms of telomere length, a marker of biological ageing. Shorter telomeres are linked with a higher risk of degenerative disease and higher mortality rate.

A 2009 US study found epidemiological evidence that multivitamin use is associated with longer telomere length among women.[46] Multivitamin supplements represent a major source of micronutrients, which may affect telomere length by modulating oxidative stress and chronic inflammation. In the analysis of micronutrients, higher intakes of vitamins C and E from foods were each associated with longer telomeres, even after adjustment for multivitamin use.

Resveratrol

Resveratrol, a polyphenol found in grapes and red wine, blueberries, cranberries, and even dark chocolate, is extremely helpful as a long-term component of the diet at this time of life. It is not just a powerful antioxidant and anti-inflammatory, but also regarded as a phytoestrogen. In experimental studies, as well as improving cognitive function in Alzheimer's disease, (being neuroprotective and reducing formation of sclerotic plaques) it has been shown to bind and activate oestrogen receptors and inhibiting the initiation and growth of tumours,

- An epidemiological study prospectively assessed the association between alcohol consumption and the onset of perimenopause. There was a suggestion that moderate amounts of red wine caused delaying of the menopause. This is more apparent in women who have never smoked. No similar association was found for beer and white wine.[47,48]
- Epidemiological evidence also suggests that traditional a Mediterranean diet, high in polyphenols derived from vegetables and red wine, is of benefit to health and reduces the incidence of cardiovascular disease and likely to benefit menopausal women.[49]

Adrenal support

As the ovaries slow down at the menopause, the adrenal glands take over the role producing the hormones. The adrenals may well need support, particularly in times of stress, so that they are working within their comfort zone, so to speak. In TCM, which has no specific term for the adrenals, the functioning of adaptogens is generally expressed in terms of Kidney *Qi*, the organ most closely connected to the adrenals. The kidneys store *Jing*, the essence of *Qi* and govern the periodic transitions of life.

It is very important to respect the designation of Kidney Yin deficiency or Kidney Yang deficiency. Kidney Yang tonics are regarded as adaptogens but have stimulant properties. It is important to watch overstimulation, particularly with *Panax ginseng*, Eleutherococcus or other more stimulating tonics, which are best for relatively short-term use and only if there is no risk of overdoing things—too little sleep, overwork, too much exercise, for example. The idea is to rest the adrenals more while doing the normal round of activities.

Glycyrrhiza glabra

Liquorice is generally regarded in western herbalism as an anti-inflammatory and adrenal tonic. The triterpenoid saponin glycyrrhizin, which has little of the intrinsic activity intrinsic of gluco- or mineralocorticoids, alters the way these compounds are metabolised and is thought to prolong their clearance. The interaction with glucocorticoids may support the adrenal cortex during prolonged stress.

Glycyrrhizin does bind to mineralocorticoid receptors, though, leading to the well-known side effects of hypertension and hypokalaemia—adverse effects unlikely at normal therapeutic dosages.

Eleutherococcus senticosus

Siberian ginseng is thought to normalise the hypothalamic-pituitary-adrenal function in times of shock or stress. Stress has a major impact on lowering oestrogen levels, therefore exacerbating menopausal symptoms. Eleutherococcus speeds recovery after operations and both animal and human studies support the theory that the effects of Siberian ginseng are due to the adrenal cortex responding more sensitively and effectively. During acute stress, more hormones are released; when stress stops, the adrenal glands switch off more quickly, so when stress is prolonged, the glands conserve their resources and do not release too much hormone.

Clinical studies

- In elderly hypertensive patients and volunteers taking digoxin, no significant difference in blood pressure control or digitalaemia was observed. It was stated that *E. senticosus* safely improves some aspects of mental health and social functioning after 4 weeks of therapy, although these differences diminish with continued use.[50]
- An old review focused on over 35 clinical trials on *Eleutherococcus senticosus* in healthy human subjects (ca. 6,000 subjects aged from 19 to 72), observed that there was an improvement of the physical and mental work capacities in all cases.[51]

Panax ginseng

Historically, the classic Chinese tonic for invigoration and fortification in times of fatigue, debility, declining capacity for work, and concentration, used for longevity, to improve general health, appetite, and restore memory. It is indicated for tonification of the vital energy, calming nerves, chronic general weakness with irritability, insomnia, and organ prolapse. Studies on patients with fatigue have shown improvements in fatigue, nervousness, anxiety, and poor concentration,[52] and in nurses' consumption of ginseng improved scores in job competencies, mood, and mental and physical performance.[53]

Astragalus membranaceus

Astragalus is a powerful immunostimulating tonic, with adaptogenic, cardiotonic, diuretic, hypotensive, antioxidant properties. It has often been used in conditions leading to immune suppression such as chemotherapy, radiotherapy, and surgery. In Chinese medicine, it is a Qi and blood tonic, used for organ prolapse and uterine bleeding. In the menopause, it is helpful for general debility, and particularly excessive, spontaneous sweating, and it may also be used in chronic fatigue syndrome, as a tonic for elderly, palpitations, but as with *Panax ginseng* and Eleutherococcus, it is important to be watchful for overstimulation—nervous excitability in particular.

Withania somnifera

Ashwagandha has a very distinctive reputation in Ayurvedic medicine for general debility, nervous exhaustion, loss of muscle strength, and brain fog, especially due to stress.[54]

Mood, hormones, and nervous function in menopausal women

Liquorice

- Glabridin has also been shown to inhibit serotonin reuptake (an action shared with oestradiol). The inhibition of serotonin reuptake was dose-dependent and suggests that liquorice may be useful for mild to moderate depression in peri- and postmenopausal women.[55]
- Liquorice and *Paeonia lactiflora* lower the LH/FSH ratio and reduce ovarian testosterone production, inducing regular ovulation in those with PCOS and increase aromatase activity, thus increasing conversion of androgen to oestrogen. In premenopausal women this increases progesterone levels. Perimenopausally, PMS symptoms are generally worse, but by making the corpus luteum more fully

functioning, the Paeonia and Glycyrrhiza combination can improve these symptoms.

Hypericum perforatum

- In trials, St John's wort has been shown to help with mild to moderate depression, leading to a significant improvement after 3 months of treatment along with amelioration of menopause-specific quality of life and significantly fewer sleep problems.[56]
- *Panax ginseng*:[57] Menopausal women reported improvements in mood and anxiety.

Cimicifuga racemosa

Perhaps the archetypal herb for the main symptoms of the menopause; significantly reduced depression and anxiety in all studies reviewed.[58]

Clinical trials using Hypericum and Cimicifuga combination

A prospective, controlled open-label observational study of 6,141 women at 1,287 outpatient gynaecologists in Germany used St John's

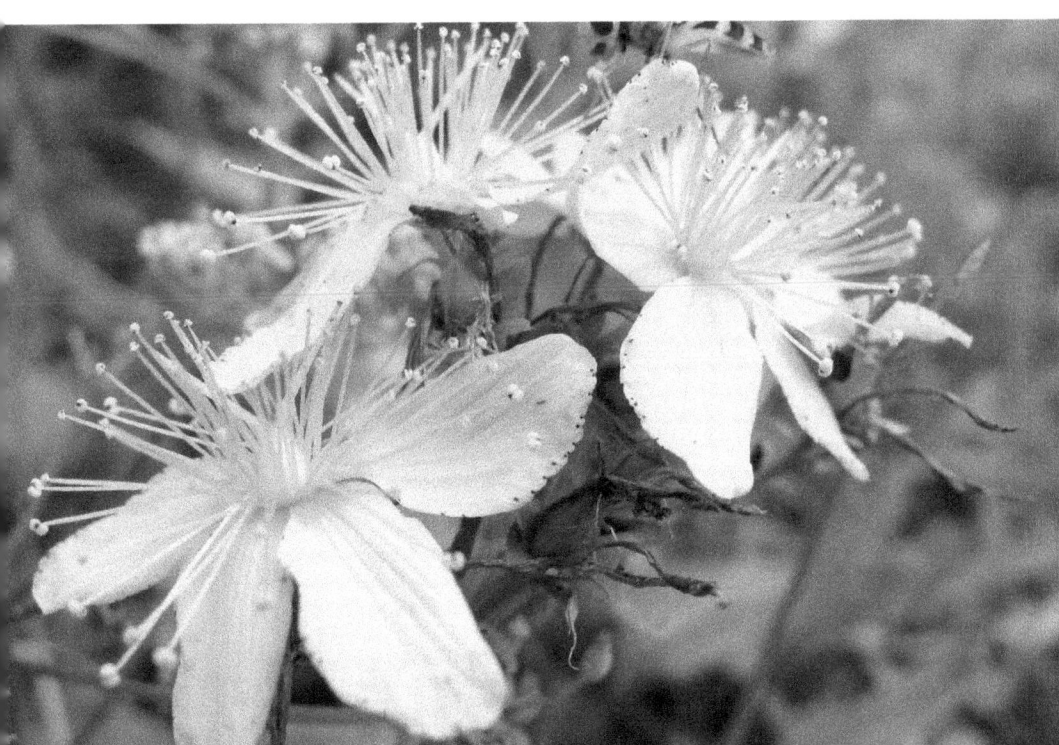

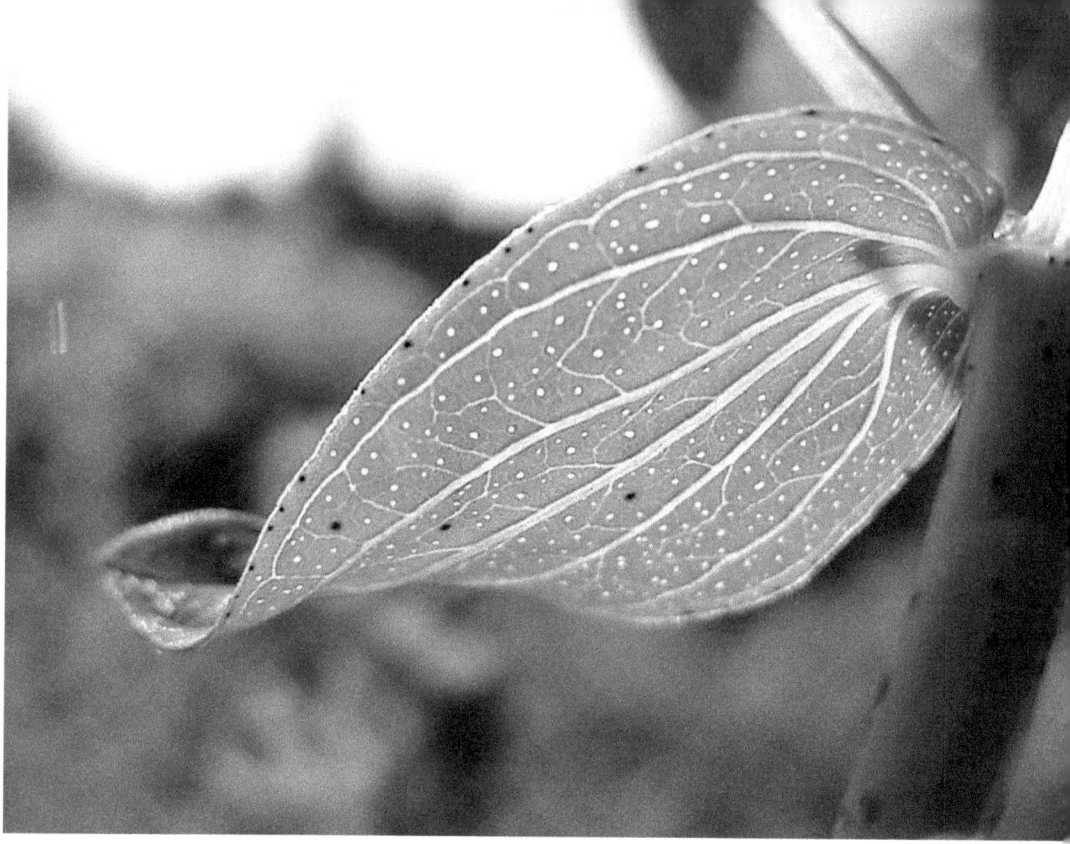

wort for neurovegetative symptoms, or a combination of Hypericum and Cimicifuga for patients with more pronounced mood complaints. The treatment was chosen by the participating physicians. The combination of black cohosh and St. John's wort was superior to black cohosh alone in alleviating climacteric mood symptoms.[59,60]

In a systematic review on *Cimicifuga racemosa*, *Hypericum perforatum*, *Vitex agnus-castus*, vitamins, and minerals, either singly or combined, for vasomotor, genital and psychological menopausal complaints found that single herbs were no better than placebo. However, the combination of *Cimicifuga racemosa* and *Hypericum perforatum* demonstrated a positive effect on climacteric complaints.[61] That is not only interesting as a detail: herbalists rarely use single herbs, and prize a well formulated prescription as conveying a combined effect that goes beyond the sum of its parts.

Vitex agnus-castus *(chaste tree/berry)*

Traditionally, Vitex has not been used in menopause-related complaints, and this use is relatively recent, so evidence from clinical trials is lacking in this context. But there is emerging pharmacological evidence for a role for alleviating menopausal symptoms, as it is effective for irregular bleeding and PMS symptoms (which tend to increase during the perimenopausal period).[62] Many medical herbalists will use *Vitex agnus-castus* in high doses when there is heavy, unopposed bleeding, and found to be very successful for this.

Diterpenes in Vitex, which are highly lipophilic, easily pass the blood-brain barrier and have dopaminergic activity in the brain and thus, like dopamine, inhibit prolactin secretion from the anterior pituitary gland. Supraphysiological release of prolactin due to stress will decrease progesterone and oestradiol secretion in the luteal phase and may hasten the onset of the menopause. The effects of Vitex on brain dopaminergic systems may also modulate locomotor unrest and behaviour instability and so be of use in restless leg syndrome.

Vitex and melatonin release

The pineal gland, through melatonin, is involved in the mechanisms that regulate the ageing process involved in the onset of menopause. It has been shown that melatonin administration was able to delay the endocrine changes that occur during the course of menopause.[63] Vitex given during the day caused a dose-dependent increase in melatonin secretion especially during the night (compared to placebo treatment, 60% higher, beginning 1 hour after the lights had turned off).[64] Together with its effect on luteal insufficiency this suggests that Vitex is a generally useful herb in the perimenopausal phase.

Hypericum perforatum *with* Vitex agnus-castus

In a trial of this combination (1g Vitex, and 5.4g Hypericum daily) in late-perimenopausal and postmenopausal women, no difference in hot flushes and other menopausal symptoms was found. However, data on PMS-like symptoms was collected from a small subgroup of late-perimenopausal women, and here this combination of herbs showed itself to be helpful in PMS-like symptoms among perimenopausal women.[65] There are no clinical trials with *Vitex agnus-castus* alone for the relief of menopausal symptoms, but studies of combinations of botanicals including chasteberry are promising.[66]

Other herbs of benefit in nervous and hormonal support in the menopause

- *Melissa officinalis*
- *Rosa damascena*
- *Verbena officinalis*
- *Avena sativa*

Reduced sexual desire

This tends to be worse with an ovariectomy as there is then even less testosterone around.

Turnera diffusa

Damiana has a long history of use by indigenous people in Mexico as general stimulant, and for muscular and nervous debility.

Constituents include β-sitosterol, an essential oil containing alpha-pinene, p-cymene, 1,8-cineol, tannins, resins, arbutin, and apigenin. Arbutin is a glycoside: a glycosylated hydroquinone extracted from the bearberry, *Arctostaphylos uva-ursi* and an important urinary antiseptic. β-sitosterol, also found in saw palmetto, has been studied for its potential to reduce benign prostatic hyperplasia.[67]

Apigenin is thought to be responsible for sedative and antinociceptive (reducing sensitivity to pain) properties.[68]

In vitro research seems to suggest that it has anti-progestogenic activity and inhibits aromatase,[69] and thus may increase tissue levels of testosterone by reducing its conversion to oestrogen.

Actions and indications in relation to reduced sexual desire

- Nervine tonic, with application to lowered libido. Antidepressant, digestive tonic, nervous dyspepsia, anxiety neurosis.
- Sexual anxiety, impotence with frigidity. Depression with physical weakness.
- *In vivo* it is found to be an anxiolytic and an aphrodisiac.[70]

ArginMax®

ArginMax® contains extracts of ginseng, Ginkgo, and damiana, L-arginine, multivitamins, and minerals. In a double-blind placebo-controlled study in women who reported a lack of sexual desire there were improvements in sexual desire, reduction of vaginal dryness, frequency of sexual intercourse and orgasm, and clitoral sensation.

The largest number of improvements was seen in premenopausal and perimenopausal women, but the level of desire was shown to increase significantly in postmenopausal women.[71] Another trial found that ArginMax® had no significant impact on sexual functioning, but patient quality of life was significantly better at 12 weeks.[72]

Other herbs

- *Panax ginseng*: Improved scores on the Female Sexual Function Index (FSFI) as improvements were shown for frequency, level and satisfaction of arousal. However, it did not have a significant effect on desire, lubrication, orgasm, global satisfaction or pain.[73]
- *Asparagus racemosus*: is prescribed as a general female tonic in Ayurvedic medicine but particularly as an aphrodisiac, 'to give the capacity to have a hundred husbands' being one translation of its name from Sanskrit.
- *Hypericum perforatum* (treating mood may have an important influence). St. John's wort in trials improved psychological and psychosomatic symptoms, as well as a feeling of sexual wellbeing.[74]
- *Foeniculum vulgare* vaginal cream has been shown to improve sexual function in postmenopausal women.[75]

Cardiovascular disease and insulin resistance

Multiple reasons for increased incidence oestrogen maintain higher HDL levels, and protecting the cardiovascular systems, and keeps LDL levels low, and slows the ageing of the arteries. HRT was supposed to reduce cardiovascular disease.

Crataegus laevigata

Cardioprotective

- Cholesterol lowering (although controversial, but nevertheless some herbs shown to have effect here)
    - *Curcuma longa, Cynara scolymus, Allium sativum, Trigonella foenum-graecum, Dioscorea villosa, Cimicifuga racemosa*, soy, and flaxseed
    - *Eleutherococcus senticosus*

Nigella sativa

A small study on menopausal women found that treatment will exert a protective effect by improving lipid profile and blood glucose in menopausal women. As an improvement was observed in total cholesterol (TC), triglycerides (TG), low-density lipoprotein cholesterol (LDL-C), high density lipoprotein cholesterol (HDL-C), and blood glucose.[76]

Panax ginseng

- Positive effect on lipid metabolism: total cholesterol and low-density lipoprotein cholesterol significantly decreased, and there was also a significant decrease in carotid intima-media thickness.[77]

Siberian ginseng

- In patients with Type 2 diabetes (oral medication 80%, insulin therapy 20%), Siberian ginseng intake resulted in a highly significant decline of fasting blood sugar and postprandial blood sugar level, and significantly lowered HbA1c, total cholesterol and triglyceride levels; it also reduced symptoms of peripheral polyneuropathy. It has been suggested that additional intake is able to fine-tune the pathological glucose metabolism, as well as reducing symptoms of peripheral polyneuropathy.[78]
- In addition, over 35 studies have focused on the effect of *Eleutherococcus senticosus* on more than 2,200 sick patients. The studies included patients with atherosclerosis, acute pyelonephritis, diabetes, hypertension, trauma, neuroses, rheumatic heart disease, chronic bronchitis, insomnia, cancer, and several other ailments. In most cases, a moderate improvement relative to the initial conditions was observed. Another clinical trial has shown beneficial effects of Eleutherococcus against oxidative stress and improved serum lipid profiles in postmenopausal women.[79]

Osteoporosis

A consequence of low oestrogen levels at menopause is an increase in osteoporosis risk.

- Isoflavones: most isoflavones are ERβ-selective ligands. Genistein has been shown to stimulate bone formation, inhibit bone resorption, and prevent bone loss in ovariectomised rat models.[80] Randomised, double-blind placebo-controlled studies have shown that genistein (54mg/day for 1 or 2 years) is effective in preventing bone loss in postmenopausal women.[81,82] Favourable effects have been demonstrated in other clinical studies. The data suggest that diets rich in isoflavones are beneficial for bone health in the long-term.
- Different studies have also analysed red clover products for prevention of osteoporosis. A patented aqueous and fermented red clover extract standardised to 37.1mg isoflavones per day it has to be noted that the actual changes were small and that the differences could also be due to the variability in bone density scanning. Studies with bisphosphonate therapy showed that reliable treatment effects can be best observed after 3 years.
- A clinical study in Korean postmenopausal women showed a significant increase in serum osteocalcin levels, suggesting improved bone remodelling, in women taking *Eleutherococcus senticosus*.[83]
- A small trial using 3.5g liquorice increased parathyroid hormone and urinary calcium levels from baseline, consistent with an oestrogen-like effect. The researchers concluded that the effect of liquorice on calcium metabolism is probably influenced by several components of the root.[84,85]
- *Astragalus membranaceus: In vivo* and *in vitro* experiments (osteoclasts were induced through a calcium-deficient diet and inhibition effects were measured) indicate that the herb may have an effect on bone metabolism.
- Sage, *Humulus lupulus, Astragalus membranaceus, Cimicifuga racemosa*, soy, *Trifolium pratense* all promising effect in osteoporosis.

Ready list of herbs for different aspects of menopause treatment

- **Hormonal:** Soy, *Trifolium pratense, Linum usitatissimum, Dioscorea villosa, Trillium erectum, Humulus lupulus, Salvia officinalis, Glycyrrhiza glabra, Vitex agnus-castus, Peaonia lactiflora* plus *Glycyrrhiza glabra, Asparagus racemosus, Cimicifuga racemosa*
- **Adrenal support:** such as the adaptogens, e.g. *Panax ginseng*, or *Eleutherococcus senticosus, Cimicifuga racemosa, Astragalus membranaceus, Salvia officinalis*

- **Sweating:** Salvia officinalis, Astragalus membranaceus, Panax ginseng, Eleutherococcus senticosus
- **Nervine:** Hypericum perforatum, Verbena officinalis (cooling), Avena sativa, Leonurus cardiaca, Melissa officinalis
- **Circulatory herbs:** Angelica sinensis (not, by the way, an oestrogenic herb), Ginkgo biloba, Achillea millefolium
- **Digestive, assimilation, gut flora:** Verbena officinalis, Berberis vulgaris, Taraxacum officinale radix, Artemisia absinthium (bitters are cooling)
- **Elimination:** Taraxacum officinale radix, Carduus marianus, Schisandra chinensis
- **Cholesterol lowering:** Curcuma longa, Cynara scolymus, Allium sativum, Trigonella foenum-graecum
- **Cardioprotective:** Crataegus laevigata
- **Maintaining bone density:** Soy, Humulus lupulus, Salvia officinalis, Cimicifuga racemosa, Panax ginseng, Equisetum arvense, Astragalus membranaceus, Trifolium pratense, Camellia sinensis
- **Protecting and moistening mucous membranes:** Cimicifuga racemosa, Chamaelirium luteum, Althea officinalis folia, Zea mays, Plantago lanceolata, Glycyrrhiza glabra, Asparagus racemosus

Patient-friendly summary

1. The perimenopause generally begins at somewhere between 41 and 51 years of age, and the menopause proper marks the end of the menstrual cycle.
2. The perimenopause is a time of big fluctuations in hormone levels and symptoms such as low mood, insomnia, worsening of PMS and irregular menstruation.
3. Oestrogens necessary for many tissue functions are then produced in the tissues by conversion of androgens such as testosterone, a process called aromatization.
4. It is a time of transition to a physiological state with similarities to before the menarche, and to male physiology, too.

5. It has come to symbolise a loss of something rather than a transformation, but it can be a time of new possibilities instead.
6. Some protective effects of oestrogen are reduced, for example on blood sugar, cholesterol, inflammation and cardiovascular disease, and it is important to adjust lifestyle and diet to take this into account.
7. Phyto-oestrogenic herbs can help to compensate for the effects of oestrogen depletion, by lessening some of the psychological and physical challenge.
8. The health of the gut flora is vital to making phytoestrogens bioavailable.
9. A healthy diet will provide many of the substances that are needed for bowel health and better hormonal and immune system balance during and after the menopause.
10. Foods such as soya, flaxseed, legumes and nuts will help hormonal balance and the health of the microbiome.
11. Initial treatment is aimed at improving symptoms, digestive system health, and inflammatory tendencies.
12. As treatment progresses, the aim is to establish through nutrition, lifestyle and tonifying herbs a balanced hormonal functioning that will persist once active treatment has finished, or will require minimal long-term support.
13. Healthy exercising will help with metabolism, thyroid function, and bone density.
14. Dealing with stress is important for the proper functioning of the adrenal glands, which have a vital function in supporting hormonal and immune function after the menopause, and also for the health of the nervous system.

Table 7.1: Overview of treatment options for menopausal problems

Diet	Lifestyle	Elimination	Assimilation
Promote healthy weight: for healthy bone density, and vaginal dryness. Avoid excess fibre as this leads to lower levels of oestrogen. Work on healthy bacterial flora to make phytoestrogens bioavailable. Lots of vegetables and fruit. Good sources of vitamins and minerals or a nutritional supplement. Probiotics to establish normal intestinal flora.	Ensure healthy exercising, as this will help with metabolism, thyroid function, and bone density. Avoid over-exercising as it leads to decreased activity of 3 beta-dehydrogenase vital for the production of oestradiol. No Smoking: it alters the metabolism so more inactive oestrogen is produced, and leads to earlier menopause and increased incidence of osteoporosis.	Important to support healthy functioning of hormones by eliminating excess oestrogens, and limiting re-entry of endogenous oestrogen in the blood stream. Constipation, if present, needs to be treated to ensure oestrogen metabolites are excreted efficiently. Often an apparent lack of progesterone is actually a relative excess of oestrogen: Gentle laxatives, such as *Taraxacum officinalis* radix, *Rumex crispus*, flaxseeds Lipotrophic factors such as choline in *Taraxacum officinalis* radix help with removal of fat and bile in the liver through interaction with fat metabolism, and have a decongesting effect on the liver. Liver involved with oestrogen clearance: use liver herbs, *Carduus marianus* as a restorative, herbs such as *Berberis vulgaris* or fumitory to stimulate. *Carduus marianus, Schisandra chinensis* in case of poor liver function or liver damage.	**Herbs to encourage healthy gut flora:** Garlic, *Verbena officinalis, Berberis vulgaris, Artemisia absinthium,* bitters in general. Slippery elm.

Hormonal	Nervous System	Circulation	Symptoms
Isoflavonoids: Soy, Trifolium, *Linum usitatissum*, *Humulus lupulus*, *Salvia officinalis*, *Glycyrrhiza glabra*, Steroidal saponins: *Tribulus terrestris Vitex agnus-castus*, Paeonia and *Glycyrrhiza*, *Dioscorea villosa*, *Asparagus racemosa* Triterpenoid saponins: *Cimicifuga racemosa* Adaptogens to bridge the transition to a low oestrogen environment: *Withania somnifera*, *Eleutherococcus senticosus*, *Astragalus membranaceus*: *Panax ginseng*, *Rhodiola rosea*, *Schisandra chinensis*, *Panax ginseng*, *Salvia officinalis*.	*Hypericum perforatum*, *Verbena officinalis* (cooling), *Avena sativa*, *Leonurus cardiaca*, *Melissa officinalis*, *Cimicifuga racemosa*, *Rosa damascena*, *Avena sativa*, *Withania somnifera*	*Ginkgo biloba*, *Achillea millefolium*, *Angelica sinensis*, (not oestrogenic), **Cholesterol-lowering**: *Curcuma longa*, *Cynara scolymus*, *Allium sativum*, *Trigonella foenum-graecum* **Cardioprotective**: *Crataegus* spp. Probably best to avoid the heating herbs such as Zingiber.	**Hot flushes**: *Salvia officinalis*, *Astragalus membranaceus*, *Panax ginseng*, *Zizyphus spinosa*, *Cimicifuga racemosa*, *Dioscorea villosa*, soy and flaxseed. **Sweating**: *Salvia officinalis*, *Astragalus membranaceus*, *Panax ginseng*, *Eleutherococcus senticosus*. **Vaginal dryness**: Vitamin E in Aloe gel, Calendula pessaries, *Cimicifuga racemosa*, Steroidal saponins (*Dioscorea villosa*, *Chamaelirium luteum*, *Trillium pendulum*), Phytoestrogen-rich diet, Omega 3 protects and moistens mucous membranes: *Cimicifuga racemosa*, *Chamaelerium luteum*, *Althea* fol., *Zea mays*, *Plantago lanceolata*, *Glycyrrhiza glabra*. **Thrush**: Pessaries: EO: Tea tree, *Thymus off.* CT linalool, *Lavandula off.* Wash: Propolis, *Commiphora molmol* and Calendula 90%. Restore mucous membranes and pH: *Cimicifuga rac.*, *Hydrastis canadensis*. Immune support increases pelvic circulation: uterine tonics/emmenagogues: *Achillea mill.*, *Angelica sinesis*, *Artemisia vulgaris*. Diet, acidophilus **Uterine prolapse**: Pelvic floor exercises and Uterine tonics: *Angelica sinensis*, *Leonurus cardiaca*, *Capsella bursa-pastoris*, *Chamaelirium luteum*, *Astragalus membranaceus*, *Panax ginseng* **Recurrent UTIs**: *Cimicifuga racemosa*, *Chamaelirium luteum*, *Equisetum arvense*, *Glycyrrhiza*, Cranberry, *Hydrastis canadensis*, demulcents plus herbs to support the immune system. Diet: Acidophilus **Reduced sexual desire**: *Panax ginseng*, *Asparagus racemosus* (aphrodisiac), *Rhodiola rosea*, *Hypericum perforatum*, *Turnera diffusa* **Insomnia**: *Humulus lupulus*, *Salvia officinalis*, *Lactuca virosa*, *Valeriana officinalis*, *Vitex agnus-castus*, *Hypericum perforatum*, *Cimicifuga racemosa* **Bone density**: Soy, Humulus, *Salvia off.*, *Cimicifuga rac.*, *Panax ginseng*, *Equisetum arvense*, *Astragalus mem.*, *Trifolium rep.*, *Camelia sinensis*.

CHAPTER EIGHT

PMS: common myths

Is PMS a problem of too much oestrogen or too much progesterone? This has been quite often a rule of thumb—is the first or the second half of the cycle longer? Luteal insufficiency is certainly one condition in which progesterone may be low, but this is the exception rather than the rule, and trying to pinpoint which hormone is 'at fault' is not actually a very practical place to start, as there is a lot more going on! It is perhaps better to look at it from the point of view of the nervous system (including the pituitary gland), immune system, ovaries and adrenals working in harmony through the month.

The menstrual cycle is a rhythm of nature and PMS indicates disruption to it. Physiological and biochemical changes are accompanied by shifts in mood, mental performance, and perspective each month in the natural order of things. There is some plausibility in the belief that the monthly cycle was originally tied to the waxing and waning of the moon, with ovulation occurring at the time of the full moon and menstruation beginning at the new moon, as melatonin release is light-dependent and varies during the cycle. There is also the reported phenomenon of women living in close proximity synchronizing their cycles but there is no real experimental support for this, nor is it necessarily a practical way to approach therapy, although if it provides an incentive for decreasing the time spent in front of LED screens or under artificial light, and for spending more quality time with other women, that could be very therapeutic indeed.

The fact that both theories are the subject of great uncertainty shows that even with so universal a feature of women's lives, much is unknown. Perhaps that lack of certainty points towards the importance of the cycle as an experience whose significance needs to be respected for itself and not 'explained away'.

Science, medicine, and the meaning of the menstrual cycle

What is known, as we have seen, is that the sex steroid hormones easily pass blood-brain barrier, and high densities of oestrogen and progesterone receptors are present in brain regions that regulate emotions, drives and perceptions: the amygdala, the hippocampus, and the hypothalamus. Sex hormones also affect the expression of neurotransmitter receptors, and the activity, of serotonin, dopamine, GABA, and glutamate.[1] As the levels of hormones, particularly oestrogen, progesterone and allopregnanolone, vary through the month, differences in feelings and inclination at different times of the month are inevitable and generally coped with well.

Premenstrual syndrome (PMS), a common cyclic disorder of young and middle-aged women, refers to emotional and physical symptoms that cause severe dysfunction in social or occupational realms, and they consistently occur during the luteal phase of the menstrual cycle. Women with more severe affective symptoms are classified as having premenstrual dysphoric disorder (PMDD). Studies report that 12.2% of women have PMS symptoms that impacted their daily lives, made up of 4.1% of women with severe PMS (six symptoms) and 8.1% moderate PMS (one to five symptoms).[2]

Traditional explanations include a 'wandering womb' and 'looking for a baby', and hysteria (from the Greek ὑστέρα: hystera, uterus) clearly associated mental/emotional phenomena with the menstrual cycle, and not very sympathetically. Cultural norms and taboos may indicate fear (restraint from sexual intercourse associated with being 'unclean')—or respect, the withdrawal from society as a time for reflection. The terms 'syndrome' and 'disorder' may reflect the medicalization of our culture—something is out of balance but is it really a matter of re-establishing harmony or adapting? It may also be it is important to try to accommodate the lifestyle to the menstrual cycle, because when the everyday outlook and competences suddenly seem irrelevant or problematic, perhaps there is an element of letting in other types of seeing or responding.

Perhaps the middle line to take is to see the potential of changes of mood or perspective as potentially a gift, but one that somehow has to be lived with!

Diagnostic criteria and diagnosis of PMS and PMDD

Prospective daily monitoring of symptoms over at least two menstrual cycles is needed. A US Dept of Health tracker is free to use for this purpose (see Figure 8.1).

The American College of Obstetricians & Gynaecologists states that at least one of the symptoms below has to occur during the 5 days before menses, in three consecutive cycles, to definitely indicate PMS:

Somatic

- Headache
- Breast tenderness
- Abdominal bloating
- Swelling of extremities

Affective

- Depression
- Anxiety
- Irritability
- Confusion

Behavioural

- Social withdrawal
- Angry outbursts
- Identifiable dysfunction in social or economic performance

Pattern of presentation

- Symptoms relieved within 4 days of the onset of menses, no recurrence until at least cycle day 13

PMS Symptom Tracter

Cycle Dates: _____

Use this chart to track your PMS symptoms.

Symptoms	Day 1	2	3	4	5	6	7	8	9	10	11	12	13	14	15	16	17	18	19	20	21	22	23	24	25	26	27	28	29	30	31	32	33	34	35	36	37	38	39	40	41	42	43	44	45
Period																																													
Acne																																													
Breast swelling and tenderness																																													
Feeling tired																																													
Having trouble sleeping																																													
Upset stomach																																													
Cramps																																													
Bloating																																													
Constipation																																													
Diarrhea																																													
Headache																																													
Backache																																													
Appetite changes or food cravings																																													
Joint or muscle pain																																													
Trouble concentrating or remembering																																													
Tension, irritability, mood swings, or crying spells																																													
Anxiety																																													
Depression																																													
Other Symptoms:																																													
Other Symptoms:																																													
Other Symptoms:																																													

Figure 8.1: US Dept of Health PMS symptom tracker, a handy way to keep a clear record and a useful research tool.

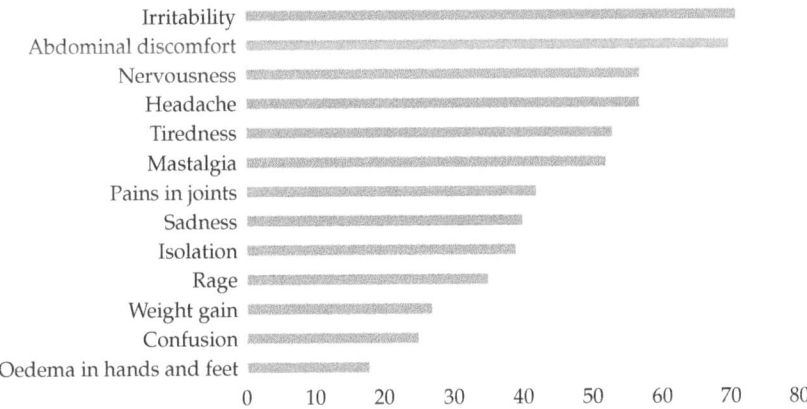

Figure 8.2: Prevalence and distribution of premenstrual symptoms (N=1,096). Pelotas, state of Rio Grande do Sul, Brazil, 2003.[3]

- Symptoms in absence of any pharmacologic therapy, hormone ingestion, or drug, or alcohol use
- Symptoms during two cycles of prospective recording.

Premenstrual dysphoric disorder (PMDD) severe cognitive and mood changes, more aggressive than seen in premenstrual syndrome (PMS).

Full symptom list

There are some 150 symptoms listed in total including:

Behavioural symptoms:
Fatigue, insomnia, dizziness, changes in sexual interest, food cravings, or overeating.

Psychological symptoms: (see Figure 8.2)
Irritability, anger, depressed mood, crying and tearfulness, anxiety, tension, mood swings, lack of concentration, confusion, forgetfulness, restlessness, loneliness, decreased self-esteem, tension.

Physical symptoms:
Headaches, breast tenderness and swelling, back pain, abdominal pain and bloating, weight gain, swelling of extremities, water retention, nausea, muscle and joint pain.

Risk factors

As the list of factors indicates, this is a multi-system, multi-level phenomenon, and causes are likewise multifactorial. What is often said of psychological or physiological dysbalances is that one predisposes to the other—it depends on perspective which is primary and which secondary. So it probably makes more sense to think in terms a whole picture containing interdependent factors.

Predisposing or contributory factors:

- Stress[4] and exogenous hormones are the most important
- Family history[5]
- Pressure of social expectation
- High body mass index[6]
- Past birth control use, alcohol use, drug use
- Traumatic events[7]
- Unhealthy or unbalanced eating habits such as fast food consumption, irregular breakfasts, and coffee and alcohol consumption[8]
- Metabolic syndrome[9]
- Times of changing hormones, i.e. menarche, pregnancy, postpartum, premenstrual, perimenopause
- Ovarian steroid fluctuation, irregular menstruation[10]
- CNS neurotransmitter levels

Particularly for PMDD:

- Prior anxiety states, traumatic events, physical threat, childhood abuse, serious accidents.
- Women with PMS have greater frequency of postpartum depression and PMS generally returns once cycles begin again.

Causes

The aetiology of PMS is poorly understood, and there are many proposed theories, reflecting the range of hormones and neurotransmitters involved in attention, alertness, and mood, and also that big range of presenting symptoms. There are almost several different causes, one of which may predominate but not exclusively, so a division into 'types' of PMS is probably going to be misleading. In any case, a holistic approach has at its centre the idea that the person needs to be perceived first, and so these subdivisions would in that context function only as indicators.

One difference in pattern is that while premenstrual symptoms tend to typically appear during the drop in progesterone concentrations in the late luteal phase, some have symptoms that start at ovulation and during the early luteal phase—i.e. before the fall in progesterone has started.[11]

The idea that the key cause is an abnormal relationship between oestrogen and progesterone now seems somewhat crude, and studies of women with or without PMS have failed to demonstrate consistent hormonal differences. However, hormones are certainly important, as bilateral oophorectomy or medical suppression of cycle stops premenstrual symptoms, and adding progesterone to hormonal contraceptives or hormone therapy (HT) leads to negative mood.[12]

The major theories involve:

- Sensitivity to the change in progesterone levels during the luteal phase, particularly as this affects GABA receptors in the brain.
- The effect of falling oestrogen concentration on serotonin levels before menstruation.
- Low dopamine/high prolactin levels in the luteal phase.
- Stress-related disturbance of endogenous opioid production.

The more these are researched, the more interdependence emerges. Trying to find a single, definite cause even for one patient is likely to be chasing the wind. There is not only the complexity of PNEI (psycho-neuro-endocrino-immunology) to take into account but also the central problem of neuropsychiatry: if our brains were simple enough for us to understand, we would be too simple to study them is one way to say it, but even that does not quite express the problem of the hand drawing itself, so to speak.

There is also the fact that we are trying to understand things of one kind using evidence of another kind—do we know actually what we are looking for? The psyche, the spirit, are not about systems or even their interactions—what we experience is what we experience, and it cannot be mapped to pharmacology experiments. It is not that these are irrelevant, just that they belong to a physicalist model, not to mention their technical limitations and the fact that the more research is done, the more complexity and the more unknowns are revealed.

In herbal medicine, traditional indications often helpfully refer to effects on the humours or spirits. Herbalists work within the pattern that presents itself. What is generally helpful for hormonal and neurological balance will always be helpful in PMS and in any case there are no purely hormonal herbs or nervine herbs to tempt one into a simple match-up between symptoms and prescribing. But thinking about oestrogen, serotonin, opioids, prolactin, or dopamine may give one indicator for treatment of symptoms such as poor sleep, feeling low, or breast tenderness.

Current theories about PMS now tend to focus on both nervous and endocrine components and it is best to think of these as aspects of one system, the neuroendocrine system. We think of neurotransmitters having local effects at synapses, whereas hormones are carried in the blood, but this does not fit the picture for endorphins or adrenaline, carried in the blood but with receptors on neuronal membranes. In some brain pathways, neurones also have receptors for progesterone and oestrogen, as shown in Figure 8.3. Many neuromodulators, including substances produced in the body or ingested, affect what happens in the synapses either by affecting receptors directly, like the adrenaline or endorphins, changing the receptor density or sensitivity, or affecting the production, reabsorption or metabolism of neurotransmitters.

It is worth noting that that two of the main herbs we concentrate in this book, *Vitex agnus-castus* and *Cimicifuga racemosa*, can be thought of equally as nervine and endocrine in function.

Neurotransmitters associated with the menstrual cycle

GABA, dopamine, serotonin and opiates

As mentioned in Chapter 2 of this book, GABA is the main inhibitory transmitter in the brain, and has a tranquillizing effect, whereas dopamine and serotonin are particularly associated with communication between the layers just under the cortex, i.e. conscious processing centres, and deeper structures to do with memory, spatial awareness, reward, and motivation, known as the limbic system, and containing the thalamus, amygdala, and hippocampus.

As mentioned, good sleep, gut health, and exercise all make serotonin levels higher. People with low serotonin levels tend to be fixated with short-term rewards rather than long-term gains, and short-term

PMS: COMMON MYTHS 223

Glutamatergic Pathways

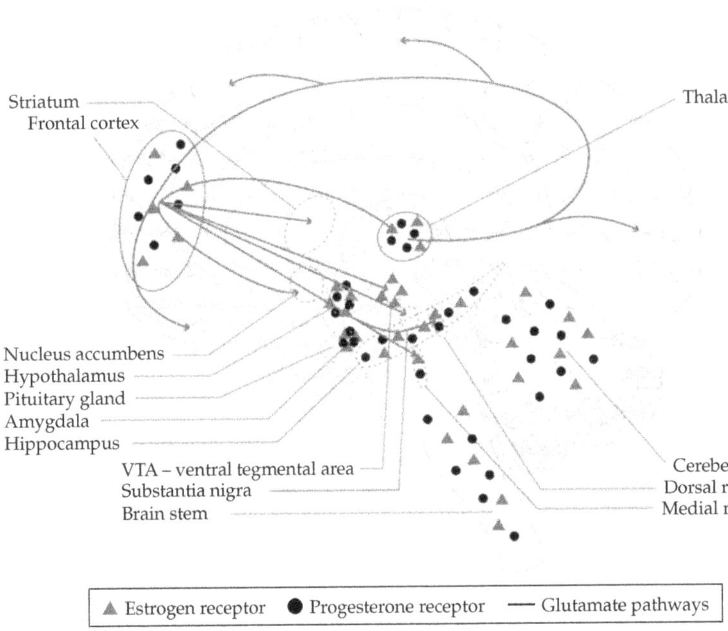

Striatum
Frontal cortex
Thalamus
Nucleus accumbens
Hypothalamus
Pituitary gland
Amygdala
Hippocampus
VTA – ventral tegmental area
Substantia nigra
Brain stem
Cerebellum
Dorsal raphe
Medial raphe

▲ Estrogen receptor   ● Progesterone receptor   — Glutamate pathways

GABA-ergic Pathways

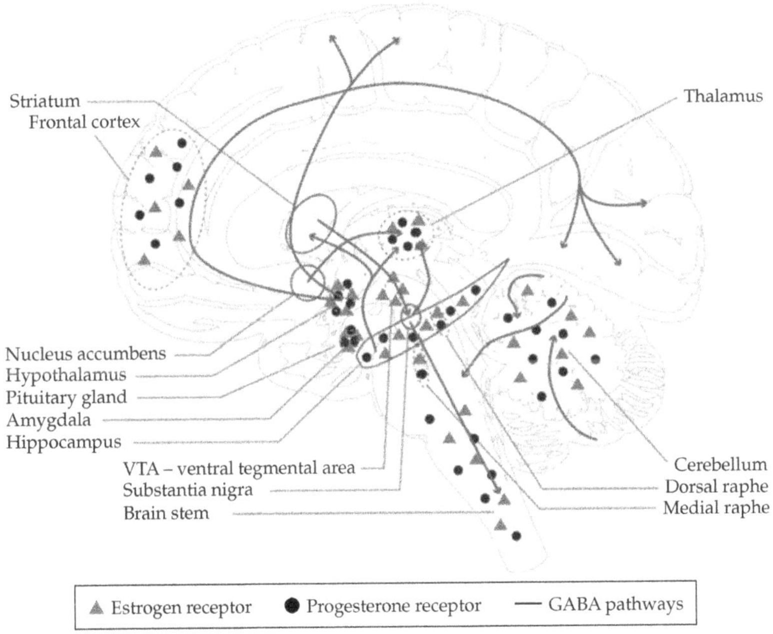

Striatum
Frontal cortex
Thalamus
Nucleus accumbens
Hypothalamus
Pituitary gland
Amygdala
Hippocampus
VTA – ventral tegmental area
Substantia nigra
Brain stem
Cerebellum
Dorsal raphe
Medial raphe

▲ Estrogen receptor   ● Progesterone receptor   — GABA pathways

Figure 8.3: (Continued)

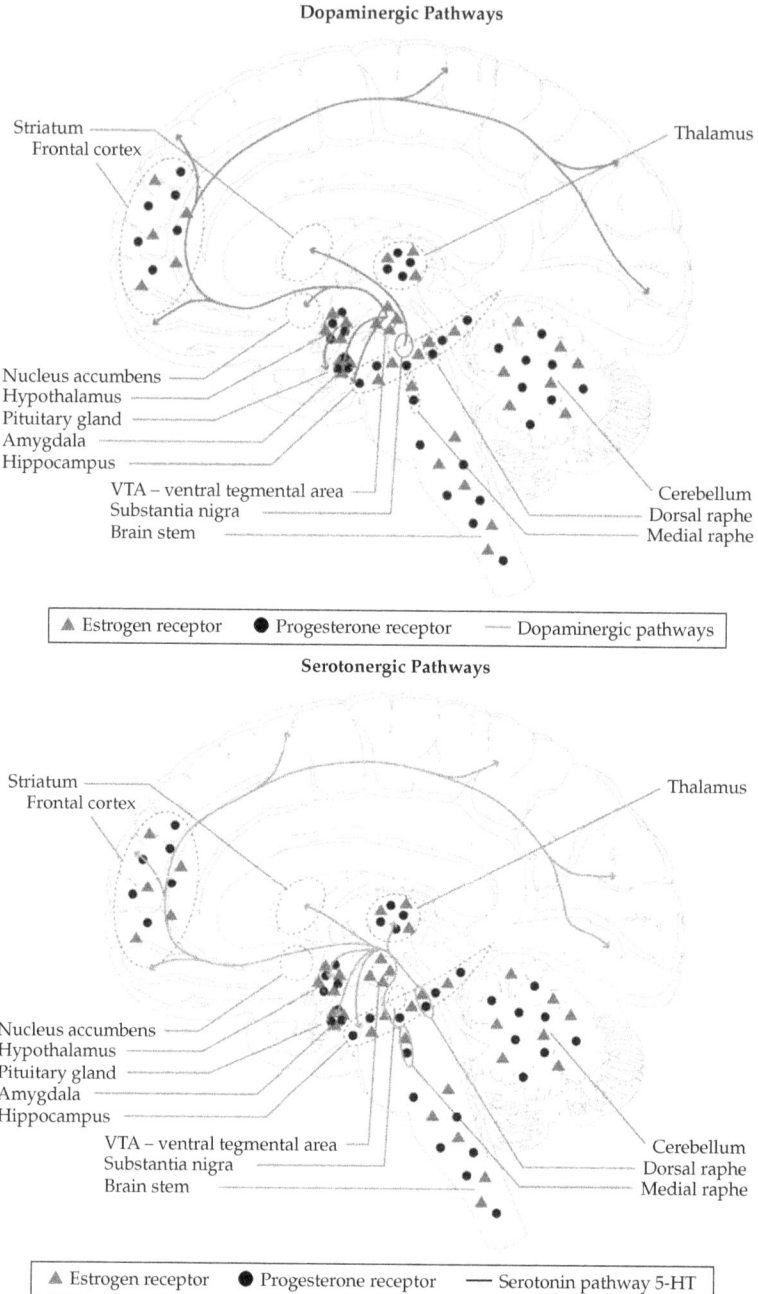

Figure 8.3: Sex hormones affect neurotransmitters and shape the adult female brain during hormonal transition periods.

fixes effectively mean addiction—to sugar, to alcohol, to gambling, and so on.

While serotonin and dopamine are associated with motivation, reward, learning and planning, natural opiates in the brain elicit a sense of wellbeing and detachment particularly familiar to endurance athletes. Likewise, people receiving morphine for pain, along with heroin addicts, know the effects of opiates intimately.

All of these neurotransmitters are affected by the levels of oestrogen and progesterone through the cycle in various ways. Figure 8.3 shows the close relationship between oestrogen and progesterone receptors and the critical pathways of these systems.

Progesterone sensitivity and GABA

The progesterone metabolite allopregnanolone has a high affinity for $GABA_A$ receptors (the main type) and facilitates GABAergic neurotransmission. So progesterone, converted to allopregnanolone, tends to have a sedative effect (as do benzodiazepines, barbiturates, and alcohol). Allopregnanolone also suppresses the excitatory glutamate response. As a result of this, progesterone normally has anxiolytic, analgesic, sedative and anaesthetic properties, and so some signs of these properties would be normal during the luteal phase. Of course, at high levels, the effect you would expect is excessive sedation and so perhaps depression.

Anxiety does indeed seem to be closely related to allopregnanolone serum concentrations, following an inverted U-shaped curve. A low concentration of allopregnalone is anxiogenic, and higher concentrations calming unless they are very high. So this could help explain anxiety levels commonly arising as progesterone levels fall in the late luteal phase.

However, progesterone does not have the same effect in all women, and some have an excessive sensitivity to the hormone. It seems likely that for women with PMS and PMDD occurring earlier in the luteal phase, $GABA_A$ receptor modulation is different for some reason, and while low concentrations of allopregnanolone are calming, the levels that are normal in the luteal phase cause high anxiety.[13] This could explain why traumatic episodes can predispose to PMS and particularly PMDD.

Acute stress increases the levels of circulating allopregnanolone. That is adaptive in short-term, restoring normal GABAergic and hypothalamic-pituitary-adrenal (HPA) function following stress.[14] The phenomenon of habituation mentioned above may explain why an elevated allopregnanolone level, as a response to a chronic stress situation then leads to lower levels of allopregnanolone and blunted allopregnanolone responses to acute stress. A clinical study confirms an altered sensitivity to allopregnanolone in PMDD patients.[15]

Anxiety is also related to heightened amygdala function. Progesterone concentrations similar to those occurring in the luteal (i.e. premenstrual) phase were associated in one trial with an increase in amygdala reactivity, whereas a still higher progesterone concentration, similar to that observed during pregnancy, led to a reduction in amygdala activity.[16] Another study found that a combination of anxiety and progesterone levels modulate amygdala reactivity across the menstrual cycle in women with PMDD.[17]

What can be taken from these studies is that it is likely that in PMDD, the brain pathways critical to emotional stability have become unstable, and so the ability to respond to stress is very limited. So, it becomes very important to help to relieve stress in women with early- or mid-luteal phase anxiety in as a practical measure of help, but also to create conditions where the paradoxical response of the progesterone/allopregnanolone/$GABA_A$ system can recover its function over time.

Oestrogen, serotonin, and melatonin

Oestrogen has a range of effects on neurotransmitters, affecting glutamate transmission, suppressing GABA inhibitory inputs, and also promoting dopamine release in the striatum, increasing serotonin levels and decreasing serotonin reuptake. So, as ovarian hormones fluctuate during the normal cycle, so do the levels of these major neurotransmitters. Oestrogen may also have the opposite effect to progesterone on amygdala reactivity, so one might expect more of an impulse to social interaction during the first half of the cycle, on a very simplistic level.

Many women who have been in a good mood during pregnancy later develop postnatal depression, suggesting that their normal hormonal cycle is causing problems with these neurotransmitter pathways. When the periods return, premenstrual depression begins. These women with reproductive depression are often progesterone/progestogen intolerant and the treatment of choice is transdermal oestrogen.[18]

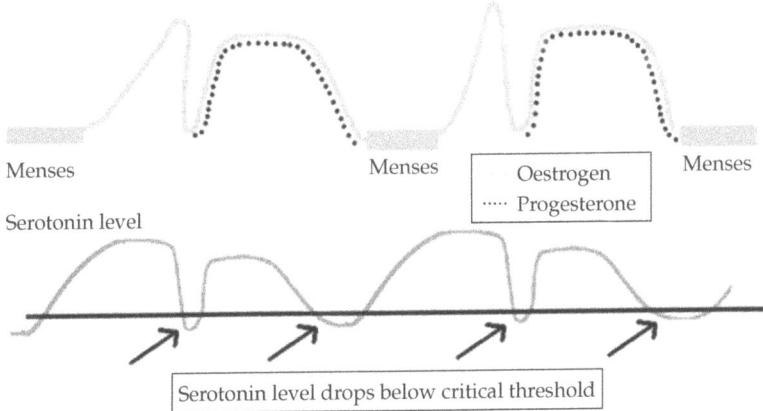

Figure 8.4: Variation of serotonin levels through the menstrual cycle, showing points where the level drops below a critical threshold.

Oestrogen medication itself also has an antidepressant effect in women with perimenopausal depression[19] and reproductive depression. It may be that oestrogen not only affects catecholamine levels in key areas, but also that it 'primes' the receptors, i.e. increases their sensitivity. There is good evidence that it does this for dopamine receptors, for example.[20]

It may well be that serotonin is the most important of these pathways in PMS. Lower serotonin can give rise to PMS-like symptoms (mood, sleep, eating behaviour, depression, suicide, aggression) and selective serotonin reuptake inhibitors are generally now the conventional treatment of choice in PMS and PMDD and have demonstrated efficacy for treating PMS in some (but not all) randomised placebo-controlled trials.

PMS worsens when on a tryptophan-free diet[21] and there is evidence that PMS sufferers have lower levels of serotonin in the blood before menstruation (see Figure 8.4).[22] However, reduced libido is a common side effect of long-term treatment with serotonin reuptake inhibitors (SSRIs),[23] again raising the question whether that is a result of habituation.

Melatonin and PMDD

An association between disturbances in menstrual function with disruption of circadian rhythms is also seen in shift workers, who are more likely to report menstrual irregularity and longer menstrual cycles, accompanied by an increased risk of breast cancer, again possibly related to altered light exposure and reduced melatonin secretion.[24]

Women with PMDD showed a decreased response to melatonin in their luteal phase as compared to the follicular phase. Decreased melatonin secretions due to hormonal fluctuations during the luteal phase of the menstrual cycle could also explain some of the sleep complaints of PMDD.[25] Possible associations with disrupted serotonergic transmission have also been proposed.[26] As mentioned previously, melatonin is derived from serotonin, and it may be that some of the functions ascribed to SSRIs are not only a result of increased serotonin levels but also due to increased production of melatonin. Likewise, foods—nuts, seeds, tofu, eggs, etc.—that provide tryptophan are not only important for serotonin production but also that of melatonin.

Endogenous opioids, the HPA axis, and cortisone

High levels of endorphins are a normal stress response, and tend to suppress the HPA axis, meaning that the pituitary stimulates the ovaries and the adrenals less, for example decreasing LH secretion.[27] Differences in beta-endorphin levels between the peri-ovulatory and premenstrual phases have been reported in women diagnosed with PMS.[28] There is not a great deal of consistent evidence for cortisol dysregulation in PMS, but PMS is known to decrease the effectiveness of the stress response, including a blunting of adrenal and cortisol response.[29] This control is altered in patients with severe PMS because of the possible hyposensitivity of opiate receptors.

In other words, over time, the inhibitory effect of endogenous opioids on the HPA axis may be reduced but this can lead to a decrease in sensitivity of the HPA axis, too.[30] So, women with PMS may have lower levels of endogenous opioids, and women with PMDD can also have lower levels of cortisol,[31] and so both the psychological and physiological damping of reactions to stress (anxiety and inflammation respectively) become less efficient. One small study concluded that hyporeactivity of the HPA axis may predict heightened PMS severity.[32]

Dopamine and latent hyperprolactinaemia

Some women with premenstrual syndrome have elevated prolactin levels, but in most the prolactin concentrations are normal, although it may be that some are abnormally sensitive to prolactin. There is evidence that prostaglandin E1 (PGE1), derived from dietary essential fatty acids, is able to attenuate the biological actions of prolactin, so deficiency of prostaglandin PGE1 could exaggerate the effects of prolactin. Nutrients that help in the metabolism of EFAs are magnesium, pyridoxine, zinc, niacin and ascorbic acid and the clinical success obtained with some of these nutrients may in part relate to their effects on essential fatty acid metabolism.

Sensitivity to prolactin is thought to be related to breast soreness and swelling. The dopamine D2 receptor agonist, bromocriptine,[33] or chasteberry,[34] which lower serum concentrations of prolactin, are effective for the treatment of premenstrual mastalgia, although bromocriptine does not help mood symptoms. Premenstrual mastalgia is also treated effectively by luteal administration of danazol[35] or an oestrogen receptor antagonist,[36] while oestradiol stimulates prolactin synthesis and release.[37]

The emotional component of prolactin and cortisol release

One fascinating trial examines the effects of emotional responses to narratives introduced under hypnosis on hormone release. When the response to the evocation of humiliating experiences was rage, it was accompanied by a prolactin surge. Cortisol surges, on the other hand, were related to surprise and shock, which were negatively associated with prolactin levels. Prolactin and cortisol may thus indicate two different coping strategies to 'psychological stress'.[38]

Clinically, high prolactin levels have been associated with certain autoimmune diseases,[39] and both higher and lower than normal prolactin levels have been shown to compromise immune responses *in vivo*.

Any process (i.e. some classes of medication) that disrupts dopamine secretion or interferes with the delivery of dopamine may cause hyperprolactinemia. Likewise, some medications can cause hyperprolactinemia: for example, tricyclic antidepressants, monoamine oxidase inhibitors, serotonin reuptake inhibitors, opiates, and cocaine and several anti-hypertensive medications.

In the postpartum period, there are elevated levels of prolactin and low levels of gonadotropins and sex steroids, and during breast feeding, this leads to postpartum amenorrhea. Women with PMS also release prolactin at greater than physiological amounts in response to stressful situations, and especially during sleep. Low thyroid function is also related to higher prolactin levels,[40] and low levels of B6, or zinc deficiency, may possibly contribute. Oestrogen increases prolactin secretions but also increases dopamine levels, and dopamine is known to be a prolactin inhibiting factor, and low levels lead to elevation of prolactin, so oestrogen by itself is not a sufficient cause of hyperprolactinaemia. Magnesium deficiency is associated with low dopamine levels

In PMS, excessive amounts of prolactin are released in response to stress, and B6 or zinc deficiency may affect prolactin levels, too.

Hypothyroidism

Some women with premenstrual syndrome have found to have thyroid hypofunction, mostly subclinical hypothyroidism,[41] although not consistently, and so it may be that for a subset of women with PMS, thyroid axis abnormalities may contribute to their disorder.[42]

Aldosterone

Some studies show increased premenstrual urinary aldosterone, so this could be the pathophysiological background to fluid-retention symptoms during the late luteal phase. In women with PMS, plasma renin activity and aldosterone levels were higher during the late luteal phase,[43] something that is likely to be a causal factor in studies that have found that diastolic blood pressure is elevated in young adult women experiencing PMS.[44] Inflammatory markers

Chronic inflammation has been implicated in the aetiology of depression, Serum levels of inflammatory markers, including interleukins IL-2, IL-4, IL-10, IL-12, and interferon (IFN)-γ have been positively associated with menstrual symptom severity and/or PMS in young women.[45]

Gut flora

Sex hormones may influence peripheral and central regulatory mechanisms of the brain-gut axis. A concept of 'microgenderome' related to the potential role of sex hormone modulation of the gut microbiota is also emerging.[46]

Other symptoms

Migraine is twice as prevalent in women as in men. Changing levels of oestrogen appear to trigger menstrual migraine. Pure menstrual migraine without aura is probably a distinct type of migraine caused by a fall in oestrogen levels before the onset of menstruation.[47] The proposed aetiology is increased sensitivity to normal cycling levels of oestrogen and progesterone, a pattern not related to different levels of the hormones but different response to normal hormonal levels.

Conventional treatment

No single treatment is universally recognised as effective. Among medications prescribed are oral contraceptives, transdermal oestrogens, nonsteroidal anti-inflammatory drugs (NSAIDs), dopamine agonists, diuretic agents, bromocriptine (for breast swelling), anxiolytic medications, induced medical menopause (plus HRT to prevent side effects), analgesics for headaches,[48] and oral contraceptives with shortened to no hormone-free interval. Selective serotonin reuptake inhibitors such as fluoxetine and sertraline are seen as a more effective treatment.[49]

Summary of aetiological factors

PMS is clearly complex and multifactorial. The next section discusses some useful treatment options, but before that it would be best to summarise the main causes and those aetiological factors that are likely to be treatable.

Predisposing causes that may be treatable include:

- Stress[50] and exogenous hormones
- Pressure of social expectation
- Past birth control use, alcohol use, drug use
- High body mass index[51]
- Unhealthy or unbalanced eating habits such as fast food consumption, irregular breakfasts, and coffee and alcohol consumption[52]
- Metabolic syndrome[53]
- Ovarian steroid fluctuation, irregular menstruation[54]
- CNS neurotransmitter levels
- Prior anxiety states, traumatic events, physical threats, childhood abuse, serious accidents

The main aetiological factors that give an insight into treatment:

- Progesterone sensitivity and paradoxical $GABA_A$ response to allopregnanolone

- Low serotonin levels in the periovulatory and late luteal phase
- Low opioid sensitivity following prolonged stress
- Possible low dopamine, excess prolactin or heightened prolactin sensitivity

Also consider:

- Hypothyroidism
- Chronic inflammation
- Gut flora imbalance or lack of diversity
- High aldosterone
- Migraine

One of the main principles of aetiology worth bearing in mind constantly is habituation and loss of resilience. In other words, if part of a complex system, that normally responds flexibly, is kept under pressure, in the end it will stop responding and just set itself into a steady state, much as a person constantly in a no-win situation will end up depressed and going through the motions of life. This we can see in terms of all the hormones and neurotransmitters. It has been a central principle in understanding drug addiction for many decades, but the same thing happens commonly in the neuroendocrine system.

Stages of treatment

How the aetiological picture helps treatment is in the second step of the treatment sequence:

- Take the pressure off (unload, treat symptoms)
- Re-establish normal function (nourish, and support function)
- As the symptom picture normalises, rebuild resilience (tonify)

The next section looks at how to do that.

Treatment principles: establishing the rationale

The treatment principles are not meant to be a formula or an 'if-then' exercise. There is certainly no one standard remedy—magnesium, B_6 and Vitex, for example. Normally, PMS will have been a long-standing condition and it is complex, so that means a pattern of disharmony and habituation, so the treatment will take time. But it is certainly useful to follow a general strategy of staged treatment that will help both psychologically and physiologically. The patient's confidence and buy-in are crucial, with the idea of enhancing the placebo aspect of treatment (once again a respectable idea) as well as the physiological effects of the nutritional, lifestyle and herbal treatment.

One way to explain the treatment is that the nervous and endocrine system are like an orchestra, and then one section, probably under stress for some reason, has started playing its own tune, out of time with the others. That affects the others, one by one, and in the end the rhythm and harmony are seriously disturbed, and that the most important thing can be to quieten things a little, in terms of stress, diet and inflammation.

This also prepares the idea that treatment will change over time, which can otherwise appear confusing or ad hoc. And finally, there are only so many changes that a patient can be expected to make at a time, and staging treatment can help with making and understanding each diet and lifestyle change.

1. Take the pressure off (unload, treat major symptoms)

The first thing is to take the stress off: to reduce the tempo and the volume so that they players can hear each other a bit more clearly, and at the same time quieten the loudest section (main symptoms). In other words, take away factors that are pro-inflammatory (poor sleep, unsuitable diet, too little exercise) and add anti-inflammatory factors (herbs and foods), and give symptomatic relief. It is a good idea at this point to set up a diary of symptoms so that the most troubling symptoms are brought into focus and progress begins to be measured. This phase may last a few weeks or a few months depending how long-standing it is. It is important not to try to change function too much early on so that there is some kind of benchmark to measure against. It may be tempting to cut corners, but it really helps when assessing a long-term strategy just to see what happens purely out of generally calming things down.

2. Re-establish normal function (nourish, and support function)

The second stage is to make sure the specific nutritional and herbal treatment are in place to restore normal function. By analogy with our orchestra, this might mean giving active support to some of the players and bringing in one or two extra. Foods that support particular functions, for example the B vitamins for neurotransmitter production. Herbs that have adjusting effects on neuroendocrine function are the key to this stage, i.e. nervine, hormonal or adaptogenic actions (although of course these are not separate). It is important of course to treat all aspects of the terrain at this point.

3. As the symptom picture normalises, rebuild resilience (tonify)

The third stage is to establish resilience, so that the body itself takes over most of the functions that had been supported by herbal treatment. It can be tempting to either stop treatment or to continue it indefinitely when symptoms are resolved, but neither is ideal. This is the time to review what long-term maintenance is needed in terms of general health and not specifically neuroendocrine, to look at trophorestoratives and permanent changes in diet and lifestyle, and to establish a minimal set of herbal standbys for emergencies or easing symptoms.

Unload, and treat symptoms

During the first few months of treatment, the aim should be to stabilise, improve symptoms, and remove triggers. Conventional medication may be left in place unless it seems to be causing problems.

Lifestyle

As we discussed earlier, obesity, habits such as fast food consumption, irregular breakfasts, and alcohol consumption increase PMS risk.[55] Coffee has nowadays been found to have some positive impacts on health, and not all studies associate caffeine intake with PMS[56] (and the supposed link with fibrocystic breast disease now seems to be spurious),[57] so that may be something to monitor rather than try to change.

Metabolic syndrome, i.e. putting weight on in the central zone (hips to chest), higher levels of low-density lipids and cholesterol, and low sensitivity to insulin, is associated with PMS,[58] and a useful pointer for general dietary advice.

General dietary advice as for PMS and for metabolic syndrome

- Regular meals
- Avoid refined sugar
- Complex carbohydrates, vegetables, fruit, nuts, seeds, fish, legumes, yoghurt
- Limit animal foods (or eat organic) as they are related to higher oestrogen levels
- Reduce alcohol intake (a moderate association with PMS risk): there is an interaction between alcohol and GABA receptors, even low amounts resulting in decreasing peripheral allopregnenolone levels (so anxiety increases).[59] Alcohol also plays a role in reactive hypoglycaemia[60]
- Reduce caffeine if symptoms of anxiety are present

And in addition

- Avoid environmental oestrogens (pesticides on food, plastics, air fresheners and cosmetics): eat organic and use non-industrial household products
- Plant foods for oestrogen excess or deficiency: nuts, seeds, legumes such as soy foods
- Tryptophan-rich foods support serotonin and melatonin production: nuts, seeds, tofu, cheese, red meat, chicken, turkey, fish, oats, beans, lentils, and eggs

Exercise

Exercise is very useful in all sorts of ways: improving energy levels, self-esteem, pain tolerance, and mood.

- Aerobic Exercise:
  - Influences endorphins and stress-coping mechanisms.
  - Improves most premenstrual symptoms.
  - Increases haemoglobin, red cell and platelet count; decreases prolactin, oestradiol and progesterone; helps fatigue and confusion.[61]
- Exercise and the thyroid:
  - Exercises is beneficial in hypothyroidism because it not only stimulates thyroid secretion, but also increases tissue sensitivity to thyroid hormone.[62]

Intestinal health

Supporting a healthy diversity of gut flora is important for all sorts of reasons including elimination of oestrogen and xeno-oestrogen metabolites, which both tend to be inflammatory and carcinogenic, avoiding recirculation of endogenous oestrogen in the blood stream, and preventing excess beta-glucuronidase, which is linked to increased cancer risk. Often the lack of progesterone is more likely due to relative excess oestrogen.

If constipation is present, it needs to be treated. Probiotics will help to establish normal intestinal flora, but ideally as part of the diet. A diverse gut flora is now acknowledged to be major factor in the control of body weight, also important to management of PMS. As an addition to the measures above, a probiotic diet will ideally include lacto-fermented foods, such as kimchi, sauerkraut or lacto-fermented pickles.

Elimination

Gentle laxatives, such as *Taraxacum radix*, *Rumex crispus*, and flaxseeds, will help directly with elimination and help to re-establish a healthy microflora. Lipotrophic factors such as choline in *Taraxacum radix* also help with removal of fat and bile in the liver through interaction with fat metabolism, and decongesting effect on liver.[63]

Hepatic stimulants in general will help with the elimination of hormonal metabolites, and foods such as turmeric, ginger, and artichoke will be useful additions to the diet.

Anti-inflammatory herbs

In the longer-term, restoring the balance of the HPA axis, ensuring gut health and good dietary balance of EFAs and antioxidants is necessary to decrease tissue damage, encourage repair but keep inflammation under control. In the shorter term, these herbs are very helpful:

Zingiber officinalis, *Chamomilla recutita*, *Curcuma longa*, *Glycyrrhiza glabra*, *Cimicifuga racemosa* (just a few of a long list).

Symptomatic relief

As the underlying neuroendocrine causes create a complex symptom picture, dealing with symptoms individually is of limited benefit, but migraines and mastalgia are two obvious targets for immediate attention.

Migraines

Avoid trigger foods.

Ginkgo biloba. Vitex agnus-castus, Cimicifuga racemosa (careful as too high a dose may result in a frontal headache), *Stachys betonica, Tanacetum parthenium.*

For menstrual migraine, there is some evidence of efficacy for magnesium, phytoestrogens (not specified), and ginkgolide B.[64]

Mastalgia

Vitex agnus-castus, Ginkgo biloba, Taraxacum officinale fol, *Paeonia lactiflora,* and *Glycyrrhiza glabra, Ruscus aculeatus.*

Fluid retention

Dandelion leaf, *Ginkgo biloba, Vitex agnus-castus.*

Pain

Magnesium, *Tanacetum parthenium.*

Clinical trials

This list of herbs is not necessarily limited to the first phase of treatment, but most of the following trials of herbs on PMS symptoms measure outcomes over the first 3 months of treatment.

- *Melissa officinalis* capsules have proven effective in reduction of PMS symptoms in high school girls.[65]
- *Chamomilla recutica* vs. mefenamic acid: the two treatments had similar efficacy on physical symptoms, but chamomile was more effective for emotional symptoms.[66]
- *Valeriana officinalis*. The crude extract has high affinity to $GABA_A$ receptors in increase of GABA (gamma-aminobutyric acid) in the synaptic cleft and could explain sedative effects.[67] Binding to $GABA_A$ receptors is a common finding in calming herbs—another example being *Leonurus cardiaca*.[68] A study showed that Valerian root extract reduces emotional, physical, and behavioural symptoms of premenstrual syndrome in students, the authors attributing the improvement in physical symptoms to inhibition of prostaglandin release.[69]

- *Foeniculum vulgare*: improvement in most PMS symptoms (stress, depression, excitement, somatic and cluster symptoms) but not bloating).[70]
- *Curcuma longa*. Curcumin led to reductions in physical, behavioural and mood scores. The total PMS score significantly decreased,[71] which the authors thought to be partly through modulation of neurotransmitters serotonin, dopamine and noradrenaline, and partly anti-inflammatory effects of curcumin. Quite large doses of turmeric powder are needed for a significant impact, so it is best treated as a food: absorption is helped by mixing it with coconut oil and adding black pepper.
- *Zingiber officinalis*: reduction of severity of mood and physical and behavioural symptoms of PMS. It is important to use a very high ethanol (minimum 90%) extract or use the powdered or fresh root.
- *Ruscus aculeatus*: reduced symptoms of mastalgia and mood disorders, and showed a trend towards improving ankle oedema.[72]
- *Ginkgo biloba*. Ginkgo has a range of cardiovascular effects, which may be synergistic with those of *Ruscus aculeatus*. It corrects capillary hyperpermeability, strengthens capillary resistance, and inhibits platelet activating factor. Trials have indicated that Ginkgo reduces congestive symptoms and ameliorates cyclic oedema.[73] It is especially helpful in mastalgia of premenstrual syndrome, but also improved neuropsychological symptoms (anxiety, depression and headaches),[74,75] a pointer to the link between inflammation and general wellbeing.

Second phase of treatment: compensate and restore function

The second phase is where the practitioner moves towards more nuanced treatment. The point of this phase is to restore neuroendocrine balance as far as possible, making sure deficiencies are remedied, but also investigating where weak tendencies lie. Nutrition aims to correct deficiencies in vitamins, minerals and essential fatty acids, ideally using diet rather than supplements. Herbal treatment moves from symptomatic and anti-inflammatory to supportive and corrective.

There is no rigid cut-off between the first and second phase of treatment but elements of the first phase should be phased out as general health improves and they are no longer necessary, and to avoid developing dependency and habituation where herbs have quite a strong effect. Care should be taken to withdraw anti-inflammatory herbs and pre-existing medication gradually and full monitoring of symptoms needs to continue.

Restoring function: nutrition: vitamins, minerals and EFAs

Thiamine (B1), riboflavin (B2), niacin (B3), pyridoxine (B6), folic acid (B9), and cobalamine (B12) are required to synthesise neurotransmitters. High intakes of B_1 and B_2 from food sources lower the risk of PMS,[76] as does a combined supplement of B_1 and B_6.

Vitamin D, calcium, and magnesium status tend to be compromised in PMS subjects.[77] These are not just necessary for skeletal health but have a profound effect on the stability of the nervous system and various aspects of neuroendocrine function, so particularly important where depression or migraines are part of the symptom picture.

Zinc has been found helpful in PMS and iron is important in the synthesis of brain neurotransmitters.

A healthy diet should be sufficient to provide all of these in sufficient quantities. Smoking, stress, and excess consumption of sugar, coffee, and alcohol can lead to depletion of these vitamins.

The recommendations to use plant foods for oestrogen excess or deficiency (nuts, seeds, legumes) along with tryptophan-rich foods to support serotonin and melatonin production (nuts, seeds, tofu, cheese, red meat, chicken, turkey, fish, oats, beans, lentils, and egg) are useful throughout treatment.

Vitamin B_1 and B_6

These, like other B vitamins, are particularly concentrated in meat such as turkey, tuna, and liver, legumes (pulses or beans), whole grains, potatoes, bananas, chilli peppers, tempeh, nutritional yeast, brewer's yeast, and molasses.

Vitamin B_1 plays an important role in the functioning of the central nervous system and neuromuscular system, and is required for the metabolism of glucose. In clinical trials it has been effective in helping with the mental and physical symptoms of PMS.[78]

Vitamin B_6 is involved in the synthesis of various neurotransmitters. It is a coenzyme in tryptophan and tyrosine metabolism, is involved in the synthesis of GABA, and increases serotonin and dopamine levels.

B_6 also normalises low intracellular magnesium levels—which are also associated with dopamine and serotonin deficiency—and it may be particularly useful in women taking either oral contraceptives or HRT.

- B_6 deficiency may lead to reduced concentrations of noradrenaline and increased prolactin levels.[79]
- The vitamin has an essential role in the synthesis of prostaglandin and fatty acids (deficiency is associated with various aetiologies causing PMS).[80]
- Deficiency might decrease dopamine in the kidneys, leading to increase sodium excretion, triggering oedema and abdominal and chest discomfort.[81]
- B_6 levels are typically low in women taking HRT and OCP.[82] B_6 supplementation improves depression and anxiety scores related to use of OCP.[83]
- *In vivo*, B_6 leads to increase tissue sensitivity to oestrogen.[84]

A systematic review found that B_6 supplementation benefits premenstrual depression[85] and reduces the overall symptoms of PMS. Studies indicate a positive effect on abdominal pain, back ache, reduced breast sensitivity, and improvements in premenstrual acne.

Vitamin D

Sources include sunlight, fish, mushrooms, egg yolk, beef, fortified products are also on the market. Vitamin D affects not only calcium levels, but also neurotransmitter function.

- Vitamin D level of serum of women with PMS in luteal phase is lower than that in women without the syndrome.[86] Higher intake of vitamin D from foods was associated with a lower prevalence of PMS.[87,88]
- Vitamin D could influence menstrual depression and symptoms related to fluid balance, and supplementation may lower the risk of unipolar depression.[89]
- Deficiency is also associated with increased renin-angiotensin-aldosterone function, contributing to increased fluid balance, blood pressure changes, and hypertension.[90]
- Link between presence of PMS, increased risk of osteoporosis after menopause in women with PMS.[91]

Vitamin E

Sources of vitamin E: Vegetable oils (such as wheatgerm, sunflower, safflower, corn, and soybean oils)—NB should be in small, dark bottles kept in a cool place and used up quickly to prevent deterioration due to light and contact with air. Nuts (such as almonds, peanuts, and hazelnuts/filberts), and seeds (such as sunflower seeds). Green leafy vegetables (such as spinach and broccoli) also contain high levels of vitamin E.

Supplemental therapy with vitamins D and E is an effective and affordable treatment for PMS.

- Vitamin E modulates production of prostaglandins, reduces inflammation, and improves oestrogen/progesterone ratio.
- Improves benign breast disorders and pain. Improves tension, irritability, incoordination. Clinical trials found improvement in the physical and mental symptoms after the treatment.[92,93]
- Wheatgerm reduces general, psychological and physical symptoms.[94]

Omega 3

Oestrogen has similar effects to the Omega 3 EFAs on hippocampal function,[95] and, as discussed before in the context of general treatment, is important in shifting the production of prostaglandins from the 2-series to the anti-inflammatory PGE:

- Omega-3 supplement (1g fish oil daily) reduced symptoms and ameliorated women's quality of life in those suffering from PMS,[96] the effects increasing over the duration (6 months) of treatment.[97,98] Not all studies have found EFA supplementation to be effective,[99] but this is almost inevitable in a multifactorial syndrome like PMS.
- Studies have demonstrated that patients suffering from depression or mood disorders had significantly lower dietary intake and serum levels of EPA and DHA.[100]

Calcium

Sources: most milk products, most types of tofu, some dark green leafy cabbage family vegetables, turnip greens and canned fish such as salmon and sardines that include bones.

Calcium is important in cell signalling, blood clotting, muscle contraction and nerve function.

- Levels of calcium in red blood cells have been found to be lower than normal in women with PMS although within the normal range,[101] with altered mid-cycle metabolism of vitamin D and calcium in PMDD. Some studies show exaggerated fluctuations of calcium-regulating hormones across the menstrual cycle in PMS, perhaps in tandem with vitamin D deficiency.[102]
- Calcium supplements have shown efficacy in reducing PMS-related mood disorders[103,104] and both physical and psychological symptoms of PMS, as well as ameliorating PMS-related migraine, early fatigability and appetite.
- In a systematic review of 62 herbs, vitamins and minerals with claims of benefit for PMS, only calcium had good quality evidence to support its use in PMS (it was noted that data suggest that chasteberry and vitamin B6 may be effective, and there were indications of benefit with Ginkgo, magnesium pyrrolidone, saffron, St. John's Wort, soy and vitamin E).[105]

Magnesium

High magnesium foods include spinach, chard, pumpkin seeds, yoghurt or kefir, almonds, black beans, avocado, figs, dark chocolate, bananas, salmon, coriander, cashews, goat's cheese, and artichokes.

Magnesium is a co-factor in over 300 enzymatic reactions and essential for many crucial physiological functions, such as heart rhythm, vascular tone, nerve function and muscle contraction and relaxation, as well as for bone formation. The mineral can be seen as a natural 'calcium antagonist'.[106]

- There is an association between very low magnesium intake and depression, especially in younger adults.[107] Low levels of magnesium are also associated with Alzheimer's disease, insulin resistance, Type-2 diabetes mellitus, hypertension, cardiovascular disease (e.g., stroke), migraine headaches, attention-deficit hyperactivity disorder (ADHD), early mortality, menstrual headaches and migraines and PMS.[108,109] Clinical studies indicate that magnesium supplements are helpful for treatment of PMS symptoms,[110] particularly reducing

anxiety-related premenstrual symptoms,[111] though not necessarily mood symptoms in women with PMDD.[112] It takes at least 2 months of administration to show an effect on PMS.[113]
- Magnesium inhibits aldosterone production. Supplement have been found to have anti-hypertensive effect. Mg deficiency and low or high progesterone elevate aldosterone levels and cause fluid retention, creating a vicious circle as aldosterone increases Mg excretion, stress raises aldosterone levels[114] (importance of managing the adrenal cortex's response to stress).[115]

Zinc

Sources include red meat and poultry, beans, nuts, certain types of seafood (such as oysters, crab, and lobster), whole grains, and dairy products.

Zinc is highly concentrated in the brain and may be involved in neuronal function and hormonal function. It is known to be important in the sense of smell and taste, and in cell reproduction and immunity, as it is involved in cell signalling and the function of calcium, iron and other metal ions involved in neuronal regulation and transmission.[116] This suggests why it might be important for neuroendocrine function in general.

- Zinc sulphate (50mg elemental zinc) was associated with improvement of PMS symptoms, need to be taken at least for 3 months (clinical trial).[117]
- There is some evidence that high zinc intake is associated with a lower risk of PMS,[118] particularly in association with hyperprolactinaemia.[119]

Iron

Sources: haem iron (derived from haemoglobin), found in animal foods that such as red meats, fish, and poultry (meat, poultry, and seafood contain both haem and non-haem iron). Most non-haem iron is from plant foods such as legumes, tofu, dried fruit (apricots, raisins, peaches, or prunes), potato, nuts and seeds, green vegetables (broccoli, spinach), and pumpernickel.

Iron is a co-factor for an enzyme that catalyses the conversion of tryptophan into 5-hydroxytryptophan (precursor of serotonin).[120] Many brain areas are rich in iron, especially those cells receiving input from the gamma-aminobutyric acid system, and in anxiety states a lack of iron could contribute to decreased production of serotonin.

- Low iron is associated with higher risk of postpartum depression,[121] and high intake of non-haem iron (above 20mg/day) is associated with lower risk of PMS.[122]

Supportive herbal therapeutics system by system

Dividing the herbs into those for symptomatic relief (e.g. valerian and ginger) and those with a more restorative character is obviously a little bit arbitrary and it is not so much the plants as the rationale for using them that is a little different, i.e. from using them for their immediate effects at the start of treatment and then using them for tonic effects.

Digestive system

The use of herbs to help with liver function, gut health and elimination was covered in the last section, and it is important to maintain that, although with an emphasis on liver and bowel support more than stimulation.

As the emphasis now is on nourishment and support, bitters are useful to assist the absorption of nutrients[123] related to PMS symptoms, e.g. *Taraxacum officinale, Gentiana lutea, Centarium erythrea, Artemisia absinthium, Chamomilla recutita*, and *Achillea millefolium*.

Circulation

There is a big overlap between anti-inflammatory and circulatory herbs, as antioxidant activity, correction of blood lipid abnormalities and PAF inhibition all affect perfusion. In addition to this, some herbs will give a little extra help, such as *Ginkgo biloba, Achillea millefolium* and *Zingiber officinalis*.

Endocrine function

The key in this phase is herbs traditionally listed as nervines and hormonal tonics, targeted towards particular dysfunctions in PMS.

Prolactin levels (NB mastalgia)

In general, stress, oestrogen dominance, low thyroid function, and low levels of dopamine increase prolactin secretion, as do B6 or Zinc deficiency. The effect of relaxation, exercise and calming herbs is something likely to have been started in the first phase of treatment. At this point the focus may shift onto adaptogens and general nervines, thyroid function and the HPA axis.

The main control for prolactin, however, is dopamine.

- Dopaminergic agents tend to be herbs that regulate ovulation and support the corpus luteum include: *Vitex agnus-castus*, and *Paeonia lactiflora* with *Glycyrrhiza glabra*—these also indirectly affect progesterone production.

Low oestrogen in perimenopause

- *Cimicifuga racemosa*
- Steroidal saponins such as *Dioscorea villosa*
- Isoflavonoids: soya, flaxseed, *Trifolium pratense*
- *Vitex agnus-castus*, and paeony and Glycyrrhiza support the corpus luteum where ovulation is still happening

Hypothalamic-pituitary-adrenal axis

The effect of some adaptogens on the HPA axis is somewhat similar to the effects of wild yam and other herbs containing steroidal saponins on the HPG (hypothalamus-pituitary-gonadal) axis, in that it tends to normalise function by mimicking hormones. In general, these herbs contain substances that mimic or potentiate the effects of stress chemicals such as cortisol, fine-tune the effects of ACTH on the adrenals, but at a lower level. *Withania somnifera, Eleutherococcus senticosus, Rhodiola rosea, Schisandra chinensis*.[124] The overall effect is to assist tissues (particularly the adrenal glands) that have become exhausted.

Thyroid support

Turnera diffusa, Glycyrrhiza glabra, Panax ginseng, *Capsicum minimum, Eleutherococcus senticosus, Avena sativa, Nigella sativa*[125]

Neuroendocrine herbs

Vitex agnus-castus

Vitex has an affinity to opiate receptors, particularly acting as an agonist at the μ-opiate receptor, and so may be particularly indicated where there is a history of stress. It is also dopaminergic and has an effect on melatonin levels—which also suggests an ability to normalise serotonin production.

Its hormonal actions include reducing prolactin secretion, normalizing a shortened luteal phase and increasing mid-luteal progesterone and 17β-oestradiol level.[126] So, in reasonable doses (not drop doses) it is a harmonizing herb for PMS for many women, having an influence on most of the patterns of disharmony looked at above. One can thus think of Vitex as generally allowing the re-establishment of normal function—provided that it is taken over a reasonable period of time. However, it is important to monitor carefully because Vitex is not a cure-all, and in cases of PMDD or low mood beginning shortly after ovulation, it is best not to introduce it until there is some sense of control of symptoms through nervine and nutritional support.

Clinical studies on Vitex in PMS

- Premenstrual syndrome (i.e. depressive symptoms, anxiety, craving, and hyperhydration, irritability, mood changes, anger, headache, and breast fullness, insomnia). Differences were more significant after 3 months of treatment.[127]
- Flaxseed and *Vitex agnus-castus* have similar efficacy in terms of the PMS score,[128] and *Vitex agnus-castus* in a systematic review is reported to consistently ameliorate PMS better than placebo.[129]
- PMDD (comparison with fluoxetine). Fluoxetine was more effective for psychological symptoms (depression and irritability) while Vitex diminished the physical symptoms (breast tenderness, cramps, food cravings, swelling).[130,131]
- Mastodynia and latent hyperprolactinemia:[132-134] effective as treatment of cyclical mastalgia,[135] comparable to flurbiprofen (nonsteroidal anti-inflammatory drugs)[136] and bromocriptine with respect to lowering serum prolactin and reducing breast pain.

- Migraine related to cycle; reduction in frequency and duration (days with headache) of monthly attacks.[137]
- Abnormal menstrual cycle, amenorrhea.
- Equally effective for women taking OCP.[138]

Cimicifuga racemosa

The effect of Cimicifuga on PMS has not been much researched—the interest has been in menopausal problems, and to an extent fertility. However, the Eclectics regarded *Cimicifuga racemosa* as a primary remedy for menstrual irregularities.

Emotional symptoms as well as physical symptoms in menopause are effectively treated with *Cimicifuga racemosa*, so it probably makes sense with what we know about this plant that it could be of use in PMS.

- Cimicifuga contains active principles that activate human μ-opiate receptors (hMOR), which may not only help alleviate menopausal symptoms, but might indicate also usefulness in PMS.[139]
- Black cohosh has also been shown to have serotonergic activity,[140] another possible underlying mechanism of PMS, and the herb also enhances the effectiveness of paroxetine.[141]

Nervines

Hypericum perforatum

St. John's wort seems to be more helpful after 2–3 months, with improvement in overall symptoms (food craving, swelling, coordination, insomnia, confusion, headaches, crying, fatigue), associated with PMS,[142,143] and particularly women experiencing mild PMS.

- Possible anxiety reduction.[144]
- Helped emotional lability, hostility or anger, and impulsivity related to premenstrual syndrome in single women.[145]

Other nervine tonics to consider include *Melissa officinalis, Avena sativa, Scutellaria lateriflora, Withania somnifera, Stachys betonica* and *Verbena officinalis*.

Hypericum and Vitex combination trial in perimenopausal women

This herbal combination improved PMS-like symptoms among perimenopausal women, along with depression, anxiety, and hydration. Not only overall PMS measurement, but all subscales improved.[146]

Third phase of treatment: long-term stability

Depending on the severity of the problem and the length of treatment, the period of compensation and support of function may be anything from 6 months to a few years, particularly if there is a history of trauma or a chronic history of ill health.

At some point, it will be time to decide that things have reached the point of maintenance rather than active treatment. That means potentially taking medicines and nutritional support regularly over the long-term and sticking to a diet and exercise plan. A 6-monthly schedule of visits is useful on a review and prevention basis, to avoid a situation where a patient lets things slide and feels too guilty or upset to ask for help.

A transition to this long-term arrangement is something ideally agreed between patient and practitioner, in which medication is reduced, in terms of the number of herbs and the amount of each, over a period of months. It is important to maintain a symptom diary. It is also good to have an 'emergency mixture' at hand for symptom relief.

PMS: patient-friendly summary

> PMS consists of a wide array of physiological symptoms that regularly attend the luteal phase of the menstrual cycle, affecting over 10% of women of reproductive age.
>
> Predisposing factors include being overweight, stress, and exogenous hormones.
>
> Alcohol, recreational drug use, and smoking are also predisposing factors, along with family history and unhealthy or unbalanced eating habits.
>
> Endogenous contributory factors include metabolic syndrome, changes in hormonal balance, e.g. menarche, pregnancy, irregular menstruation, and perimenopause.

Symptoms commonly include headaches, bloating, breast tenderness, poor sleep, irritability, and water retention.

- During the late luteal phase, levels of both oestrogen and progesterone fall and the change in oestrogen levels or in the ratio of the hormones is implicated in PMS.
- High densities of oestrogen and progesterone receptors are present in brain regions that regulate emotions, drives and perceptions and this explains the range of emotional and psychological effects of the menopause.
- The symptoms of PMS are closely tied to serotonin and dopamine levels (monoamines with a strong influence on mood) in the brain, and also to opioid and GABA pathways.

Some women suffer extreme anxiety and agitation, known as PMDD, typically in the early luteal phase as progesterone rises, a part of the menstrual cycle that is not unpleasant for most women. Many of these women have experienced very traumatic phases earlier in their lives.

Herbal treatment deals at first with the
- Symptoms (sleep, anxiety, bloating, breast tenderness and so on)
- Predisposing factors (diet and exercise particularly to reduce inflammation)
- Elimination, liver function and healthy gut flora

Subsequent treatment ensures that there are
- Healthy conditions, particularly digestive, to support neuroendocrine function
- Adequate nutrition to ensure balanced production of neurotransmitters and anti-inflammatory prostaglandins

Herbal treatment includes phyto-oestrogenic herbs, nervines, anti-inflammatories, liver tonics, and adaptogens according to need (see the Table 8.1 below for more details).

Table 8.1: Summary of diet, lifestyle and herbal treatment for PMS/PMDD

Condition	Diet	Lifestyle	Elimination
PMS	Regular meals Complex carbohydrates, avoid refined sugar. vegetables, fruit, nuts, seeds (flaxseed), fish, legumes, (soya), yoghurt. Limit animal foods (and eat organic) Avoid environmental oestrogens (eat organic if possible to avoid pesticides in food, avoid clingwrap and other soft plastics, avoid synthetic aerosols, cleaning products and cosmetics). Low alcohol intake Food rich in (or supplement, preferably only temporarily) omega 3, magnesium, calcium, zinc, iron. Vitamins B, D and E. Reduce caffeine if anxiety is a problem. Control body weight. Support healthy gut flora: excess beta-glucuronidase linked to increased cancer risk, especially oestrogen-linked cancer. Probiotics, lacto-fermented vegetables, beans, pulses and root vegetables to establish normal intestinal flora. Support using bitter and perhaps warming, carminative herbs.	Exercise: Reduces the effect of stress Aerobic exercise improves most premenstrual symptoms. increases haemoglobin, haematocrit, red cell count and platelet count, and decreases levels of prolactin, oestradiol and progesterone. It results in improvement of fatigue, impaired concentration, decreased confusion. Relaxation, absorption in a relaxing hobby.	Supporting healthy functioning of hormones, eliminating excess oestrogens, avoiding re-entering of endogenous oestrogen in the blood stream. Constipation, if present, needs to be treated. Often an apparent lack of progesterone is actually a relative excess of oestrogen due to reabsorption of metabolites: Gentle laxatives, such as *Taraxacum officinalis* radix, *Rumex crispus*, flaxseeds Lipotrophic factors such as choline in *Taraxacum officinalis* radix help with removal of fat and bile in the liver through interaction with fat metabolism and have a decongesting effect on liver. The liver is involved with oestrogen clearance: use liver herbs, *Carduus marianus* as a restorative, herbs such as *Berberis vulgaris* or fumitory to stimulate.

Assimilation	Hormonal	Nervous System	Circulation	Symptoms
Bitters for absorption of nutrients: *Taraxacum offinalis*, *Artemisia absinthium*, *Chamomilla recutita*, *Achillea millefolium*, etc. Herbs to encourage healthy gut flora: garlic, *Berberis vulgaris*, *Artemisia absinthium*, bitters in general. Slippery elm.	Reduce prolactin levels (zinc, B_6, stress, stimulate thyroid, adaptogens, nervines, relaxation, exercise, etc.) Dopaminergic agents: *Vitex agnus-castus*, *Cimicifuga racemosa*, Paeony and Glycyrrhiza combination. Hypothalamic-pituitary-adrenal (HPA) axis: adaptogens *Withania somnifera*, *Eleutherococcus senticosus*, *Rhodiola rosea*, *Schisandra chinensis*, Thyroid support: *Turnera diffusa*, *Glycyrrhiza glabra*, *Panax ginseng*, *Capsicum minimum*, *Eleutherococcus senticosus*, *Avena sativa*, *Nigella sativa*.	*Hypericum perforatum*, *Chamomilla recutita*, *Foeniculum vulgare*, *Lavandula officinalis*, *Betonica officinalis*, *Scutellaria lateriflora*, *Valeriana officinalis*, *Melissa officinalis*, *Withania somnifera*, *Verbena officinalis*…	*Ginkgo biloba*, *Ruscus aculeatus*, *Achillea millefolium*, *Zingiber officinalis*	Fluid retention: dandelion leaf, *Ginkgo biloba*, *Vitex agnus-castus* Pain: magnesium, *Tanacetum parthenium* Inflammation: *Zingiber officinalis*, *Chamomilla recutita*, Turmeric, *Glycyrrhiza glabra*, *Cimicifuga racemosa*… Migraines: Avoid trigger foods, *Ginkgo biloba*, *Vitex agnus-castus*, *Cimicifuga racemosa* (careful as also in high doses will give frontal headache), *Stachys betonica*, *Tanacetum parthenium* Mastalgia: *Vitex agnus-castus*, *Ginkgo biloba*, *Taraxacum officinalis* fol, *Paeonia lactiflora* & *Glycyrrhiza glabra*, *Ruscus aculeatus*. **Perimenopausal PMS:** PMS related to low oestrogen levels (also seen in menarche and after childbirth). *Vitex agnus-castus*, peony and liquorice when still ovulating (supporting corpus luteum, so promoting both oestrogen and progesterone) Steroidal saponins such as *Dioscorea villosa*, *Asparagus racemosus*. Isoflavonoids: soya, flaxseed, *Trifolium pratense* Triterpenoid saponins: *Cimicifuga racemosa* Adaptogens important to adapt body to new hormonal levels.

CHAPTER NINE

Some other gynaecological conditions

The aims of this book have been to set out general principles for treating hormonal conditions, give some kind of physiological rationale underlying the actions and the effect of diet, lifestyle, and above all herbs for menopausal conditions and premenstrual syndrome. We did not set out to create an exhaustive guide to the treatment of gynaecological conditions, and two things are missing. Firstly, there is very little in this book about the human side of the interaction. Treatment for chronic conditions is a partnership between patient and practitioner, and the soft side is very important to make that work, especially as there are questions about relationships, roles, and sexual history and identity. We will touch on these in the next book, the companion to this one, which will also put right the second gap in this one, namely our focus on the two most general presentations of PMS and the menopause, at the expense of reviewing a wider range of problems including osteoporosis, uterine fibroids, polycystic ovarian syndrome, infertility, endometriosis, and other menstrual irregularities.

In the meantime, here is a brief guide linking the treatment of some of these problems to the general hormonal picture and principles of treatment described in this book rather than a complete picture of aetiology or therapeutics for these conditions.

Uterine fibroids

Hormonal picture

Oestrogen dominance, poor clearance of xeno-oestrogens and hormone metabolites.

Management principles

The main factors are supporting healthy functioning of hormones, eliminating excess oestrogens, avoiding re-entering of endogenous oestrogen in the blood stream. This can be a worrying and psychologically distressing condition, and management of that side of it will also help the hormonal picture—but will also be helped by the diet and lifestyle changes. Not all the treatment suggestions below will apply to every patient but there should be enough to be a help.

Diet

- Vegetable and fruit-rich
- Include soy, flaxseed, nuts, seeds, probiotics for microbiome health and to moderate oestrogen dominance
- Nutritional support: Nutrient rich diet, including B vitamins, organic foods (minerals including calcium, magnesium)

Exercise and lifestyle

- Aerobic exercise will increase haemoglobin and red cell count and decrease levels of free oestradiol. Healthy exercising will stimulate thyroid function and metabolism, and improve bone density.
- Calmness is very helpful. Yoga or other gentle, meditative pursuits, a daily walk and/or absorption in a relaxing hobby can be of great benefit.
- No smoking: it alters metabolism of oestrogen.
- Health of the pelvic area is improved through belly dancing, pelvic floor exercises, hula hoop.

Herbal treatment

Bitters will help with the absorption of nutrients: *Taraxacum offinale, Gentiana lutea, Centaurium erythraea, Artemisia absinthium, Chamomilla recutita, Achillea millefolium,* etc.

Herbs that encourage healthy gut flora include garlic, *Berberis vulgaris, Artemisia absinthium,* bitters in general and slippery elm, and of course flaxseeds.

Assist oestrogen clearance with liver herbs: *Carduus marianus* as a restorative if there is a concern over possible liver damage, herbs such as *Taraxacum officinale* radix, *Berberis vulgaris* or *Fumaria officinalis* (among many) to stimulate. Lipotrophic factors such as choline in *Taraxacum officinalis* radix help with removal of fat and bile in the liver through interaction with fat metabolism, and have a decongesting effect on the liver.

Constipation needs to be treated. Often an apparent lack of progesterone is actually a relative excess of oestrogen and can be related to the reabsorption of oestrogen metabolites from the colon: gentle laxatives, such as *Taraxacum officinalis* radix, *Rumex crispus,* flaxseeds are indicated.

Specific herbs for oestrogen dominance include *Vitex agnus-castus,* Paeonia and Glycyrrhiza combination.

Uterine decongestants/tonics include *Achillea millefolium, Angelica sinensis* (avoid this herb during period in the case of heavy bleeding)

Lymphatics: *Thuja occidentalis*

Antihaemorrhagic herbs: *Capsella bursa-pastoris, Alchemilla vulgaris, Achillea millefolium*

Endometriosis, adenomyosis

Hormonal picture

Oestrogen dominance, poor clearance of xeno-oestrogens and hormone metabolites. The level of oestrogen and relative lack of progesterone create a pro-inflammatory background.[1]

Management principles

The main factors are supporting healthy functioning of hormones, eliminating excess oestrogens, avoiding the re-entering of endogenous oestrogen into the blood stream, promoting oestrogen-progesterone balance and managing inflammation. Pain management and managing extreme menstrual discomfort are also a priority.

Diet

- Omega 3 oils are particularly useful, so fatty fish
- Vegetable and fruit-rich, particularly dark green and red/purple foods
- Include soy, flaxseed, nuts, seeds, probiotics for microbiome health and to moderate oestrogen dominance
- Nutritional support: Nutrient rich diet, including the vitamins B (particularly B_6), C, E

Exercise and lifestyle

- Aerobic exercise to increase haemoglobin and red cell count, and decrease levels of free oestradiol. Healthy exercising will help with metabolism, thyroid function, and bone density.
- Calmness is so helpful. Yoga or other gentle, meditative pursuits, a daily walk and/or absorption in a relaxing hobby help to regain psychological balance.
- No smoking: it alters metabolism of oestrogen.
- Health of the pelvic area is improved through belly dancing, pelvic floor exercises, hula hoop.

Herbal treatment

As for the management of fibroids, bitters for absorption: *Taraxacum officinale, Gentiana lutea, Centaurium erythraea, Artemisia absinthium, Chamomilla recutita, Achillea millefolium*, etc.

Herbs that encourage healthy gut flora include garlic, *Berberis vulgaris, Artemisia absinthium*, bitters in general and slippery elm, and of course flaxseeds.

Assist oestrogen clearance including *Taraxacum officinale* radix, *Berberis vulgaris* or *Fumaria officinalis* (among many). Lipotrophic factors such as choline in *Taraxacum officinalis* radix to help with removal of fat and bile.

Treat constipation to correct relative oestrogen excess using gentle laxatives such as *Taraxacum officinalis* radix, *Rumex crispus*; flaxseeds are also indicated.

Cimicifuga racemosa is extremely useful, not only for its oestrogen-balancing effect but also its anti-inflammatory, nervine and anodyne properties. *Vitex agnus-castus* may help to regularise the menstrual cycle and correct luteal phase deficiency.

Pelvic pain and inflammation: *Anenome pulsatilla, Viburnum prunifolium, Cimicifuga racemosa*

Lymphatics: *Calendula officinalis*

Against scarring: *Hydrocotyle asiatica*, vitamin E

Anti-inflammatory: *Zingiber officinalis, Cimicifuga racemosa, Curcuma longa*, resveratrol

Bleeding: *Panax notoginseng, Capsella bursa-pastoris, Alchemilla vulgaris, Achillea millefolium*

Infertility/ovulation: *Chamaelirium luteum* (if obtainable from sustainable sources), *Alchemilla vulgaris, Tribulus terrestris, Angelica sinensis, Vitex agnus-castus*. NB treatment of the hormonal and inflammatory picture itself should help greatly.

PCOS

Hormonal picture

A complex disease closely related to metabolic syndrome, i.e. insulin resistance, difficulty controlling weight, and low-grade chronic inflammation associated with cardiovascular risk factors. Symptoms result from disturbed ovarian function and androgen excess. The tendency to put on weight except under carbohydrate restriction is hypothesised by some to have had an evolutionary value in earlier times during famine, in which more women with the characteristic genotype would have maintained fertility better than others.[2]

Management principles

Control weight, reduce inflammatory intermediates and thus normalise ovarian function, increase fertility (if that is what the patient wants!) and improve cardiovascular health.

Diet

- Low carbohydrate diet (less than 30% of calories consumed)
- Omega 3 oils are particularly useful, so fatty fish (also for vitamin D content)
- Nuts and seeds
- Gut biome-friendly diet including soluble fibre (flaxseeds, beans and pulses in particular)
- Vegetable and fruit-rich, particularly dark green and red/purple foods
- Folic acid is important but an organic, vegetable-rich diet should provide enough

Exercise

Exercise has a triple benefit of reducing the effect of stress, which tends to exacerbate inflammation and the production of glucocorticoids, helping the circulation and consuming excess energy.

Herbal treatment

Lipotrophic factors such as choline in *Taraxacum officinale* radix help with removal of fat and bile in the liver through interaction with fat metabolism, and have a decongesting effect on the liver. Liver herbs in general help with hormonal balance such as *Berberis vulgaris* or *Fumaria officinalis* to stimulate and *Carduus marianus* as a restorative if there are reasons to suspect liver debility.

Herbs to encourage healthy gut flora: garlic, *Verbena officinalis*, *Berberis vulgaris*, *Taraxacum officinalis* radix, Artemisia absinthium, bitters in general, and slippery elm powder.

For the hormonal aspects, Vitex agnus-castus (low dosage) helps normalise ovarian function. Cimicifuga is both nervine and normalises high LH levels, and Paeonia and Glycyrrhiza combination, *Serenoa repens* may help with reducing free androgens. Flaxseed and soy increase SHBG and so reduce the level of free testosterone, and nettle root might potentially be useful in this way, too. *Humulus lupulus* may help as both oestrogenic, bitter, and helpful with stress.

Other herbs to help with stress include *Hypericum perforatum*, *Verbena officinalis* (cooling), *Avena sativa*, *Leonurus cardiaca*, *Melissa officinalis*,

Cimicifuga racemosa, *Rosa damascena*, and *Withania somnifera*. *Withania* is traditionally used to help with weight gain, so should be used with caution, but it has adrenal-sparing properties and is calming. *Angelica sinensis* is anti-inflammatory as well as being an emmenagogues and uterine tonic.

For insulin resistance: *Cinnamonum cassia*, *Gymnema sylvestris*, *Glycyrrhiza* spp., *Galega officinalis*, *Trigonella foenum-graecum*, *Curcuma longa*, and a high intake of beans and pulses.[3]

In clinical trials of fertility in women with PCOS, *Cimicifuga racemosa* has performed well. A number of steroidal plants may also be indicated, e.g. *Chamaelirium luteum*, *Tribulus terrestris*, *Dioscorea villosa*, and *Asparagus racemosus*. Some practitioners also recommend using these for 10 days in the early follicular phase, or 10 days every month. Another potentially useful herb is *Serenoa repens*, as it is antiandrogenic. A number of successful trials have been done with fennel cream for hirsutism.[4]

Fibrocystic breasts

Hormonal picture

As with PMS, the cause is not clear as the components, including lumps, cysts, hyperplasia of cells in the milk ducts or lobules, and adenosis can be related to both prolactin and oestrogen secretion.

Management: tissue health

Part of the treatment consists of a generally anti-inflammatory strategy with a focus on this area:

- Restrict saturated fats, increase omega 3, dietary fibre, phytoestrogens (e.g. linseeds), brassicas, avoid alcohol.
- Vitamins E, B_1, B_6, and B_{12}.
- Arm exercises, and a cold shower to finish off in the arm and breast area will support circulation.
- Lymphatics are also extremely useful, including *Calendula officinalis*, *Phytolacca americana*, *Galium aparine*, and circulatory and anti-inflammatory herbs such as *Ginkgo biloba* and *Zingiber officinalis*.
- Iodine has been shown to help with fibrocystic breast disease. Sources include *Fucus vesiculosis* and other seaweeds, and also *Taraxacum officinalis* fol.

Management: hormonal health

Longer-term treatment involves supporting healthy functioning of hormones, eliminating excess oestrogens, and avoiding the re-entry of endogenous oestrogen metabolites into the blood stream.

- Constipation, if present, needs to be treated. Often an apparent lack of progesterone is actually a relative excess of oestrogen and enterohepatic recirculation is a potential factor. Gentle laxatives include *Taraxacum officinalis* radix, *Rumex crispus*, and flaxseeds.
- To support the role of the liver in oestrogen clearance use *Carduus marianus* as a restorative and herbs such as *Berberis vulgaris* or fumitory to stimulate. Lipotrophic factors such as choline in *Taraxacum officinalis* radix help with removal of fat and bile and support the elimination of excess oestrogen.
- Encourage healthy gut flora: garlic, *Berberis vulgaris*, *Artemisia absinthum*, *Taraxacum officinalis* radix and folia, slippery elm, and bitters in general.
- *Paeonia lactiflora* and *Glycyrrhiza glabra* combination and *Vitex agnus-castus* will promote a healthy oestrogen/progesterone balance.

NOTES

Foreword

1. Block KI, Mead MN. (2003). Immune system effects of Echinacea, Ginseng, and Astragalus: A review. *Integrative Cancer Therapies*, 247–67. https://doi.org/10.1177/1534735403256419

Chapter one

1. Abdull Razis AF, Bagatta M, De Nicola GR, Iori R, Ioannides C. (2010). Intact glucosinolates modulate hepatic cytochrome P450 and phase II conjugation activities and may contribute directly to the chemopreventive activity of cruciferous vegetables. *Toxicology*. 9;277(1–3):74–85.
2. Michnovicz JJ, Bradlow HL. (1990). Induction of estradiol metabolism by dietary indole-3-carbinol in humans. *J Natl Cancer Inst*. 6;82(11):947–9.
3. Chow HH, Garland LL, Hsu CH, Vining DR, Chew WM, Miller JA, et al. (2010). Resveratrol modulates drug- and carcinogen-metabolizing enzymes in a healthy volunteer study. *Cancer Prev Res (Phila)*. 3(9):1168–75.

4. Bradlow HL, Sepkovic DW, Telang N, Tiwari R. (2011). Adipocyte-derived factor as a modulator of oxidative estrogen metabolism: implications for obesity and estrogen-dependent breast cancer. *In Vivo.* 25(4):585–8.
5. Knudsen JG, Bertholdt L, Gudiksen A, Gerbal-Chaloin S, Rasmussen MK. (2018). Skeletal muscle interleukin-6 regulates hepatic cytochrome P450 expression; effects of 16 weeks high fat diet and exercise. *Toxicol Sci.* 162(1):309–17
6. Smith AJ, Phipps WR, Thomas W, Schmitz KH, Kurzer MS. (2013). The effects of aerobic exercise on estrogen metabolism in healthy premenopausal women. *Cancer Epidemiol Biomarkers Prev.* 22(5): 756–64.
7. Agbor LN, Wiest EF, Rothe M, Schunck WH, Walker MK. (2014). Role of CYP1A1 in modulating the vascular and blood pressure benefits of omega-3 polyunsaturated fatty acids. *J Pharmacol Exp Ther.* 351(3):688–98.
8. Dikshit A, Hales K, Hales DB. (2017). Whole flaxseed diet alters estrogen metabolism to promote 2-methoxtestradiol-induced apoptosis in hen ovarian cancer. *J Nutr Biochem.* 42:117–25.
9. Kall MA, Vang O, Clausen J. (1996). Effects of dietary broccoli on human in vivo drug metabolizing enzymes: evaluation of caffeine, oestrone and chlorzoxazone metabolism. *Carcinogenesis.* 17(4):793–9.
10. Walters DG, Young PJ, Agus C, Knize MG, Boobis AR, Gooderham NJ, et al. (2004). Cruciferous vegetable consumption alters the metabolism of the dietary carcinogen 2-amino-1-methyl-6-phenylimidazo[4,5-b] pyridine (PhIP) in humans. *Carcinogenesis.* 25(9):1659–69.
11. Hakooz N. (2007). Effects of dietary broccoli on human *in vivo* caffeine metabolism: a pilot study on a group of Jordanian volunteers. *Curr Drug Metab.* 8(1):9–15.
12. Peterson S, Schwarz Y, Li SS, Li L, King IB, Chen C, et al. (2009). CYP1A2, GSTM1, and GSTT1 polymorphisms and diet effects on CYP1A2 activity in a crossover feeding trial. *Cancer Epidemiol Biomarkers Prev.* 18(11):3118–25.
13. Chen Y, Xiao P, Ou-Yang DS, Fan L, Guo D, Wang YN, et al. (2009). Simultaneous action of the flavonoid quercetin on cytochrome P450 (CYP) 1A2, CYP2A6, N-acetyltransferase and xanthine oxidase activity in healthy volunteers. *Clin Exp Pharmacol Physiol.* 36(8):828–33.
14. Peng WX, Li HD, Zhou HH. (2003). Effect of daidzein on CYP1A2 activity and pharmacokinetics of theophylline in healthy volunteers. *Eur J Clin Pharmacol.* 59(3):237–41.

15. Fuhr U, Klittich K, Staib AH. (1993). Inhibitory effect of grapefruit juice and its bitter principal, naringenin, on CYP1A2 dependent metabolism of caffeine in man. *Br J Clin Pharmacol.* 35(4):431–6.
16. Hodges RE, Minich DM. (2015). Modulation of metabolic detoxification pathways using foods and food-derived components: A scientific review with clinical application. *J Nutr Metab.* 2015:760689.
17. Cho HJ, Yoon IS. (2015). Pharmacokinetic Interactions of Herbs with Cytochrome P450 and P-Glycoprotein. *Evid Based Complement Alternat Med.* 2015:736431.
18. Patri M, Padmini A, Babu PP. (2009). Polycyclic aromatic hydrocarbons in air and their neurotoxic potency in association with oxidative stress; a brief perspective. *Annals of Neurosciences.* 16:1.
19. Bretveld RW, Thomas CMG, Scheepers PTJ, Zielhuis GA, Roeleveld N. (2006). Pesticide exposure: the hormonal function of the female reproductive system disrupted? *Reprod Biol Endocrinol.* 4:30.
20. Tanaka S, Uchida S, Miyakawa S. (2013). Comparison of inhibitory duration of grapefruit juice on organic anion-transporting polypeptide and cytochrome P450 3A4. *Biological and Pharmaceutical Bulletin.* 36(12):1936–41.
21. Chow HHS, Garland L, Hsu CH, Vining DR, Chew WM, Miller JA, et al. (2010). Resveratrol modulates drug and carcinogen metabolizing enzymes in a healthy volunteer study. *Cancer Prevention Research (Philadelphia, PA.).* 3(9): 1168–75.
22. Al-Jenoobi F, Al-Thukair A, Alam M. (2014). Effect of garden cress seeds powder and its alcoholic extract on the metabolic activity of CYP2D6 and CYP3A4. *Evidence-Based Complementary and Alternative Medicine.* 2014, Article ID 634592.
23. Bogacz A, Bartkowiak-Wieczorek J, Mikołajczak PL, Rakoska-Mrozikiewicz B., Grzeskowiak E, Wolksi H, et al. (2014). Phe influence of soybean extract on the expression level of selected drug transporters, transcription factors and cytochrome P450 genes encoding phase I drug-metabolizing enzymes. *Ginekologia Polska.* 85(5):348–53.
24. Yamasaki I, Yamada M, Uotsu N, Teramoto S, Takayanagi R, Yamada Y. (2012). Inhibitory effects of kale ingestion on metabolism by cytochrome P450 enzymes in rats. *Biomedical Research.* 33(4):235–42.
25. Li C, Lim SC, Kim J, Choi JS. (2011). Effects of myricetin, an anticancer compound, on the bioavailability and pharmacokinetics of tamoxifen and its main metabolite, 4-hydroxytamoxifen, in rats. *Eur J of Drug Metabolism and Pharmacokinetics.* 36(3):175–82.

26. Obi N, Vrieling A, Heinz J, Chang-Claude J. (2011). Estrogen metabolite ratio: Is the 2-hydroxyestrone to 16α-hydroxyestrone ratio predictive for breast cancer? *Int J Womens Health.* 8;3:37–5.

Nishida CR, Everett S, Ortiz de Montellano PR. (2013). Specificity Determinants of CYP1B1 Estradiol Hydroxylation. *Molecular Pharmacology.* 84(3):451–8.

Eliassen H, Spiegelman D, Xia Xu K, Keefer L, Veenstra T, Barbieri R, et al. (2012). Urinary estrogens and estrogen metabolites and subsequent risk of breast cancer among premenopausal women. *Cancer Res.* 72(3): 696–706.

27. Schendzielorz N, Rysa A, Reenila I, Raasmaja A, Mannisto PT. (2011). Complex estrogenic regulation of catechol-O-methyltransferase (COMT) in rats. *J Physiol Pharmacol.* 62(4):483–90.

28. Zhou T, Chen Y, Huang C, Chen G. (2012). Caffeine induction of sulfotransferases in rat liver and intestine. *Journal of Applied Toxicology.* 32(10):804–9.

29. Maiti S, Chen X, Chen G. (2005). All-trans retinoic acid induction of sulfotransferases. *Basic and Clinical Pharmacology and Toxicology.* 96(1): 44–53.

30. Chang JL, Bigler J, Schwarz Y, Li SS, Li L, King IB, et al. (2007). UGT1A1 polymorphism is associated with serum bilirubin concentrations in a randomized, controlled, fruit and vegetable feeding trial. *Journal of Nutrition.* 137(4):890–7.

31. Navarro SL, Peterson S, Chen C, Makar KW, Schwarz Y, King IB, et al. (2009). Cruciferous vegetable feeding alters UGT1A1 activity: diet- and genotype-dependent changes in serum bilirubin in a controlled feeding trial. *Cancer Prevention Research (Philadelphia, Pa.).* 2(4):345–52.

32. Chow HHS, Garland L, Hsu CH, Vining DR, Chew WM, Miller JA, et al. (2010). Resveratrol Modulates Drug and Carcinogen Metabolizing Enzymes in a Healthy Volunteer Study. *Cancer Prevention Research.* 3(9):1168–75.

33. Saracino MR, Bigler J, Schwarz Y, Chang JL, Li S, Li L. et al. (2009). Citrus Fruit Intake Is Associated with Lower Serum Bilirubin Concentration among Women with the UGT1A1*28 Polymorphism. *The Journal of Nutrition.* 139(3):555–60.

34. Maliakal PP, Wanwimolruk S. (2001). Effect of herbal teas on hepatic drug metabolizing enzymes in rats. *J of Pharmacy and Pharmacology.* 53(10):1323–9.

35. Kosmala M, Zduńczyk Z, Kołodziejczyk K, Klimczak E, Jukiewicz J, Zduńczyk P. (2014). Chemical composition of polyphenols extracted from strawberry pomace and their effect on physiological properties of diets supplemented with different types of dietary fibre in rats. *Eur J of Nutr*. 53(2):521–32.
36. Kwa M, Plottel CS, Blaser MJ, Adams S. (2016). The Intestinal Microbiome and Estrogen Receptor–Positive Female Breast Cancer. *J Natl Cancer Inst*. 108(8).
37. De Preter V, Raemen H, Cloetens L, Houben E, Rutgeerts P, Verbeke K. (2008). Effect of dietary intervention with different pre- and probiotics on intestinal bacterial enzyme activities. *Eur J Clin Nutr*. 62(2):225–31.
38. Krishnan S, Tryon RR, Horn WF, Welch L, Keim NL. (2016). Estradiol, SHBG and leptin interplay with food craving and intake across the menstrual cycle. *Physiol Behav*. 165:304–12.
39. Park CY, Weaver CM. (2012). Vitamin D Interactions with Soy Isoflavones on Bone after Menopause: A Review. *Nutrients*. 4(11):1610–21.
40. Sáez-López C, Soriguer F, Hernandez C, Rojo-Martinez G, Rubio-Martín E, Simó R, et al. (2014). Oleic acid increases hepatic sex hormone binding globulin production in men. *Mol Nutr Food Res*. 58(4):760–7.
41. Huang M, Liu J, Lin X, Goto A, Song Y, Tinker LF, et al. (2017). Relationship between dietary carbohydrates intake and circulating sex hormone-binding globulin levels in postmenopausal women. *J Diabetes*. 10(6):467–77.
42. Longcope C, Feldman HA, McKinlay JB, Araujo AB. (2000). Diet and Sex Hormone-Binding Globulin. *J of Clin End & Met*. 85:1:293–6.
43. Brinkman MT, Baglietto L, Krishnan K, English DR, Severi G, Morris HA, et al. (2010). Consumption of animal products, their nutrient components and postmenopausal circulating steroid hormone concentrations. *Eur J Clin Nutr*. 64(2):176–83.
44. Sinha D, Sarkar N, Biswas J, Bishayee A. (2016). Resveratrol for breast cancer prevention and therapy: Preclinical evidence and molecular mechanisms. *Semin Cancer Biol*. 40–1:209–32.
45. McCann SE, Edge SB, Hicks DG. (2014). A pilot study comparing the effect of flaxseed, aromatase inhibitor, and the combination on breast tumor biomarkers. *Nutr Cancer*. 66(4):566–75.
46. Grube BJ, Eng ET, Kao YC, Kwon A, Chen S. (2001). White button mushroom phytochemicals inhibit aromatase activity and breast cancer cell proliferation. *J Nutr*. 131(12):3288–93.

47. Eng ET, Ye J, Williams D, Phung S, Moore RE, Young MK, Gruntmanis U, Braunstein G, Chen S. (2003). Suppression of estrogen biosynthesis by procyanidin dimers in red wine and grape seeds. *Cancer Res.* 63(23):8516–22.
48. Balunas MJ, Su B, Brueggemeier RW, Kinghorn AD. (2008). Xanthones from the botanical dietary supplement mangosteen (Garcinia mangostana) with aromatase inhibitory activity. *J Nat Prod.* 71(7):1161–6.
49. Park YJ, Choo WH, Kim HR, Chung KH, Oh SM. (2015). Inhibitory aromatase effects of flavonoids from *Ginkgo Biloba* Extracts on estrogen biosynthesis. *Asian Pac J Cancer Prev.* 16(15):6317–25.
50. Li F, Ye L, Lin SM, Leung LK. (2011). Dietary flavones and flavonones display differential effects on aromatase (CYP19) transcription in the breast cancer cells MCF-7. *Mol Cell Endocrinol.* 344(1–2):51–8.
51. Satoh K, Sakamoto Y, Ogata A, Nagai F, Mikuriya H, Numazawa M, Yamada K, Aoki N. (2002). Inhibition of aromatase activity by green tea extract catechins and their endocrinological effects of oral administration in rats. *Food Chem Toxicol.* 40(7):925–33.
52. Balunas MJ, Su B, Brueggemeier RW, Kinghorn AD. (2008). Natural products as aromatase inhibitors. *Anticancer Agents Med Chem.* 8(6):646–82.
53. Brown K, DeCoffe D, Molcan E, Gibson DL. (2012). Diet-Induced Dysbiosis of the Intestinal Microbiota and the Effects on Immunity and Disease. *Nutrients.* 4(8): 1095–119.
54. Khodarahmi M, Azadbakht L. (2014). The association between different kinds of fat intake and breast cancer risk in women. *Int J Prev Med.* 5(1): 6–15.
55. Heard ME, Melnyk SB, Simmen FA, Yang Y, Pabona JMP, Simmen RCM. (2016). High-Fat Diet Promotion of Endometriosis in an Immunocompetent Mouse Model is Associated With Altered Peripheral and Ectopic Lesion Redox and Inflammatory Status. *Endocrinology.* 157(7):2870–82.
56. Flores R, Shi J, Gail MH, Gajer P, Ravel J, Goedert JJ. (2012). Association of Fecal Microbial Diversity and Taxonomy with Selected Enzymatic Functions. *PLoS ONE.* 7(6):e39745.
57. Gaskins AJ, Mumford SL, Zhang C, Wactawski-Wende J, Hovey KM, Whitcomb BW, et al. (2009). Effect of daily fiber intake on reproductive function: the BioCycle Study. *Am J Clin Nutr.* 90(4):1061–1069.
58. Kwa M, Plottel CS, Blaser MJ, Adam S. (2016). The Intestinal Microbiome and Estrogen Receptor–Positive Female Breast Cancer. *J Natl Cancer Inst.* 108(8):djw029.

59. Maggio M, de Vita F, Lauretani F, Bandinelli S, Semba RD, Bartali B, et al. (2015). Relationship between carotenoids, retinol, and estradiol levels in older women. *Nutrients.* 7(8):6506–19.
60. Hoch AZ, Papanek P, Szabo A, Widlansky ME, Schimke JE, Gutterman DD. (2011). Association between the female athlete triad and endothelial dysfunction in dancers. *Clin J Sport Med.* 21(2):119–25.
61. Oboni JB, Marques-Vidal P, Bastardot F, Vollenweider P, Waeber G. (2016). Impact of smoking on fertility and age of menopause: a population-based assessment. *BMJ Open.* 6(11): e012015.
62. Var C, Keller S, Tung R, Freeland D, Bazzano AN. (2014). Supplementation with vitamin B6 reduces side effects in Cambodian women using oral Contraception. *Nutrients.* 26;6(9):3353–62.
   Bailey LB, Gregory JF. (1999). 3rd Folate metabolism and requirements. *J Nutr.* 129:779–82.
63. Gavaler JS, Deal SR, Van Thiel DH, Arria A, Allan MJ. (1993). Alcohol and estrogen levels in postmenopausal women: the spectrum of effect. *Alcohol Clin Exp Res.* 17(4):786–90.
64. Roy JR, Chakraborty S, Chakraborty TR. (2009). Estrogen-like endocrine disrupting chemicals affecting puberty in humans – A review. *Med Sci Monit.* 15:RA137–45.
65. Gibson DA, Saunders PT. (2014). Endocrine disruption of oestrogen action and female reproductive tract cancers. *Endocr Relat Cancer.* 21(2):T13–31.
66. Trabert B, Chen Z, Kannan K, Peterson CM, Pollack AZ, Sun L, et al. (2015). Persistent organic pollutants (POPs) and fibroids: results from the ENDO Study. *J Expo Sci Environ Epidemiol.* 25(3): 278–85.
67. Ganmaa D, Sato A. (2005). The possible role of female sex hormones in milk from cows in the development of breast, ovarian and corpus uteri cancers. *Medical Hypothesis.* 65:1028–37
68. Li MY, Liu Y, Liu LZ, et al. (2015). Estrogen receptor alpha promotes smoking-carcinogen-induced lung carcinogenesis via cytochrome P450 1B1. *J Mol Med.* 93:1221.
69. Majidi M, Al-Wadel HA, Takahashi T, Schuller HM. (2007). Nongenomic beta estrogen receptor enchance beta1 adrenergic signaling induced by the nicotine-derived carcinogen 4-(methylnitrosamino)-1-(3-pyridyl)-1-butanone in human small airway epithelial cells. *Cancer Res.* 67:6863–74.
70. Misaki K, Suzuki M, Nakamura M, Handa H, Iida M, Kato T, et al. (2008). Aryl hydrocarbon receptor and estrogen receptor ligand activity

of organic extracts from road dust and diesel exhaust particulates. *Arch Environ Contam Toxicol.* 55:199–209.

71. Henson MC, Chedrese PJ. (2004). Endocrine disruption by cadmium, a common environmental toxicant with paradoxical effects on reproduction. *Exp Biol Med.* 229:383–92.
72. Fucic A, Gamulin M, Ferencic Z, Katic J, Krayer von Krauss M, Bartonova A, Merlo DF. (2012). Environmental exposure to xenoestrogens and oestrogen related cancers: reproductive system, breast, lung, kidney, pancreas, and brain. *Environmental Health: A Global Access Science Source.* 11(Suppl 1):S8. doi:10.1186/1476-069X-11-S1-S8.
73. Bonner MR, Han D, Nie J, Rogerson P, Vena JE, Muti P, et al. (2005). Breast cancer risk and exposure in early life to polycyclic aromatic hydrocarbons using total suspended particulates as a proxy measure. *Cancer Epidemiol Biomarkers Prev.* 14(1):53–60.
74. Ohayama K, Magai F, Tsuchiya Y. (2001). Certain styrene oligomers have proliferative activity on MCF-7 cells and binding affinity for human estrogen receptor alpha. *EHP.* 109:699–703.
75. Darbre PD. (2009). Underarm antiperspirants/deodorants and breast cancer. *Breast Cancer Res.* 11(Suppl 3):S5.
76. Wada H, Tarumi H, Imazato S, Narimatsu M, Ebisu S. (2004). In vitro estrogenicity of resin composites. *Journal of Dental Research.* 83;3:222–6.
77. Schrader TJ, GM Cooke. (2000). Examination of selected food additives and organochlorine food contaminants for androgenic activity in vitro. *Toxicological Sciences.* 53;2:278–88.
78. Henley DV, Korach KS. (2006). Endocrine-disrupting chemicals use distinct mechanisms of action to modulate endocrine system function. *Endocrinology.* 147;6: S25–32.

    Barlow NJ, McIntyre BS, Foster PM. (2004). Male reproductive tract lesions at 6, 12, and 18 months of age following in utero exposure to di(n-butyl) phthalate. *Toxicologic Pathology.* 32;1: 79–90.
79. DG Environment, Delft, Netherlands: RPS BKH Consulting Engineers (2002).

    Towards the establishment of a priority list of substances for further evaluation of their role in endocrine disruption, *Final Report to European Commission.* http://ec.europa.eu/environment/endocrine/documents/bkh_report.pdf.
80. DG Environment, Delft, Netherlands: RPS BKH Consulting Engineers. (2000). Study on Gathering Information on 435 Substances with Insufficient Data. Final Report to European Commission. http://ec.europa.eu/environment/docum/pdf/bkh_annex_13.pdf.

NOTES   269

81. Griffin S. (2007). *CancerSmart 3.0: The Consumer Guide* (Vancouver: Labour Environmental Alliance Society, 2007).
82. Engeli R, Rohrer S, Vuorinen A, Herdlinger S, Kaserer T, Leugger S, et al. (2017). Interference of Paraben Compounds with Estrogen Metabolism by Inhibition of 17β-Hydroxysteroid Dehydrogenases. *International Journal of Molecular Sciences*. 18(9):2007. doi:10.3390/ijms18092007
83. Darbre PD, Aljarrah A, Miller WR, Coldham NG, Sauer MJ, Pope GS. (2004). Concentrations of parabens in human breast tumours. *Journal of Applied Toxicology*. 24:5–13.
84. Darbre PD, Harvey PW. (2008). Paraben esters: review of recent studies of endocrine toxicity, absorption, esterase and human exposure, and discussion of potential human health risks. *Journal of Applied Toxicology*. 28;5:561–78.
85. DHI Water and Environment. (2007). Study on Enhancing the Endocrine Disrupter Priority List with a Focus on Low Production Volume Chemicals. *Revised Report to DG Environment*. Hersholm, Denmark: DHI. http://ec.europa.eu/environment/endocrine/documents/final_report_2007.pdf.
86. Moss T, Howes D, Williams FM. (2000). Percutaneous penetration and dermal metabolism of triclosan (2,4,4'-trichloro-2'-hydroxydiphenyl ether). *Food Chem Toxicol*. 38:361–70.
87. Erler C, Novak J. (2010). Bisphenol a exposure: Human risk and health policy. *J Pediatr Nurs*. 25:400–7.
88. Meert Meerts IA, Letcher RJ, Hoving S, Marsh G, Bergman A, Lemmen JG, et al. (2001). In vitro estrogenicity of polybrominated diphenyl ethers, hydroxylated PDBEs, and polybrominated bisphenol A compounds. *Environ Health Perspect*. 109(4):399–407.
89. Bretveld RW, Thomas CM, Scheepers PT, Zielhuis GA, Roeleveld N. (2006). Pesticide exposure: the hormonal function of the female reproductive system disrupted. *Reprod Biol Endocrinol*. 4:30.
90. Morito K, Aomori T, Hirose T, Kinjo J, Hasegawa J, Ogawa S, et al. (2002). Interaction of phytoestrogens with estrogen receptors alpha and beta (II). *Biol Pharm Bull*. 25(1):48–52.

Chapter two

1. Cani PD, Knauf C. (2016). How gut microbes talk to organs: The role of endocrine and nervous routes. *Molecular metabolism*. 5(9):743–52. doi:10.1016/j.molmet.2016.05.011.

2. Rastelli M, Knauf C, Cani PD. (2018). Gut Microbes and Health: A Focus on the Mechanisms Linking Microbes, Obesity, and Related Disorders. *Obesity (Silver Spring, Md.)*. 26(5):792–800.
3. Browning S, Verheijden S, Boeckxstaens G. (2017). The Vagus nerve in appetite regulation, mood, and intestinal inflammation. *Gastroenterology*. 152(4):730–44. https://doi.org/10.1053/j.gastro.2016.10.046.
4. Neuman H, Debelius J, Knight R, Koren O. (2015). Microbial endocrinology: the interplay between the microbiota and the endocrine system. *FEMS Microbiology Reviews*. 39(4):509–21. https://doi.org/10.1093/femsre/fuu010.
5. Greiner TU, Bäckhed F. (2016). Microbial regulation of GLP-1 and L-cell biology. *Molecular Metabolism*. 5(9):753–8. doi:10.1016/j.molmet.2016.05.012.
6. Rea K, Dinan T, Cryan J. (2016). The microbiome: A key regulator of stress and neuroinflammation. *Neurobiology of Stress*. 4:23–33. https://doi.org/10.1016/j.ynstr.2016.03.001.
7. Walsh C, Guinane C, O'Toole P, Cotter P. (2014). Beneficial modulation of the gut microbiota. *FEBS Letters*. 588(22):4120–30. https://doi.org/10.1016/j.febslet.2014.03.035.
8. DiPatrizio NV, Piomelli D. (2012). The thrifty lipids: endocannabinoids and the neural control of energy conservation. *Trends in Neurosciences*. 35(7):403–11.
9. Watkins BA, Kim J. (2015). The endocannabinoid system: directing eating behavior and macronutrient metabolism. *Frontiers in Psychology*. 5:1506. doi:10.3389/fpsyg.2014.01506.
10. Raduner S, et al. (2006). Alkylamides from Echinacea are a new class of cannabinomimetics. Cannabinoid type 2 receptor-dependent and -independent immunomodulatory effects. *J Biol Chem*. 281:14192–206.
11. Bhathena SJ. (2006). Relationship between fatty acids and the endocrine and neuroendocrine system. *Nutr Neurosci*. 9(1–2):1–10.
12. Seo D, Patrick CJ, Kennealy PJ. (2008). Role of serotonin and dopamine system interactions in the neurobiology of impulsive aggression and its comorbidity with other clinical disorders. *Aggression And Violent Behavior*. 13(5):383–95.
13. Bennesch MA, Picard D. (2015). Minireview: Tipping the balance: ligand-independent activation of steroid receptors. *Mol Endocrinol*. 29(3):349–63.
14. Au A, Feher A, McPhee L, Jessa A, Oh S, Einstein G. (2016). Estrogens, inflammation and cognition. *Frontiers in Neuroendocrinology*. 40:87–100.

15. Catanzaro M, Corsini E, Rosini M, Racchi M, Lanni C. (2018). Immunomodulators Inspired by Nature: A Review on Curcumin and Echinacea. *Molecules (Basel, Switzerland)*. 23(11):2778. doi:10.3390/molecules2311 2778.
16. Lin TW, Kuo YM. (2013). Exercise benefits brain function: the monoamine connection. *Brain Sciences*. 3(1):39–53. doi:10.3390/brainsci3010039.
17. Woods JA, Wilund KR, Martin SA, Kistler BM. (2011). Exercise, inflammation and aging. *Aging and Disease*. 3(1):130–40.
18. Allen JM, Mailing LJ, Niemiro GM, Moore R, Cook MD, White BA, Holscher HD, Woods JA. (2018). Exercise Alters Gut Microbiota Composition and Function in Lean and Obese Humans. *Med Sci Sports Exerc*. 50(4):747–57. doi:10.1249/MSS.0000000000001495.
19. Münger E, Montiel-Castro AJ, Langhans W, Pacheco-López G. (2018). Reciprocal Interactions Between Gut Microbiota and Host Social Behavior. *Frontiers in Integrative Neuroscience*. 12:21. doi:10.3389/fnint.2018.00021.
20. Pellizzon MA, Billheimer JT, Bloedon LT, Szapary PO, Rader DJ. (2007). Flaxseed reduces plasma cholesterol levels in hypercholesterolemic mouse models. *J Am Coll Nutr*. 26:66–75.
21. Goyal A, Sharma V, Upadhyay N, Gill S, Sihag M. (2014). Flax and flaxseed oil: an ancient medicine & modern functional food. *J Food Sci Technol*. 51(9):1633–53.
22. Kilkkinen A, Stumpf K, Pietinen P, Valsta LM, Tapanainen H, Adlercreutz H. (2001). Determinants of serum enterolactone concentration. *Am J Clin Nutr*. 73:1094–100.
23. Adlercreutz H, Höckerstedt K, Bannwart C, Bloigu S, Hämäläinen E, Fotsis T, et al. (1987). Effect of dietary components, including lignans and phytoestrogens, on enterohepatic circulation and liver metabolism of estrogens and on sex hormone binding globulin (SHBG). *Journal of Steroid Biochemistry*. 27;4–6:1135–44.
24. Martin ME, Haourigui M, Pelissero C, Benassayag C, Nunez EA. (1996). Interactions between phytoestrogens and human sex steroid binding protein. *Life Sci*. 58(5):429–36.
25. McCann SE, Muti P, Vito D, Edge SB, Trevisan M, Freudenheim JL. (2004). Epidemiology. Dietary lignan intakes and risk of pre- and postmenopausal breast cancer. *International Journal of Cancer*. 111;3: 440–3.

26. Kreydin EI, Kim MM, Barrisford GW, Rodriguez D, Sanchez A, Santiago-Lastra Y, et al. (2015). Urinary Lignans Are Associated With Decreased Incontinence in Postmenopausal Women. *Urology.* 86(4):716–20.
27. Wang C, Mäkelä T, Hase T, Adlercreutz H, Kurzer MS. (1994). Lignans and flavonoids inhibit aromatase enzyme in human preadipocytes. *Steroid Biochem Mol Biol.* 50(3–4):205–12.
28. Cristoni A, Di Pierro F, Bombardelli E. (2000). Botanical derivatives for the prostate. *Fitoterapia.* 71(1)1:S21–S28.
29. Brooks JD, Thompson LU. (2005). Mammalian lignans and genistein decrease the activities of aromatase and 17beta-hydroxysteroid dehydrogenase in MCF-7 cells. *J Steroid Biochem Mol Biol.* 94(5):461–7.
30. Cetisli NE, Saruhan A, Kivcak B. (2015). The effects of flaxseed on menopausal symptoms and quality of life. *Holist Nurs Pract.* 29(3):151–7.
31. Colli MC, Bracht A, Soares AA, de Oliveira AL, Bôer CG, de Souza CG, et al. (2012). Evaluation of the efficacy of flaxseed meal and flaxseed extract in reducing menopausal symptoms. *J Med Food.* 15(9):840–5.
32. Hutchins AM, Martini MC, Olson BA, Thomas W, Slavin JL. (2001). Flaxseed consumption influences endogenous hormone concentrations in postmenopausal women. *Nutr Cancer.* 39(1):58–65.
33. Hutchins AM, Martini MC, Olson BA, Thomas W, Slavin JL. (2001). Flaxseed consumption influences endogenous hormone concentrations in postmenopausal women. *Nutr Cancer.* 39(1):58–65.
34. Brooks JD, Ward WE, Lewis JE, Hilditch J, Nickell L, Wong E, Thompson LU. (2004). Supplementation with flaxseed alters estrogen metabolism in postmenopausal women to a greater extent than does supplementation with an equal amount of soy. *The Am J of Clin Nutr.* 79(2):318–25.
35. Nowak DA, Snyder DC, Brown AJ, Denmark-Wahnefried W. (2007). The Effect of Flaxseed Supplementation on Hormonal Levels Associated with Polycystic Ovarian Syndrome: A Case Study. *Curr Top Nutraceutical Res.* 5(4):177–81.
36. Dodin S, Lemay A, Jacques H, Légaré F, Forest JC, Mâsse B. (2005). The effects of flaxseed dietary supplement on lipid profile, bone mineral density, and symptoms in menopausal women: a randomized, double-blind, wheat germ placebo-controlled clinical trial. *J Clin Endocrinol Metab.* 90(3):1390–7.
37. Dodin S, Cunnane SC, Mâsse BR, Forest JC. (2008). Flaxseed on cardiovascular disease markers in healthy menopausal women: A randomized, double-blind, placebo-controlled trial. *Nutrition.* 24(1):23–30.

38. Lemay A, Dodin S, Kadri N, Jacques H, Forest JC. (2002). Flaxseed dietary supplement versus hormone replacement therapy in hypercholesterolemic menopausal women. *Obstet Gynecol.* 100(3):495–504.
39. Mirghafourvand M, Mohammad-Alizadeh-Charandabi S, Ahmadpour P, Javadzadeh Y. (2016). Effects of Vitex agnus and Flaxseed on cyclic mastalgia: A randomized controlled trial. *Complement Ther Med.* 24:90–5.
40. Goyal A, Sharma V, Upadhyay N, Gill S, Sihag M. (2014). Flax and flaxseed oil: an ancient medicine & modern functional food. *J Food Sci Technol.* 51(9):1633–53.
41. Thompson LU, Rickard SE, Cheung F. (1997). Variability in anticancer lignan levels in flaxseed. *Nutr Cancer.* 27:26–30.
42. Thompson LU, Rickard SE, Orcheson LJ, Seidl MM. (1997). Flaxseed and its lignan and oil components reduce mammary tumor growth at a late stage of carcinogenesis. *Carcinogenesis.* 17:1373–6.
43. Saggar JK, Chen J, Corey P, Thompson LU. (2010). Dietary flaxseed lignan or oil combined with tamoxifen treatment affects MCF-7 tumor growth through estrogen receptor- and growth factor-signaling pathways. *Mol Nutr Food Res.* 54(3):415–25.
44. Mason JK, Thompson LU. (2014). Flaxseed and its lignan and oil components: can they play a role in reducing the risk of and improving the treatment of breast cancer? *Appl Physiol Nutr Metab.* 39(6):663–78.
45. Mason JK, Chen J, Thompson LU. (2010). Flaxseed oil–trastuzumab interaction in breast cancer. *Food and Chem Toxicol.* 48(8–9):2223–6.
46. Chen J, Hui E, Ip T, Thompson LU. (2004). Dietary flaxseed enhances the inhibitory effect of tamoxifen on the growth of estrogen-dependent human breast cancer (mcf-7) in nude mice. *Clin Cancer Res.* 10:7703–11.
47. Saarinen NM, Tuominen J, Santti R, Pylkkänen L. Yagasaki K, Yamazaki M. (2008). Anticarcinogenic effects of lignans in breast and prostate – a critical review of the current knowledge. Kerala, India: Research Signpost. pp. 1–44. *Bromacology: Pharmacology of Foods and Their Components.*
48. Sonestedt E, Borgquist S, Ericson U. (2008). Enterolactone is differently associated with estrogen receptor beta-negative and -positive breast cancer in a Swedish nested case-control study. *Cancer Epidemiol Biomarkers Prev.* 17:3241–51.
49. Flower G, Fritz H, Balneaves LG, Verma S, Skidmore B, Fernandes R, et al. (2014). Flax and Breast Cancer: A Systematic Review. *Integr Cancer Ther.* 13(3):181–92.

50. Sturgeon SR, Heersink JL, Volpe SL, Bertone-Johnson ER, Puleo E, Stanczyk FZ, et al. (2008). Effect of Dietary Flaxseed on Serum Levels of Estrogens and Androgens in Postmenopausal Women. *Nutrition and Cancer*. 60(5):612–8.
51. Azrad M, Vollmer RT, Madden J, Dewhirst M, Polascik TJ, Snyder DC, et al. (2013). Flaxseed-Derived Enterolactone Is Inversely Associated with Tumor Cell Proliferation in Men with Localized Prostate Cancer. *J Med Food*. 16(4):357–60.
52. He J, Wang S, Zhou M, Yu W, Zhang, He X. (2015). Phytoestrogens and risk of prostate cancer: a meta-analysis of observational studies. *World J Surg Oncol*. 13:231.
53. Cotterchio M, Boucher BA, Manno M, Gallinger S, Okey A, Harper P. (2006). Dietary phytoestrogen intake is associated with reduced colorectal cancer risk. *J Nutr*. 136:3046–53.
54. Adlercreutz H. (1995). Phytoestrogens: Epidemiology and a Possible Role in Cancer Protection. *Environ Health Perspect*. 103(S7):103–12.
55. Prasad K, Mantha SV, Muir AD, Westcott ND. (2000). Protective effect of secoisolariciresinol diglucoside against streptozotocin-induced diabetes and its mechanism. *Mol Cell Biochem*. 206:141–9.
56. Lemay A, Dodin S, Kadri N, Jacques H, Forest JC. (2002). Flaxseed dietary supplement versus hormone replacement therapy in hypercholesterolemic menopausal women. *Obstet Gynecol*. 100:495–504.
57. Rhee Y, Brunt. (2011). A Flaxseed supplementation improved insulin resistance in obese glucose intolerant people: a randomized crossover design. *Nutr J*. 10:44.
58. Mani UV, Mani I, Biswas M, Kumar SN. (2011). An open-label study on the effect of flax seed powder (Linum usitatissimum) supplementation in the management of diabetes mellitus. *J Diet Suppl*. 8:257–65.
59. Ibrügger S, Kristensen M, Mikkelsen MS, Astrup A. (2012). Flaxseed dietary fiber supplements for suppression of appetite and food intake. *Appetite*. 58:490–5.
60. McCullough RS, Edel AL, Bassett CM, Lavallée R, Dibrov E, Blackwood DP, Ander BP, Pierce GN. (2011). The alpha linolenic acid content of flaxseed is associated with an induction of adipose leptin expression. *Lipids*. 46(11):1043–52.
61. Edel AL, Rodriguez-Leyva D, Maddaford TG, Caligiuri SP, Austria JA, Weighell W, et al. (2015). Dietary flaxseed independently lowers circulating cholesterol and lowers it beyond the effects of cholesterol-lowering medications alone in patients with peripheral artery disease. *J Nutr*. 145(4):749–57.

62. Prasad K. (2009). Flaxseed and cardiovascular health. *J Cardiovasc Pharmacol.* 54(5):369–77.
63. Lucas EA, Wild RD, Hammond LJ, Khalil DA, Juma S, Daggy BP, et al. (2002). Flaxseed improves lipid profile without altering biomarkers of bone metabolism in postmenopausal women. *J Clin Endocrinol Metab.* 87(4):1527–32.
64. Campbell SC, Bakhshalian N, Sadaat RL, Lerner MR, Lightfoot SA, Brackett D, et al. (2013). Flaxseed reverses atherosclerotic lesion formation and lowers lipoprotein(a) in ovarian hormone deficiency. *Menopause.* 20(11):1176–83.
65. Khalesi S, Irwin C, Schubert M. (2015). Flaxseed consumption may reduce blood pressure: a systematic review and meta-analysis of controlled trials. *J Nutr.* 145(4):758–65.
66. Clark WF, Parbtani A, Huff MW, Spanner E, de Salis H, Chin-Yee I, et al. (1995). Flaxseed: a potential treatment for lupus nephritis. *Kidney Int.* 48(2):475–80.
67. Khalatbari Soltani S, Jamaluddin R, Tabibi H, Mohd Yusof BN, Atabak S, Loh SP, et al. (2014). Effects of flaxseed consumption on systemic inflammation and serum lipid profile in hemodialysis patients with lipid abnormalities. *Hemodial Int.* 17(2):275–81.
68. Dodin S, Lemay A, Jacques H, Légaré F, Forest JC, Mâsse B. (2005). The effects of flaxseed dietary supplement on lipid profile, bone mineral density, and symptoms in menopausal women: a randomized, double-blind, wheat germ placebo-controlled clinical trial. *J Clin Endocrinol Metab.* 90(3):1390–7.
69. Inoguchi S, Ohashi Y, Narai-Kanayama A, Aso K, Nakagaki T, Fujisawa T. (2012). Effects of non-fermented and fermented soybean milk intake on faecal microbiota and faecal metabolites in humans. *Int J Food Sci Nutr.* 63:402–10.
70. Suarez FL. Springfield J. Furne JK, Lohrmann TT, Kerr PS, Levitt MD. (1999). Gas production in human ingesting a soybean flour derived from beans naturally low in oligosaccharides. *Am J Clin Nutr.* 69:135–9.
71. Tang AL, Walker KZ, Wilcox G, Strauss BJ, Ashton JF, Stojanovska L. (2010). Calcium absorption in Australian osteopenic post-menopausal women: An acute comparative study of fortified soymilk to cows milk. *Asia Pac J Clin Nutr.* 19:243–9.
72. Lonnerdal B, Bryant A, Liu X, Theil EC. (2006). Iron absorption from soybean ferritin in nonanemic women. *Am J Clin Nutr.* 83:103–7.
73. Katsuyama H, Ideguchi S, Fukunaga M, Saijoh K, Sunami S. (2002). Usual dietary intake of fermented soybeans (Natto) is associated with

bone mineral density in premenopausal women. *J Nutr Sci Vitaminol.* 48:207–15.

74. Murphy PA, Barua K, Hauck CC. (2002). Solvent extraction selection in the determination of isoflavones in soy foods. *J Chromatogr B Anal Technol Biomed Life Sci.* 777:129–38.

75. Adlercreutz H, Fotsis T, Bannwart C, Wähälä K, Mäkelä T, Brunow G, et al. (1986). Determination of urinary lignans and phytoestrogen metabolites, potential antiestrogens and anticarcinogens, in urine of women on various habitual diets. *J Steroid Biochem.* 25:791–7.

76. Van der Velpen V, Hollman PC, van Nielen M, Schouten EG, Mensink M, Van't Veer P, et al. (2014). Large inter-individual variation in isoflavone plasma concentration limits use of isoflavone intake data for risk assessment. *Eur J Clin Nutr.* 68:1141–7.

77. Taku K, Melby MK, Kronenberg F, Kurzer MS, Messina M. (2012). Extracted or synthesized soybean isoflavones reduce menopausal hot flash frequency and severity: Systematic review and meta-analysis of randomized controlled trials. *Menopause.* 19:776–90.

78. Hooper L, Ryder JJ, Kurzer MS, Lampe JW, Messina MJ, Phipps WR, et al. (2009). Effects of soy protein and isoflavones on circulating hormone concentrations in pre- and post-menopausal women: A systematic review and meta-analysis. *Hum Reprod Update.* 15:423–40.

79. Shahin AYIA, Zahran KM, Makhlouf AM. (2008). Adding phytoestrogens to clomiphene induction in unexplained infertility patients—a randomized trial. *Reprod Biomed.* 16:580–8.

Unfer VCM, Gerli S, Costabile L, Mignosa M, Di Renzo GC. (2004). Phytoestrogens may improve the pregnancy rate in in vitro fertilization-embryo transfer cycles: a prospective, controlled, randomized trial. *Fertil Steril.* 82:1509–13.

80. Muhlhauser A, Susiarjo M, Rubio C, Griswold J, Gorence G, Hassold T, et al. (2009). Bisphenol A effects on the growing mouse oocyte are influenced by diet. *Biol Reprod.* 80:1066–71.

81. Koh WP, Wu AH, Wang R, Ang LW, Heng D, Yuan JM, et al. (2009). Gender-specific associations between soy and risk of hip fracture in the Singapore Chinese Health Study. *Am J Epidemiol.* 170: 901–9.

Matthews VL, Knutsen SF, Beeson WL, Fraser GE. (2011). Soy milk and dairy consumption is independently associated with ultrasound attenuation of the heel bone among postmenopausal women: The Adventist Health Study-2. *Nutr Res.* 31:766–75.

Ma DF, Qin LQ, Wang PY, Katoh R. (2008). Soy isoflavone intake increases bone mineral density in the spine of menopausal women: Meta-analysis of randomized controlled trials. *Clin Nutr*. 27:57–64.

Ma DF, Qin LQ, Wang PY, Katoh R. (2008). Soy isoflavone intake inhibits bone resorption and stimulates bone formation in menopausal women: Meta-analysis of randomized controlled trials. *Eur J Clin Nutr*. 62:155–61.

Taku K, Melby MK, Takebayashi J, Mizuno S, Ishimi Y, Omori T, et al. (2010). Effect of soy isoflavone extract supplements on bone mineral density in menopausal women: Meta-analysis of randomized controlled trials. *Asia Pac J Clin Nutr*. 19:33–42.

82. Marini H, Bitto A, Altavilla D, Burnett BP, Polito F, Di Stefano V, et al. (2008). Breast safety and efficacy of genistein aglycone for postmenopausal bone loss: A follow-up study. *J Clin Endocrinol Metab*. 93:4787–96.
83. Korde LA, Wu AH, Fears T, Nomura AM, West DW, Kolonel LN, et al. (2009). Childhood soy intake and breast cancer risk in Asian American women. *Cancer Epidemiol Biomark Prev*. 18:1050–9.
84. Baglia ML, Zheng W, Li H, Yang G, Gao J, Gao YT, et al. (2016). The association of soy food consumption with the risk of subtype of breast cancers defined by hormone receptor and HER2 status. *Int J Cancer*. 139:742–8.
85. Russo J, Mailo D, Hu YF, Balogh G, Sheriff F, Russo IH. (2005). Breast differentiation and its implication in cancer prevention. *Clin Cancer Res*. 11:931s–936s.
86. Nechuta SJ, Caan BJ, Chen WY, Lu W, Chen Z, Kwan ML, et al. (2012). Soy food intake after diagnosis of breast cancer and survival: An in-depth analysis of combined evidence from cohort studies of US and Chinese women. *Am J Clin Nutr*. 96:123–32.
87. Chi F, Wu R, Zeng YC, Xing R, Liu Y, Xu ZG. (2013). Post-diagnosis soy food intake and breast cancer survival: A meta-analysis of cohort studies. *Asian Pac J Cancer Prev*. 14:2407–12.
88. Zhang GQ, Chen JL, Liu Q, Zhang Y, Zeng H, Zhao Y. (2015). Soy intake is associated with lower endometrial cancer risk: A systematic review and meta-analysis of observational studies. *Medicine*. 94:e2281.
89. Bitto A, Granese R, Triolo O, Villari D, Maisano D, Giordano D, et al. (2010). Genistein aglycone: A new therapeutic approach to reduce endometrial hyperplasia. *Phytomedicine*. 17:844–50.
90. Zhang Q, Feng H, Qluwakemi B, Wang J, Yao S, Cheng G, et al. (2016). Phytoestrogens and risk of prostate cancer: An updated meta-analysis of epidemiologic studies. *Int J Food Sci Nutr*. 2016:1–15.

91. Kwan W, Duncan G, Van Patten C, Liu M, Lim J. (2010). A phase II trial of a soy beverage for subjects without clinical disease with rising prostate-specific antigen after radical radiation for prostate cancer. *Nutr Cancer.* 62:198–207.
92. (Messina et al. 2006).
93. Zhou J, Yuan WJ. (2015). Effects of soy protein containing isoflavones in patients with chronic kidney disease: A systematic review and meta-analysis. *Clin Nutr.* 35:117–24.

    Fourtounas C. (2011). Phosphorus metabolism in chronic kidney disease. *Hippokratia.* 15:50–2.
94. Atteritano M, Mazzaferro S, Bitto A, Cannata ML, D'Anna R, Squadrito F, et al. (2014). Genistein effects on quality of life and depression symptoms in osteopenic postmenopausal women: A 2-year randomized, double-blind, controlled study. *Osteoporos Int.* 25:1123–9.
95. Hirose A, Terauchi M, Akiyoshi M, Owa Y, Kato K, Kubota T. (2016). Low-dose isoflavone aglycone alleviates psychological symptoms of menopause in Japanese women: A randomized, double-blind, placebo-controlled study. *Arch Gynecol Obstet.* 293:609–15.
96. Estrella RE, Landa AI, Lafuente JV, Gargiulo PA. (2014). Effects of antidepressants and soybean association in depressive menopausal women. *Acta Pol Pharm.* 71:323–7.
97. Draelos ZD, Blair R, Tabor A. (2007). Oral soy supplementation and dermatology. *Cosmet Dermatol.* 20:202–4.
98. Jenkins G, Wainwright LJ, Holland R, Barrett KE, Casey J. (2013). Wrinkle reduction in post-menopausal women consuming a novel oral supplement: A double-blind placebo-controlled randomised study. *Int J Cosmet Sci.* 36:22–31.
99. Izumi T, Makoto S, Obata A, Masayuki A, Yamaguchi H, Matsuyama A. (2007). Oral intake of soy isoflavone aglycone improves the aged skin of adult women. *J Nutr Sci Vitaminol.* 53:57–62.
100. Lou D, Li Y, Yan G, Bu J, Wang H. (2016). Soy consumption with risk of coronary heart disease and stroke: A meta-analysis of observational studies. *Neuroepidemiology.* 46:242–52.
101. Pase MP, Grima NA, Sarris J. (2011). The effects of dietary and nutrient interventions on arterial stiffness: A systematic review. *Am J Clin Nutr.* 93:446–54.
102. Zhan S, Ho SC. (2005). Meta-analysis of the effects of soy protein containing isoflavones on the lipid profile. *Am J Clin Nutr.* 81:397–408.
103. Lammi C, Zanoni C, Arnoldi A, Vistoli G. (2015). Two peptides from soy beta-conglycinin induce a hypocholesterolemic effect in HepG2

cells by a statin-like mechanism: Comparative in vitro and in silico modeling studies. *J Agric Food Chem.* 63:7945–51.

104. Li SH, Liu XX, Bai YY, Wang XJ, Sun K, Chen JZ, et al. (2010). Effect of oral isoflavone supplementation on vascular endothelial function in postmenopausal women: A meta-analysis of randomized placebo-controlled trials. *Am J Clin Nutr.* 91:480–6.

105. Dong JY, Tong X, Wu ZW, Xun PC, He K, Qin LQ. (2011). Effect of soya protein on blood pressure: A meta-analysis of randomised controlled trials. *Br J Nutr.* 106:317–26.

106. Gunther AL, Karaolis-Danckert N, Kroke A, Remer T, Buyken AE. (2010). Dietary protein intake throughout childhood is associated with the timing of puberty. *J Nutr.* 140:565–71.

107. Segovia-Siapco G, Pribis P, Messina M, Oda K, Sabate J. (2014). Is soy intake related to age at onset of menarche? A cross-sectional study among adolescents with a wide range of soy food consumption. *Nutr J.* 2014;13:54.

108. Panel on Food Additives and Nutrient Sources added to Food Scientific opinion on the risk assessment for peri- and post-menopausal women taking food supplements containing isolated isoflavones. (2015). *EFSA J.* 13:4246.

109. Divi RL, Chang HC, Doerge DR. (1997). Anti-thyroid isoflavones from soybean: Isolation, characterization, and mechanisms of action. *Biochem Pharmacol.* 54:1087–96.

110. Messina M, Redmond G. (2006). Effects of soy protein and soybean isoflavones on thyroid function in healthy adults and hypothyroid patients: A review of the relevant literature. *Thyroid.* 16:249–58.

111. Bell DS, Ovalle F. (2001). Use of soy protein supplement and resultant need for increased dose of levothyroxine. *Endocr Pract.* 7:193–4.

112. García-Mantrana I, Monedero V, Haros M. (2015). Reduction of Phytate in Soy Drink by Fermentation with Lactobacillus casei Expressing Phytases From Bifidobacteria. *Plant Foods Hum Nutr.* 70(3):269–74.

113. Zhao Y, Martin BR, Weaver CM. (2005). Calcium bioavailability of calcium carbonate fortified soymilk is equivalent to cow's milk in young women. *J Nutr.* 135:2379–82.

114. Armah SM, Boy E, Chen D, Candal P, Reddy MB. (2015). Regular consumption of a high-phytate diet reduces the inhibitory effect of phytate on nonheme-iron absorption in women with suboptimal iron stores. *J Nutr.* 145:1735–9.

115. Katz Y, Gutierrez-Castrellon P, Gonzalez MG, Rivas R, Lee BW, Alarcon PA. (2014). A comprehensive review of sensitization and allergy to soy-based products. *Clin Rev Allergy Immunol.* 46:272–81.

Chapter three

1. Felter HW. (1922). *The Eclectic Materia Medica, Pharmacology and Therapeutics*. Medical College of Cincinnati, Ohio.
2. Felter HW, Lloyd JU. (1898). *King's American Dispensatory*. Cincinnati: Ohio Valley Co.
3. Scudder JM. (1875). *Specific Medication and Specific Medicines*. Cincinnati, Wilstach, Baldwin & Co., Printers, 1875.
4. Cook W. (1869). *The Physiomedical Dispensatory*. Published by W.H. Cook.
5. Tolleson WH, Doerge DR, Churchwell MI, Marques MM, Roberts DW. (2002). Metabolism of biochanin A and formononetin by human liver microsomes in vitro. *J Agric Food Chem*. 50(17):4783–90.
6. Howes J, Waring M, Huang L, Howes LG. (2002). Long-term pharmacokinetics of an extract of isoflavones from red clover (Trifolium pratense). *J Altern Complement Med*. 8(2):135–42.
7. Thomas AJ, Ismail R, Taylor-Swanson L, Cray L, Schnall JG, Mitchell ES, et al. (2014). Effects of isoflavones and amino acid therapies for hot flashes and co-occurring symptoms during the menopausal transition and early postmenopause: a systematic review. *Maturitas*. 78:263–76.
8. Geller SE, Shulman LP, van Breemen RB, Banuvar S, Zhou Y, Epstein G, et al. (2009). Safety and efficacy of black cohosh and red clover for the management of vasomotor symptoms: a randomized controlled trial. *Menopause*. 16:1156–66.
9. Nissan HP, Lu J, Booth NL, Yamamura HI, Farnsworth NR, Wang ZJ. (2007). A red clover (Trifolium pratense) phase II clinical extract possesses opiate activity. *J Ethnopharmacol*. 30;112(1):207–10.
10. Myers SP, Vigar V. (2017). Effects of a standardised extract of Trifolium pratense (Promensil) at a dosage of 80 mg in the treatment of menopausal hot flushes: A systematic review and meta-analysis. *Phytomedicine*. 24(15):141–7.
11. Ghazanfarpour M, Sadeghi R, Roudsari RL, Khorsand I, Khadivzadeh T, Muoio B. (2015). Red clover for treatment of hot flashes and menopausal symptoms: a systematic review and meta-analysis. *J Obstet Gynaecol*. 36:301–11.
12. Lipovac M, Chedraui P, Gruenhut C, Gocan A, Kurz C, Neuber B, et al. (2011). Effect of Red Clover Isoflavones over Skin, Appendages, and Mucosal Status in Postmenopausal Women. *Obstet Gynecol Int*. 2011:949302.

13. Piersen CE, Booth NL, Sun Y, Liang W, Burdette JE, van Breemen RB, et al. (2004). Chemical and biological characterization and clinical evaluation of botanical dietary supplements: a phase I red clover extract as a model. *Curr Med Chem.* 11:1361–74.
14. Clifton-Bligh PB, Baber RJ, Fulcher GR, Nery ML, Moreton T. (2001). The effect of isoflavones extracted from red clover (Rimostil) on lipid and bone metabolism. *Menopause.* 8:259–65.
15. Atkinson C, Compston JE, Day NE, Dowsett M, Bingham SA. (2004). The effects of phytoestrogen isoflavones on bone density in women: a double-blind, randomized, placebo-controlled trial. *Am J Clin Nutr.* 79:326–33.
16. Działo M, Mierziak J, Korzun U, Preisner M, Szopa J, Kulma A. (2016). The Potential of Plant Phenolics in Prevention and Therapy of Skin Disorders. *Int J Mol Sci.* 17(2):160.
17. Chedraui P, San Miguel G, Hidalgo L, Morocho N, Ross S. (2008). Effect of Trifolium pratense-derived isoflavones on the lipid profile of postmenopausal women with increased body mass index. *Gynecological Endocrinology.* 24;11:620–4.
18. Howes JB, Tran D, Brillante D, Howes LG. (2003). Effects of dietary supplementation with isoflavones from red clover on ambulatory blood pressure and endothelial function in postmenopausal type 2 diabetes. *Diabetes Obes Metab.* 5(5):325–32.
19. Geller SE, Studee L. (2006). Soy and red clover for mid-life and aging. *Climacteric.* 9(4):245–63.
20. Engelhardt PF, Riedl CR. (2008). Effects of one-year treatment with isoflavone extract from red clover on prostate, liver function, sexual function, and quality of life in men with elevated PSA levels and negative prostate biopsy findings. *Urology.* 71(2):185–90.
21. Jarred RA, Keikha M, Dowling C, McPherson SJ, Clare AM, Husband AJ, et al. (2002). Induction of apoptosis in low to moderate-grade human prostate carcinoma by red clover-derived dietary isoflavones. *Cancer Epidemiol Biomarkers Prev.* 11(12):1689–96.
22. Domon OE, McGarrity LJ, Bishop M, Yoshioka M, Chen JJ, Morris SM. (2001). Evaluation of the genotoxicity of the phytoestrogen, coumestrol, in AHH-1 TK(+/−) human lymphoblastoid cells. *Mutat Res.* 1;474(1–2):129–37.
23. Atkinson C, Warren RM, Sala E, Dowsett M, Dunning AM, Healey CS, et al. (2004). Red clover-derived isoflavones and mammographic

breast density: a double-blind, randomized, placebo-controlled trial [ISRCTN42940165]. *Breast Cancer Res.* 6:R170–R179.

24. Powles TJ, Howell A, Evans DG, McCloskey EV, Ashley S, Greenhalgh R, et al. (2008). Red clover isoflavones are safe and well tolerated in women with a family history of breast cancer. *Menopause Int.* 14(1):6–12.

25. Fritz H, Seely D, Flower G, Skidmore B, Fernandes R, Vadeboncoeur S, et al. (2013). Soy, Red Clover, and Isoflavones and Breast Cancer: A Systematic Review. *PLoS One.* 8(11):e81968.

26. Hale GE, Hughes CL, Robboy SJ, Agarwal SK, Bievre M. (2001). A doubleblind randomized study on the effects of red clover isoflavones on the endometrium. *Menopause.* 8:338–46.

27. Bone K. (2003). *A Clinical Guide to Blending Liquid Herbs.* London; Churchill Livingstone.

28. Avicenna (Ibn Sina) (2014a). *The Canon of Medicine (al-Qānūn fī'l-tibb). The Law of Natural Healing.* Pharmacopeia. Compiled by Laleh Bakhtiar, Vol. 5. Chicago, IL: Great Books of the Islamic World Inc.

29. Biendl M, Pinzl C. (2007). *Arzneipflanze Hopfen. Anwendungen, Wirkungen, Geschichte.* Wolznach: Deutsches Hopfenmuseum Wolznach.

30. Madaus G. (1938). *Lehrbuch der Biologischen Heilmittel.* Leipzig: Georg Thieme Verlag.

31. Braungart R. (1901). *Der Hopfen als Braumaterial.* München: Verlag von R. Oldenbourg.

32. Kahnt K. (1906). Die Phytotherapie, eine Methode innerlicher Krankheitsbehandlung mit giftfreien, pflanzlichen Heilmitteln. 4th ed. Berlin S.W. 47: Verlag von Otto Nahmmacher.

33. Moerman DE. (1981) *Geraniums for the Iroquois. A Field Guide to American Indian Medicinal Plants.* 1st ed. Algonac, MI: Algonac, Michigan, USA, Reference Publications.

34. Chopra RN, Nayar SL, Chopra IC. (1958). *Glossary of Indian Medicinal Plants.* Calcutta: Council of Scientific and Industrial Research.

35. Duke JA, Castleman M. (2001). The Green Pharmacy Anti-Aging Prescriptions: Herbs, Foods, and Natural Formulas to Keep You Young. Emmaus, PA: Rodale Books.

36. Schiller H, Forster A, Vonhoff C, Hegger M, Biller A, Winterhoff H. (2006). Sedating effects of Humulus lupulus L. extracts. *Phytomedicine.* 13(8):535–41.

37. Franco L, Sánchez C, Bravo R, Rodriguez A, Barriga C, Juánez JC. (2012). The sedative effects of hops (Humulus lupulus), a component of beer, on the activity/rest rhythm. *Acta Physiol Hung.* 99(2):133–9.

38. Wohlfart R, Wurm G, Hansel R, Schmidt H. (1982). Nachweis sedativ-hypnotischer Wirkstoffe im Hopfen, 5. Mitt.—Der Abbau der Bittersaeuren zum 2-Methyl-3-buten-2-ol, einem Hopfeninhaltsstoff mit sedativ-hypnotischer Wirkung. *Archiv der Pharmazie.* 315(2):132–7.
39. Butterweck V, Brattstroem A, Grundmann O, Koetter U. (2007). Hypothermic effects of hops are antagonized with the competitive melatonin receptor antagonist luzindole in mice. *J Pharm Pharmacol.* 59(4):549–52.
40. Füssel A, Wolf A, Brattström A. (2000). Effect of a fixed valerian-Hop extract combination (Ze 91019) on sleep polygraphy in patients with non-organic insomnia: a pilot study. *Eur J Med Res.* 5(9):385–90.
41. Salter S, Brownie S. (2010). Treating primary insomnia—the efficacy of valerian and hops. *Aust Fam Physician.* 39(6):433–7.
42. Morin CM, Koetter U, Bastien C, Ware JC, Wooten V. (2005). Valerian-hops combination and diphenhydramine for treating insomnia: a randomized placebo-controlled clinical trial. *Sleep.* 28:1465–71.
43. Schmitz M, Jäckel M. (1998). Comparative study for assessing quality of life of patients with exogenous sleep disorders (temporary sleep onset and sleep interruption disorders) treated with a hops-valarian preparation and a benzodiazepine drug. *Wien Med Wochenschr.* 148: 291–8.
44. Müller-Limmroth W, Ehrenstein W. (1977). Untersuchungen über die Wirkung von Seda-Kneipp auf den Schlaf schlafgestörter Menschen: Bedeutung von Seda-Kneipp in der Therapie verschiedener Schlafstörungen. *Medizinische Klinik.* 72(25):1119–1125.
45. Koetter U, Schrader E, Käufeler R, Brattström A. (2007). A randomized, double blind, placebo-controlled, prospective clinical study to demonstrate clinical efficacy of a fixed valerian hops extract combination (Ze 91019) in patients suffering from non-organic sleep disorder. *Phytother Res.* 21(9):847–51.
46. Dimpfel W, Suter A. (2008). Sleep improving effects of a single dose administration of a valerian/hops fluid extract—a double blind, randomized, placebo-controlled sleep-EEG study in a parallel design using electrohypnograms. *Eur J Med Res.* 26;13(5):200–4.
47. Schellenberg R, Sauer S, Abourashed EA, Koetter U, Brattström A. (2004). The fixed combination of valerian and hops (Ze91019) acts via a central adenosine mechanism. *Planta Med.* 70(7):594–7.
48. Bone K. (2003). *A Clinical Guide to Blending Liquid Herbs: Herbal Formulations for the Individual Patient.* London: Churchill Livingstone.

49. Rad M, Hümpel M, Schaefer O, Schoemaker RC, Schleuning WD, Cohen AF, et al. (2006). Pharmacokinetics and systemic endocrine effects of the phyto-oestrogen 8-prenylnaringenin after single oral doses to postmenopausal women. *Br J Clin Pharmacol.* 62:288–96.
50. Heyerick A, Vervarcke S, Depypere H, Bracke M, De Keukeleire D. (2006). A first prospective, randomized, double-blind, placebo-controlled study on the use of a standardized hop extract to alleviate menopausal discomforts. *Maturitas.* 54(2):164–75.
51. Erkkola R, Vervarcke S, Vansteelandt S, Rompotti P, De Keukeleire D, Heyerick A. (2010). A randomized, double-blind, placebo-controlled, cross-over pilot study on the use of a standardized hop extract to alleviate menopausal discomforts. *Phytomedicine.* 17(6):389–96.
52. Aghamiri V, Mirghafourvand M, Mohammad-Alizadeh-Charandabi S, Nazemiyeh H. (2015). The effect of Hop (Humulus lupulus L.) on early menopausal symptoms and hot flashes: A randomized placebo-controlled trial. *Complement Ther Clin Pract.* pii: S1744–3881(15)00039-0.
53. Morali G, Polatti F, Metelitsa EN, Mascarucci P, Magnani P, Marre GB. (2006). Open, non-controlled clinical studies to assess the efficacy and safety of a medical device in form of gel topically and intravaginally used in postmenopausal women with genital atrophy. *Arzneimittelforschung.* 56(3):230–8.
54. Sehmisch S, Hammer F, Christoffel J, Seidlova-Wuttke D, Tezval M, Wuttke W, et al. (2008). Comparison of the phytohormones genistein, resveratrol and 8-prenylnaringenin as agents for preventing osteoporosis. *Planta Medica.* 74(8):794–801.
55. Pedrera-Zamorano JD, Lavado-Garcia JM, Roncero-Martin R, Calderon-Garcia JF, Rodriguez-Dominguez T, Canal-Macias ML. (2009). Effect of beer drinking on ultrasound bone mass in women. *Nutrition.* 25(10):1057–63.
56. Cermak P, Paleckova V, Houska M, Strohalm J, Novotna P, Mikyska A, Jurkova M, Sikorova M. (2015). Inhibitory effects of fresh hops on Helicobacter pylori strains. *Czech J Food Sci.* 33(4):302–7.
57. Schmid H. (1951). *Statistische Untersuchungen über das Vorkommen von Tuberkulose im Braugewerbe und in-vitro Versuche über tuberkulostatische Wirkungen einzelner Hopfenbitterstoffe.* München: Universität München. Stepp W Bier, (1954). *Wie es der Arzt sieht.* München: Gerber Verlag.
58. Serkani JE, Isfahani N, Safaei HGh, Kermanshahi K, Asghari Gh. (2012). Evaluation of the effect of Humulus lupulus alcoholic extract on rifampin-sensitive and resistant isolates of Mycobacterium tuberculosis. *Res Pharm Sci.* 7(4):235–242.

59. Cermak P, Olsovska J, Mikyska A, Dusek M, Kadleckova Z, Vanicek J, et al. (2017). Strong antimicrobial activity of xanthohumol and other derivatives from hops (Humulus lupulus L.) on gut anaerobic bacteria. *APMIS*. 125(11):1033–8.
60. Yamaguchi N, Satoh-Yamaguchi K, Ono M. (2009). In vitro evaluation of antibacterial, anticollagenase, and antioxidant activities of hop components (Humulus lupulus) addressing acne vulgaris. *Phytomedicine*. 16(4):369–76.
61. Gerhauser C. (2005). Broad spectrum anti-infective potential of xanthohumol from hop (Humulus lupulus L.) in comparison with activities of other hop constituents and xanthohumol metabolites. *Mol Nutr Food Res*. 49(9):827–31.
62. Van Cleemput M, Heyerick A, Libert C, Swerts K, Philippé J, De Keukeleire D, et al. (2009). Hop bitter acids efficiently block inflammation independent of GRα, PPARα, or PPARγ. *Mol Nutr Food Res*. 53: 1143–55.
63. Tripp ML, Konda VR, Darland G, Desai A, Chang J, Carroll BJ, et al. (2009). Rho-iso-alpha acids and tetrahydro-iso-alpha acids are selective protein kinase inhibitors which potently reduce inflammation in macrophages in vitro and in the collagen-induced rheumatoid arthritis model in vivo. *Acta Hortic*. 848:221–34.
64. Hall AJ, Babish JG, Darland GK, Carroll BJ, Konda VR, Lerman RH, et al. (2008). Safety, efficacy and anti-inflammatory activity of rho isoalpha-acids from hops. *Phytochemistry*. 69(7):1534–47.
65. Dostálek P, Karabín M, Lukáš J. (2017). Hop Phytochemicals and Their Potential Role in Metabolic Syndrome Prevention and Therapy. *Molecules*. 22(10):1761.
66. Obara K, Mizutani M, Hitomi Y, Yajima H, Kondo K. (2009). Isohumulones, the bitter component of beer, improve hyperglycemia and decrease body fat in Japanese subjects with prediabetes. *Clin Nutr*. 28(3):278–84.
67. Lopez-Jaen AB, Codoñer-Franch P, Martínez-Álvarez JR, Villarino-Marín A, Valls-Bellés V. (2010). Effect on health of non-alcohol beer and hop supplementation in a group of nuns in a closed order. *Proceedings of the Nutrition Society* (OCE3):26.
68. Karabín M, Hudcová T, Jelínek L, Dostálek, P. (2016), Biologically Active Compounds from Hops and Prospects for Their Use. *Comprehensive Reviews in Food Science and Food Safety*. 15:542–67.
69. Franziska Ferk, Wolfgang W. Huber, Metka Filipič, Julia Bichler, Elisabeth Haslinger, Miroslav Mišík, Armen Nersesyan, Bettina Grasl-Kraupp, Bojana Žegura, Siegfried Knasmüller. (2010). Xanthohumol, a

prenylated flavonoid contained in beer, prevents the induction of preneoplastic lesions and DNA damage in liver and colon induced by the heterocyclic aromatic amine amino-3-methyl-imidazo[4,5-f]quinoline (IQ). *Mutation Research/Fundamental and Molecular Mechanisms of Mutagenesis.* 691(1–2):17–22.

70. Ferk F, Mišk M, Nersesyan A, Pichler C, Jäger W, Szekeres T, et al. (2016). Impact of xanthohumol (a prenylated flavonoid from hops) on DNA stability and other health-related biochemical parameters: Results of human intervention trials. *Mol Nutr Food Res.* 60(4):773–86.

71. Weiskirchen R, Mahli A, Weiskirchen S, Hellerband C. (2015). The Hop Constituent Xanthohumol Exhibits Hepatoprotective Effects and Inhibits the Activation of Hepatic Stellate Cells at Different Levels. *Frontiers in Physiology.* 6:140. PMC. Web. 12 Aug. 2018.

72. Wang S, Dunlap TL, Howell CE, Mbachu OC, Rue EA, Phansalkar R, et al. (2016). Hop (*Humulus lupulus* L.) Extract and 6-Prenylnaringenin Induce P450 1A1 Catalyzed Estrogen 2-Hydroxylation. *Chemical Research in Toxicology.* 29(7):1142–50.

73. van Breemen, Yuan Y, Banuvar S, Shulman LP, Qiu X, Alvarenga RF, et al. (2014). Pharmacokinetics of prenylated hop phenols in women following oral administration of a standardized extract of hops. *Mol Nutr Food Res.* 58(10):1962–9.

74. Madhubhani LP, Hemachandra P, Esala R, Chandrasena P, Chen SN, Main M, et al. (2012). Hops (Humulus lupulus) inhibits Oxidative Estrogen Metabolism and Estrogen-Induced Malignant Transformation in Human Mammary Epithelial cells (MCF-10A). *Cancer Prev Res (Phila).* 5(1):73–81.

75. Liu Y, Nguyen N, Colditz GA. (2015). Links between alcohol consumption and breast cancer: a look at the evidence. *Women's health (London, England).* 11(1):65–77.

76. Dweck A. C. (2000). Introduction to the folklore and cosmetic use of various Salvia species. In: *Medicinal and Aromatic Plants Industrial Profiles*: Vol. 14, Sage, the genus Salvia (Kintzios SE, ed). UK: Harwood Academic, pp. 10–11.

77. Iuvone T, De Filippis D, Esposito G, D'Amico A, Izzo AA. (2006). The spice sage and its active ingredient rosmarinic acid protect PC12 cells from amyloid-beta peptide-induced neurotoxicity. *J Pharmacol Exp Ther.* 317(3):1143–9.

78. Miroddi M, Navarra M, Quattropani MC, Calapai F, Gangemi S, Calapai G. (2014). Systematic review of clinical trials assessing

pharmacological properties of Salvia species on memory, cognitive impairment and Alzheimer's disease. *CNS Neurosci Ther.* 20:485–95.
79. Akhondzadeh S, Noroozian M, Mohammadi M, Ohadinia S, Jamshidi AH, Khani M. (2003). Salvia officinalis extract in the treatment of patients with mild to moderate Alzheimer's disease: a double blind, randomized and placebo-controlled trial. *J Clin Pharm Ther.* 28:53–9.
80. Rahte S, Evans R, Eugster PJ, Marcourt L, Wolfender JL, Kortenkamp A, et al. (2013). Salvia officinalis for hot flushes: towards determination of mechanism of activity and active principles. *Planta Med.* 79(9):753–60.
81. Moss L, Rouse M, Wesnes KA, Moss M. (2010). Differential effects of the aromas of Salvia species on memory and mood. *Hum Psychopharmacol.* 25:388–96.
82. Moss M, Rouse M, Moss L. (2014). Aromas of salvia species enhance everyday prospective memory performance in healthy young adults. *Adv Chem Eng Sci.* 4:339–46.
83. Kennedy DO, Pace S, Haskell C, Okello EJ, Milne A, Scholey AB. (2006). Effects of cholinesterase inhibiting sage (Salvia officinalis) on mood, anxiety and performance on a psychological stressor battery. *Neuropsychopharmacology.* 31:845–52.
84. Scholey AB, Tildesley NT, Ballard CG. (2008). An extract of Salvia (sage) with anticholinesterase properties improves memory and attention in healthy older volunteers. *Psychopharmacology.* 198:127–39.
85. Eidi M, Eidi A, Bahar M. (2006). Effects of Salvia officinalis L. (sage) leaves on memory retention and its interaction with the cholinergic system in rats. *Nutrition.* 22:321–6.
86. Hasanein P, Felehgari Z, Emamjomeh A. (2016). Preventive effects of Salvia officinalis L. against learning and memory deficit induced by diabetes in rats: possible hypoglycaemic and antioxidant mechanisms. *Neurosci Lett.* 622:72–7.
87. Gomar A, Hosseini A, Mirazi N. (2014). Evaluation of Salvia officinalis L. (sage) leaves on morphine-induced memory impairment in adult male rats. *Focus Altern Complement Ther.* 19:156–162.
88. Bommer S, Klein P, Suter A. (2011). First time proof of sage's tolerability and efficacy in menopausal women with hot flushes. *Adv Ther.* 28: 490–500.
89. Rad SK, Forouhari S, Dehaghani AS, Vafaei H, Sayadi M, Asadi M. (2016). The effect of salvia officinalis tablet on hot flashes, night sweating, and estradiol hormone in postmenopausal women. *International Journal of Medical Research & Health Sciences.* 5(8):257–63.

90. Gallagher J. (2010). Salvia officinalis for menopausal hot flushes: a pilot study. *Focus on Alternative and Complementary Therapies.* 7:92–3.
91. De Leo V, Lanzetta D, Cazzavacca R, Morgante G. (1998). Treatment of neurovegetative menopausal symptoms with a phytotherapeutic agent. *Minerva Ginecol.* 50(5):207–11.
92. Vandecasteele K, Ost P, Oosterlinck W, Fonteyne V, Neve WD, Meerleer GD. (2012). Evaluation of the efficacy and safety of Salvia officinalis in controlling hot flashes in prostate cancer patients treated with androgen deprivation. *Phytother Res.* 26:208–13.
93. European Medicine Agency. (2015). Assessment report on Salvia officinalis L., folium and Salvia officinalis L., aetheroleum. EMA/HMPC/150801/2015.
94. Khattab HAH, Mohamed RA, Hashemi JM. (2012). Evaluation of hypoglycemic activity of Salvia officinalis L. (Sage) infusion on streptozotocin-induced diabetic rats. *J Am Sci.* 8:411–6.
95. Hernandez-Saavedra D, Perez-Ramirez IF, Ramos-Gomez M, Mendoza-Diaz S, Loarca-Pina G, Reynoso-Camacho R. (2016). Phytochemical characterization and effect of Calendula officinalis, Hypericum perforatum, and Salvia officinalis infusions on obesity associated cardiovascular risk. *Med Chem Res.* 25:163–72.
96. Kianbakht S, Dabaghian FH. (2013). Improved glycemic control and lipid profile in hyperlipidemic type 2 diabetic patients consuming Salvia officinalis L. leaf extract: a randomized placebo. Controlled clinical trial. *Complement Ther Med.* 21(5):441–6.
97. Kianbakht S, Abasi B, Perham M, Hashem Dabaghian F. (2011). Antihyperlipidemic effects of Salvia officinalis L. leaf extract in patients with hyperlipidemia: a randomized double-blind placebo-controlled clinical trial. *Phytother Res.* 25(12):1849–53.
98. Behradmanesh S, Derees F, Rafieian-kopaei M. (2013). Effect of Salvia officinalis on diabetic patients. *J Ren Inj Prev.* 2:51–4.
99. Mühlbauer RC, Lozano A, Palacio S, Reinli A, Felix R. (2003). Common herbs, essential oils, and monoterpenes potently modulate bone metabolism. *Bone.* 32(4):372–80.
100. Hubbert M, Sievers H, Lehnfeld R, Kehrl W. (2006). Efficacy and tolerability of a spray with Salvia officinalis in the treatment of acute pharyngitis—a randomised, double-blind, placebo-controlled study with adaptive design and interim analysis. *Eur J Med Res.* 11(1):20–6.
101. Ghorbania A, Esmaeilizadehb M. (2017). Pharmacological properties of Salvia officinalis and its components. *J Tradit Complement Med.* 7(4):433–40.

102. Pedro DF, Ramos AA, Lima CF, Baltazar F, Pereira-Wilson C. (2016). Colon cancer chemoprevention by sage tea drinking: decreased DNA damage and cell proliferation. *Phytother Res*. 30:298–305.
103. Horváthová E, Srančíková A, Regendová-Sedláčková E. (2016). Enriching the drinking water of rats with extracts of Salvia officinalis and Thymus vulgaris increases their resistance to oxidative stress. *Mutagenesis*. 31:51–9.
104. Jasicka-Misiak I, Poliwoda A, Petecka M, Buslovych O, Shlyapnikov VA, Wieczorek PP. (2018). Antioxidant Phenolic Compounds in Salvia officinalis L. and Salvia sclarea L., *Ecological Chemistry and Engineering S*. 25(1):133–42.
105. Qnais EY, Abu-Dieyeh M, Abdulla FA, Abdalla SS. (2010). The antinociceptive and anti-inflammatory effects of Salvia officinalis leaf aqueous and butanol extracts. *Pharm Biol*. 48:1149–56.
106. Abad NAA, Nouri MHK, Tavakkoli F. (2011). Effect of Salvia officinalis hydroalcoholic extract on vincristine-induced neuropathy in mice. *Chin J Nat Med*. 9:354–8.
107. Hubbert M, Sievers H, Lehnfeld R, Kehrl W. (2006). Efficacy and tolerability of a spray with Salvia officinalis in the treatment of acute pharyngitis—a randomised, double-blind, placebo-controlled study with adaptive design and interim analysis. *Eur J Med Res*. 11:20–6.
108. Delamare APL, Moschen-Pistorello IT, Artico L, Atti-Serafini L, Echeverrigaray S. (2007). Antibacterial activity of the essential oils of Salvia offcinalis L. and Salvia triloba L. cultivated in South Brazil. *Food Chem*. 100:603–8.
109. Horiuchi K, Shiota S, Hatano T, Yoshida T, Kuroda T, Tsuchiya T. (2007). Antimicrobial activity of oleanolic acid from Salvia officinalis and related compounds on vancomycin-resistant enterococci. *Biol Pharm Bull*. 30:1147–9.
110. Martins N, Barros L, Santos-Buelga C, Henriques M, Silva S, Ferreira IC. (2015). Evaluation of bioactive properties and phenolic compounds in different extracts prepared from Salvia officinalis L. *Food Chem*. 1:170:378–85.
111. Ghorbania A, Esmaeilizadehb M. (2017). Pharmacological properties of Salvia officinalis and its components. *J Tradit Complement Med*. 7(4): 433–40.
112. Bone K. (2005). *The Essential Guide to Herbal Safety*. London: Churchill Livingstone.
113. Walch SG, Kuballa T, Stühlinger W, Lachenmeier DW. (2011). Determination of the biologically active flavour substances thujone and

camphor in foods and medicines containing sage (*Salvia officinalis* L.). *Chemistry Central Journal.* 5:44.

Chapter four

1. Felter HW, Lloyd JU. (1898). *King's American Dispensatory.* Cincinnati, OH: Ohio Valley Co.
2. Ellingwood F (ed). (1908). *Ellingwood's Therapeutist.* Vol. 2. Chicago, IL: F. Ellingwood.
3. Sautour M, Miyamoto T, Lacaille-Dubois MA. (2006). Steroidal saponins and fla-van-3-ol glycosides from Dioscorea villosa. *Biochem Syst Ecol.* 34:60–3.
4. Chhatre S, Nesari T, Somani G, Kanchan D, Sathaye S. (2014). Phytopharmacological overview of Tribulus terrestris. *Pharmacognosy Reviews.* 8(15):45–51.
5. Bone K, Mills S. (2012). *Principles and Practice of Phytotherapy.* 2nd ed. London: Churchill Livingstone.
6. Milanov S, Maleeva A, Tashkov M. (1981). *Tribestan Effect on the Concentration of Some Hormones in the Serum of Healthy Subjects.* Sofia, Bulgaria: Chemical Pharmaceutical Research Institute.
7. Zarkova S. (1985). *Tribestan: Experimental and Clinical Investigations.* Sofia, Bulgaria: Chemical Pharmaceutical Research Institute.
8. Tabakova, P, Dimitrov M, Tashkov B. (1984–87). Kirkoua-Sofia Clinical studies on the preparation Tribestan in women with endocrine infertility or menopausal syndrome. (1984–87) Available from: http://www.scicompdf.se/tiggarnot/tabakova-HerbPharmUSA.pdf.
9. Akhtari E, Raisi F, Keshavarz M, Hosseini H, Sohrabvand F, Bioos S, et al. (2014). Tribulus terrestris for treatment of sexual dysfunction in women: randomized double-blind placebo—controlled study. *Daru.* 22(1):40.
10. Vale FBC, Zanolla Dias de Souza K, Rezende CR, Geber S. (2018). Efficacy of Tribulus Terrestris for the treatment of premenopausal women with hypoactive sexual desire disorder: a randomized double-blinded, placebo-controlled trial. *Gynecol Endocrinol.* 34(5):442–5.
11. Wu WH, Liu LY, Chung CJ, Jou HJ, Wang TA. (2005). Estrogenic effect of yam ingestion in healthy postmenopausal women. *J Am Coll Nutr.* 24(4):235–43.
12. Park MK, Kwon HY, Ahn WS, Bae S, Rhyu MR, Lee Y. (2009). Estrogen activities and the cellular effects of natural progesterone from wild yam extract in mcf-7 human breast cancer cells. *Am J Chin Med.* 37(1):159–67.

13. Komesaroff PA, Black CV, Cable V, Sudhir K. (2001). Effects of wild yam extract on menopausal symptoms, lipids and sex hormones in healthy menopausal women. *Climacteric.* 4(2):144–50.
14. McKoy ML, Thomas PG, Asemota H, Omoruyi F, Simon O. (2014). Effects of Jamaican bitter yam (Dioscorea polygonoides) and diosgenin on blood and fecal cholesterol in rats. *J Med Food.* 17(11):1183–8.
15. Lv YC, Yang J, Yao F, Xie W, Tang YY, Ouyang XP, et al. (2015). Diosgenin inhibits atherosclerosis via suppressing the MiR-19b-induced downregulation of ATP-binding cassette transporter A1. *Atherosclerosis.* 240(1):80–9.
16. Wu WH, Liu LY, Chung CJ, Jou HJ, Wang TA. (2005). Estrogenic effect of yam ingestion in healthy postmenopausal women. *J Am Coll Nutr.* 24(4):235–43.
17. Liu J, Chen J, Tan Z, Yang Q, Lan H, Zhao Y, et al. (2014). Effects of a dioscorea-modified pill on cognitive impairment of patients with VCIND: a preliminary study of proton magnetic resonance spectroscopy. *Zhonghua Yi Xue Za Zhi.* 94(39):3075–8.
18. Araghiniknam M, Chung S, Nelson-White T, Eskelson C, Watson RR. (1996). Antioxidant activity of dioscorea and dehydroepiandrosterone (DHEA) in older humans. *Life Sci.* 59(11):PL147–57.
19. Lima CM, Lima AK, Melo MG, Serafini MR, Oliveira DL, de Almeida EB, et al. (2013). Bioassay-guided evaluation of Dioscorea villosa—an acute and subchronic toxicity, antinociceptive and anti-inflammatory approach. *BMC Complement Altern Med.* 28;13:195.
20. Yamada T, Hoshino M, Hayakawa T, Ohhara H, Yamada H, Nakazawa T, Inagaki T, Iida M, Ogasawara T, Uchida A, Hasegawa C, Murasaki G, Miyaji M, Hirata A, Takeuchi T. (1997). Dietary diosgenin attenuates subacute intestinal inflammation associated with indomethacin in rats. *American Journal of Physiology.* 273:G355–64.
21. Accatino L, Pizarro M, Solís N, Koenig CS. (1998). Effects of diosgenin, a plant-derived steroid, on bile secretion and hepatocellular cholestasis induced by estrogens in the rat. *Hepatology.* 28(1):129–40.
22. Jesus M, Martins APJ, Gallardo E, Silvestre S. (2016). Diosgenin: Recent Highlights on Pharmacology and Analytical Methodology. *J Anal Methods Chem.* 2016:4156293.
23. Zhang ZG, Chen YJ, Xiang LH, Pan JH, Wang Z, Xiao GG, et al. (2017). Protective effect of Rhizoma Dioscoreae extract against alveolar bone loss in ovariectomized rats via regulation of IL-6/STAT3 signaling. *Int J Mol Med.* 40(5):1602–10.

24. Bone K. (2003). A Clinical Guide to Blending Liquid Herbs, 1st Edition, *Herbal Formulations for the Individual Patient*. London: Churchill Livingstone.
25. 'At-risk' forum. (2003). *J Med Plant Savers*. Winter :13.
26. *NatureServe Explorer: An Online Encyclopedia of Life*, Version 7.1. Arlington, VA: NatureServe, 2010.
27. Felter HW. (1922). *The Eclectic Materia Medica, Pharmacology and Therapeutics*. Cincinnati, OH: Medical College of Cincinnati.
28. Felter HW, Lloyd JU. (1898). *King's American Dispensatory*. Cincinnati, OH: Ohio Valley Co.
29. Challinor VL, Stuthe JM, Parsons PG, Lambert LK, Lehmann RP, Kitching W, et al. (2012). Structure and bioactivity of steroidal saponins isolated from the roots of Chamaelirium luteum (false unicorn). *J Nat Prod*. 75(8):1469–79.
30. Matovic NJ, Stuthe JM, Challinor VL, Bernhardt PV, Lehmann RP, Kitching W, et al. (2011). The truth about false unicorn (Chamaelirium luteum): total synthesis of 23R,24S-chiograsterol B defines the structure and stereochemistry of the major saponins from this medicinal herb. *Chemistry*. 17(27):7578–91.
31. Felter HW, Lloyd JU. (1898). *King's American Dispensatory*. Cincinnati, OH: Ohio Valley Co.
32. Cook W. (1869). *The Physiomedical Dispensatory*. Cincinnati, OH: WH Cook.
33. Culpeper, Nicholas. (1653) reprinted 1850. *The Complete Herbal*. London: Kelly.
34. John M. Scudder, MD. (1870). *Specific Medication and Specific Medicines*. Cincinnati, OH: Wilstach.
35. Petcu P, et al. (1979). Treatment of juvenile meno-metrorrhagia with *Alchemilla vulgaris* fluid extract. *Clujul Med*. 52(3);266–70.
36. Kalia V, Jadav AN, Bhuttani KK. (2003). In vivo effect of Asparagus racemosus on serum gonadotrophin levels in immature female wistar rats. *2nd World Congress of Biotech. Dev of Herbal Med*. Lucknow: NBRI, 2003;40.
37. Pandey SK, Sahay A. (2001). Effect of *Asparagus racemosus* on the liver of non-pregnant And pregnant rats. *Indian Drugs*. 38:132–6.
38. Sharma S, Ramji S, Kumari S, Bapna JS. (1996). Randomized controlled trial of *Asparagus racemosus* (Shatavari) as a lactogogue in lactational inadequacy. *Indian Pediatr*. 33(8):675–7.
39. Gupta M, and Shaw B. (2011). A Double-Blind Randomized Clinical Trial for Evaluation of Galactogogue Activity of *Asparagus racemosus* Willd. *Iran J Pharm Res*. 10(1):167–72.

40. Shashi Alok, Sanjay Kumar Jain, Amita Verma, Mayank Kumar, Alok Mahor, and Monika Sabharwal. (2013). Plant profile, phytochemistry and pharmacology of *Asparagus racemosus* (Shatavari): A review. *Asian Pac J Trop Dis.* 3(3):242–51.
41. Singh KP, Singh RH. (1986). Clinical trial on Satavari (*Asparagus racemosus* Willd.) in duodenal ulcer disease. *J Res Ay Sid.* 7:91–100.
42. Sairam K, Priyambada S, Aryya NC, Goel RK. (2003). Gastroduodenal ulcer protective activity of Asparagus racemosus: an experimental, biochemical and histological study. *J Ethnopharmacol.* 6(1):1–10.
43. Dalvi SS, Nadkarni PM, Gupta KC. (1990). Effect of *Asparagus racemosus* (Shatavari) on gastric emptying time in normal healthy volunteers. *J Postgrad Med.* 36(2):91–4.
44. Mandal SC, Kumar CKA, Mohana Lakshmi S, Sinha S, Murugesan T, Saha BP, et al. (2000). Antitussive effect of *Asparagus racemosus* root against sulfur dioxide-induced cough in mice. *Fitoterapia.* 71(6): 686–9.
45. Rege NN, Nazareth HM, Isaac A, Karandikar SM, Dahanukar SA. (1989). Immunotherapeutic modulation of intraperitoneal adhesions by Asparagus racemosus. *J Postgrad Med.* 35(4):199–203.
46. Jetmalani MH, Sabins PB, Gaitonde BB. (1967). A study on the pharmacology of various extracts of Shatavari-Asparagus racemosus (Willd). *J Res Indian Med.* 2:1–10.
47. Pandey SK, Sahay A, Pandey RS, Tripathi YB. (2005). Effect of *Asparagus racemosus* rhizome (Shatavari) on mammary gland and genital organs of pregnant rat. *Phytother Res.* 19(8):721–4.
48. Zhu X, Zhang W, Zhao J, Wang J, Qu W. (2010). Hypolipidaemic and hepatoprotective effects of ethanolic and aqueous extracts from Asparagus officinalis L. by-products in mice fed a high-fat diet. *J Sci Food Agric.* 90(7):1129–35.
49. Thakur M, Chauhan NS, Bhargava S, Dixit VK. (2009). A comparative study on aphrodisiac activity of some ayurvedic herbs in male albino rats. *Arch Sex Behav.* 38(6):1009–15.
50. Rao AR. (1981). Inhibitory action of *Asparagus racemosus* on DMBA-induced mammary carcinogenesis in rats. *Int J Cancer.* 28:607–10.
51. Narumalla J, Somashekara S, Chikkannasetty, Damodaram G, Golla D. (2012). Study of antiurolithiatic activity of *Asparagus racemosus* on albino rats. *Indian J Pharmacol.* 44(5):576–9.
52. Parihar MS, Hemnani T. (2004). Experimental excitotoxicity provokes oxidative damage in mice brain and attenuation by extract of Asparagus racemosus. *J Neural Transm (Vienna).* 111(1):1–12.

53. Singh GK, Garabadu D, Muruganandam AV, Joshi VK, Krishnamurthy S. (2009). Antidepressant activity of *Asparagus racemosus* in rodent models. *Pharmacol Biochem Behav.* 91(3):283–90.
54. Dahanukar S, Thatte U, Pai N, Mose PB, Karandikar SM. (1986). Protective effect of Asparagus racemosus against induced abdominal sepsis. *Indian Drugs.* 24:125–8.
55. Gautam M, Saha S, Bani S, Kaul A, Mishra S, Patil D, et al. (2009). Immunomodulatory activity of *Asparagus racemosus* on systemic Th1/Th2 immunity: implications for immune adjuvant potential. *J Ethno Pharmacol.* 121(2):241–7.
56. Ojha R, Sahu AN, Muruganandam AV, Singh GK, Krishnamurthy S. (2010). *Asparagus recemosus* enhances memory and protects against amnesia in rodent models. *Brain Cogn.* 74(1):1–9.
57. Kanwar AS, Bhutani KK. (2010). Effects of Chlorophytum arundinaceum, Asparagus adscendens and Asparagus racemosus on pro-inflammatory cytokine and corticosterone levels produced by stress. *Phytother Res.* 24(10):1562–6.
58. Pandey SK, Sahay A. (2001). Effect of Asparagus racemosus on the liver of non-pregnant And pregnant rats. *Indian Drugs.* 38:132–6.
59. Hannan JM, Marenah L, Ali L, Rokeya B, Flatt PR, Abdel-Wahab YH. (2007). Insulin secretory actions of extracts of Asparagus racemosus root in perfused pancreas, isolated islets and clonal pancreatic beta-cells. *J Endocrinol.* 192(1):159–68.
60. Karmakar UK, Sadhu SK, Biswas SK, Chowdhury A, Shill MC, Das J. (2012). Cytotoxicity, analgesic and antidiarrhoeal activities of Asparagus racemosus. *J Appl Sci.* 12:581–6.
61. Alok S, Jain SK, Verma A, Kumar M, Mahor A, Sabharwal M. (2013). Plant profile, phytochemistry and pharmacology of Asparagus racemosus(Shatavari): A review. *Asian Pac J Trop Dis.* 3(3):242–51.

Chapter five

1. Foster S, Black Cohosh. (1999). A Literature Review *HerbalGram.* 45: 35–50. American Botanical Council.
2. King John. (1813–93). *The Eclectic Dispensatory of the United States of America.* Cincinnati, OH: H.W. Derby & Co., 1852.
3. Cook W. (1869). *The Physiomedical Dispensatory.* Published by WH Cook.
4. Scudder (1883).
5. Webster (1893).

6. Jarry H, Metten M, Spengler B, Christoffel V, Wuttke W. (2003). In vitro effects of the *Cimicifuga racemosa* extract BNO 1055. *Maturitas.* 44(1) S31–8.
7. Viereck V, Grundker C, Friess SC, Frosch KH, Raddatz D, Schoppet M, et al. (2005). Isopropanolic extract of black cohosh stimulates osteoprotegerin production by human osteoblasts. *Journal of Bone and Mineral Research.* 20:2036–43.
8. Wuttke W, Jarry H, Haunschild J, Stecher G, Schuh M, Seidlova-Wuttke D. (2014). The non-estrogenic alternative for the treatment of climacteric complaints: Black cohosh (*Cimicifuga* or *Actaea racemosa*). *J Steroid Biochem Mol Biol.* 139:302–10.
9. Wuttke W, Jarry H, Becker T, Schultens A, Christoffel V, Gorkow C, et al. (2008). Phytoestrogens: endocrine disrupters or replacement for hormone replacement therapy? *Maturitas.* 61(1–2):159–70.
10. Shahin AY, Mohammed SA. (2014). Adding the phytoestrogen *Cimicifugae Racemosae* to clomiphene induction cycles with timed intercourse in polycystic ovary syndrome improves cycle outcomes and pregnancy rates – a randomized trial. *Gynecol Endocrinol.* 30(7):505–10.
11. Düker EM, Kopanski L, Jarry H, Wuttke W. (1991). Effects of extracts from *Cimicifuga racemosa* on gonadotropin release in menopausal women and ovariectomized rats. *Planta Med.* 57(5):420–4.
12. Wuttke W, Jarry H, Seidlová-Wuttke D. (2006). Cimicifuga extract for the treatment of climacteric complaints. *J Endocrinol Reprod.* 10(2):106–10.
13. Wuttke W, Seidlová-Wuttke D. (2015). Black cohosh (*Cimicifuga racemosa*) is a non-estrogenic alternative to hormone replacement therapy. *Clinical Phytoscience.* 1:12.
14. Ruhlen RL, Sun GY, Sauter ER. (2008). Black Cohosh: Insights into its Mechanism(s) of Action. *Integr Med Insights.* 3:21–32.
15. Barth, Claudia, Arno Villringer, and Julia Sacher. (2015). Sex hormones affect neurotransmitters and shape the adult female brain during hormonal transition periods. Frontiers in *Neuroscience.* 9:37. PMC. Web. 16 Oct. 2018.
16. Reame NE, Lukacs JL, Padmanabhan V, Eyvazzadeh AD, Smith YR, Zubieta JK. (2008). Black cohosh has central opioid activity in postmenopausal women: evidence from naloxone blockade and positron emission tomography neuroimaging. *Menopause.* 15(5):832–40.
17. van Breemen RB, Liang W, Banuvar S, et al. (2009). Pharmacokinetics of 23-epi-26-deoxyactein in women after oral administration of a standardized extract of black cohosh. *Clin Pharmacol Ther.* 87(2):219–25.

18. Wuttke W, Gorkow C, Seidlová-Wuttke D. (2006). Effects of black cohosh (*Cimicifuga racemosa*) on bone turnover, vaginal mucosa, and various blood parameters in postmenopausal women: a double-blind, placebo-controlled, and conjugated oestrogens-controlled study. *Menopause*. 13(2):185–96.
19. Shahin AY, Ismail AM, Zahran KM, Makhlouf AM. (2008). Adding phytoestrogens to clomiphene induction in unexplained infertility patients – a randomized trial. *Reprod Biomed Online*. 16(4):580–8.
20. Kamel HH. (2013). Role of phyto-oestrogens in ovulation induction in women with polycystic ovarian syndrome. *Eur J Obstet Gynecol Reprod Biol*. 168(1):60–3.
21. Shahin AY, Mohammed SA. (2014). Adding the phytoestrogen *Cimicifugae racemosae* to clomiphene induction cycles with timed intercourse in polycystic ovary syndrome improves cycle outcomes and pregnancy rates-a randomized trial. *Gynecol Endocrinol*. 30(7):505–10.
22. Frei-Kleiner S, Schaffner W, Rahlfs VW, Bodmer Ch, Birkhäuser M. (2005). *Cimicifuga racemosa* dried ethanolic extract in menopausal disorders: a double-blind placebo-controlled clinical trial. *Maturitas*. 51(4):397–404.

    Osmers R, Friede M, Liske E, Schnitker J, Freudenstein J, Henneicke-von Zepelin HH. (2005). Efficacy and safety of isopropanolic black cohosh extract for climacteric symptoms. *Obstet Gynecol*. 105(5):1074–83.
23. Jacobson JS, Troxel AB, Evans J, Klaus L, Vahdat L, Kinne D, et al. (2001). Randomised trial of black cohosh for the treatment of hot flushes among women with a history of breast cancer. *Journal of Clinical Oncology*. 19:2739–45.
24. Hernández Muñoz G, Pluchino S. (2003). *Cimicifuga racemosa* for the treatment of hot flushes in women surviving breast cancer. *Maturitas*. 14;44(Suppl 1):S59–65.

    Rostock M, Fischer J, Mumm A, Stammwitz U, Saller R, Bartsch HH. (2011). Black cohosh (*Cimicifuga racemosa*) in tamoxifen-treated breast cancer patients with climacteric complaints – a prospective observational study. *Gynaecol Endocrinol*. 27(10):844–8.
25. Al-Akoum M, Dodin S, Akoum A. (2007). Synergistic cytotoxic effects of tamoxifen and black cohosh on MCF-7 and MDA-MB-231 human breast cancer cells: an in vitro study. *Can J Physiol Pharmacol*. 85(11):1153–9.
26. Xi S, Liske E, Wang S, Liu J, Zhang Z, Geng L, et al. (2014). Effect of isopropanolic *Cimicifuga racemosa* extract on uterine fibroids in comparison with tibolone among patients of a recent randomized, double blind, parallel-controlled study in chinese women with menopausal symptoms. *Evid Based Complement Alternat Med*. 717686.

27. Ruhlen RL, Sun GY, Sauter ER. (2008). Black cohosh: insights into its mechanism(s) of action. *Integr Med Insights*. 3:21–32.
28. Rachoń D, Vortherms T, Seidlová-Wuttke D, Wuttke W. (2008). Effects of black cohosh extract on body weight gain intra-abdominal fat accumulation, plasma lipids and glucose tolerance in ovariectomized Sprague-Dawley rats. *Maturitas*. 60(3–4):209–15.
29. Salerno G. (1955). *Cimicifuga racemosa* in otology; experimental study. *Minerva Otorinolaringologica*. 5(3):140–7.
30. Teschke R. (2010). Black cohosh and suspected hepatotoxicity: inconsistencies, confounding variables, and prospective use of a diagnostic causality algorithm. A critical review. *Menopause*. 17(2):426–40.
31. Nasr A, Nafeh H. (2009). Influence of black cohosh (*Cimicifuga racemosa*) use by postmenopausal women on total hepatic perfusion and liver functions. *Fertil Steril*. 92(5):1780–2.
32. *Canadian Adverse Reaction Newsletter*. 2010;20(1):1–2.
33. Shams T, Setia MS, Hemmings R, McCusker J, Sewitch M, Ciampi A. (2010). Efficacy of black cohosh-containing preparations on menopausal symptoms: a meta-analysis. *Alternative Therapies in Health and Medicine*. 16(1):36–44.
34. Liske E. (1998). Therapeutic efficacy and safety of *Cimicifuga racemosa* for gynecological disorders. *Advances in Therapy*. 15:45–53.
35. Duncan A. (1789). *The Edinburgh New Dispensatory*. Edinburgh: Bell & Bradfute.
36. Javan R, Javadi B, Feyzabadi Z. (2017). Breastfeeding: A Review of Its Physiology and Galactogogue Plants in View of Traditional Persian Medicine. *Breastfeed Med*. 12(7):401–9.
37. Azadbakht M, Baheddini A, Shorideh SM, Naserzadeh A. (2005). Effect of Vitex agnus-castus L. leaf and fruit flavonoidal extracts on serum prolactin concentration. *J Med Plants*. 4:56–61.
38. King J. Felter HW, Lloyd JU. (1909). *King's American dispensatory*. Cincinnati, OH: Ohio Valley Co., 19th ed., 4th rev.
39. Mohr H. (1954). Clinical investigations of means to increase lactation. *Deutsche Medizin Wochenschrift*. 79:1513–6.
40. Probst V, Roth OA. (1954). On A Plant Extract With A Hormone-like Effect. *Dtsch Med Wschr*. 79(35):1271–4.
41. Boon H, Smith M. (1996). *The Botanical Pharmacy: The Pharmacology of 47 Common Herbs*. Kingston, ON: Quarry Press, Inc.; 1999, pp. 76–81.

    British Herbal Pharmacopeia 4th ed. Exeter, UK: British Herbal Medicine Association, pp. 19–20.

42. Jarry H, Leonhardt S, Gorkow C, Wuttke W. (1994). In vitro prolactin but not LH and FSH release is inhibited by compounds in extracts of agnus castus: direct evidence for a dopaminergic principle by the dopamine receptor assay. *Exp Clin Endocrinol.* 102(6):448–54.
43. Winterhoff H, Münster C, Gorkow C. (1991). Die Hemmung der Laktation bei Ratten als indirekter Beweis für die Senkung von Prolaktin durch Agnus castus. *Zeitschrift für Phytotherapie.* 12:175–9.
44. Merz PG, Gorkow C, Schrodter A, Rietbrock S, Sieder C, Loew D, et al. (1996). The effects of a special Agnus castus extract (BP1095E1) on prolactin secretion in healthy male subjects. *Exp Clin Endocrinol Diabetes.* 104:447–53.
45. Chan EWC, Wong SK, Chan HT. (2018). Casticin from Vitex species: a short review on its anticancer and anti-inflammatory properties. *J Integr Med.* 16(3):147–52.
46. Rasul A, Zhao B, Liu J, Liu B, Sun J, Li J, Li X. (2014). Molecular mechanisms of casticin action: an update on its antitumor functions. *Asian Pacific journal of cancer prevention: APJCP.* 15:9049–58. 10.7314/APJCP.2014.15.21.9049.
47. Choudhary MI, Azizuddin, Jalil S, Nawaz SA, Khan KM, Tareen RB, et al. (2009). Antiinflammatory and lipoxygenase inhibitory compounds from Vitex agnus-castus. *Phytother Res.* 23:1336–9.
48. Alimohammadi R, Naderi S, Imani E, Shamsizadeh A, Mobini M, Razazadeh MH, et al. (2015). The effects of the ethanolic extract of Vitex agnus castus on stroke outcomes in ovariectomized mice. *J Babol Univ Med Sci.* 16:20–7.
49. Carmichael AR. (2008). Can Vitex agnus castus be used for the treatment of mastalgia? What is the current evidence? *Evidence-based Complementary and Alternative Medicine: ECAM.* 5(3):247–50.
50. Milewicz A, Gejdel E, Sworen H, Sienkiewicz K, Jedrzejak J, Teucher T, Schmitz H. (1993). Vitex agnus castus extract in the treatment of luteal phase defects due to latent hyperprolactinemia. Results of a randomized placebo-controlled double-blind study. *Arzneimittelforschung.* 43(7):752–6.
51. Dericks-Tan JS, Schwinn P, Hildt C. (2003). Dose-dependent stimulation of melatonin secretion after administration of Agnus castus. *Exp Clin Endocrinol Diabetes.* 111(1):44–6.

   Diaz BL, Llaneza PC. (2008). Endocrine regulation of the course of menopause by oral melatonin: first case report. *Menopause.* 15(2):388–92.

52. Webster DE, Lu J, Chen SN, Farnsworth NR, Wang ZJ. (2006). Activation of the mu-opiate receptor by Vitex agnus-castus methanol extracts: implication for its use in PMS. *J Ethnopharmacol.* 106(2):216–21.
53. Webster DE, He Y, Chen SN, Pauli GF, Farnsworth NR, Wang ZJ, et al. (2011). Opioidergic mechanisms underlying the actions of Vitex agnus-castus L. *Biochem Pharmacol.* 81:170–7.
54. Nasri S1, Oryan S, Rohani AH, Amin GR. (2007). The effects of *Vitex agnus castus* extract and its interaction with dopaminergic system on LH and testosterone in male mice. *Pak J Biol Sci.* 10(14):2300–7.
55. Wuttke W, Jarry H, Christoffel V, et al. (2003). *Phytomed.* 10:348–57.
56. Sehmisch et al. (2009). Vitex agnus castus as prophylaxis for osteopenia after orchidectomy in rats compared with estradiol and testosterone supplementation. *Phytother Res.* 23(6):851–8. doi: 10.1002/ptr.2711.
57. Allahtavakoli M, Honari N, Pourabolli I, Kazemi Arababadi M, Ghafarian H, Roohbakhsh A, et al. (2015). Vitex agnus castus extract improves learning and memory and increases the transcription of estrogen receptor α in hippocampus of ovariectomized rats. *Basic Clin Neurosci.* 6:185–92.
58. Moreno FN, Campos-Shimada LB, da Costa SC, Garcia RF, Cecchini AL, Natali MR, et al. (2015). Vitex agnus-castus L. (Verbenaceae) improves the liver lipid metabolism and redox state of ovariectomized rats. *Evid Based Complement Alternat Med.* 2015:212–378.
59. Oroojan AA, Ahangarpour A, Khorsandi L, Najimi SA. (2016). Effects of hydro-alcoholic extract of Vitex agnus-castus fruit on kidney of D-galactose-induced aging model in female mice. *Iran J Vet Res.* 17(3): 203–6.
60. Ahangarpour A, Oroojan AA, Khorsandi L, Najimi SA. (2017). Pancreatic protective and hypoglycemic effects of Vitex agnus-castus L. fruit hydroalcoholic extract in D-galactose-induced aging mouse model. *Res Pharm Sci.* 12(2):137–43.
61. Saberi M, Rezvanizadeh A, Bakhtiarian A. (2008). The antiepileptic activity of *Vitex agnus-castus* extract on amygdala kindled seizures in male rats. *Neurosci Lett.* 441:193–6.
62. Rani A and Sharma A. (2013). The genus Vitex: A review. *Pharmacogn Rev.* 7(14):188–98.
63. van Die, Burger HG, Teede HJ, Bone KM. (2013). Vitex agnus-castus extracts for female reproductive disorders: a systematic review of clinical trials. *Planta Med.* 79(7):562–75.

64. Verkaik S, Kamperman AM, van Westrhenen R, Schulte PFJ. (2017). The treatment of premenstrual syndrome with preparations of Vitex agnus castus: a systematic review and meta-analysis. *Am J Obstet Gynecol.* 217(2):150–66.
65. Schellenberg R. (2001). Treatment for the premenstrual syndrome with agnus castus fruit extract: prospective, randomised, placebo controlled study. *BMJ.* 20;322(7279):134–7.
66. He Z, Chen R, Zhou Y, Geng L, Zhang Z, Chen S, et al. (2009). Treatment for premenstrual syndrome with Vitex agnus castus: A prospective, randomized, multi-center placebo controlled study in China. *Maturitas.* 20;63(1):99–103.
67. Zamani M, Neghab N, Torabian S. (2012). Therapeutic effect of Vitex agnus castus in patients with premenstrual syndrome. *Acta Med Iran.* 50(2):101–6.
68. Berger D, Schaffner W, Schrader E, Meier B, Brattström A. (2000). Efficacy of Vitex agnus castus L. extract Ze 440 in patients with premenstrual syndrome (PMS). *Arch Gynecol Obstet.* 264(3):150–3.
69. van Die MD, Bone KM, Burger HG, Reece JE, Teede HJ. (2009). Effects of a combination of Hypericum perforatum and Vitex agnus-castus on PMS-like symptoms in late-perimenopausal women: findings from a subpopulation analysis. *J Altern Complement Med.* 15(9):1045–8.
70. Ambrosini A, Di Lorenzo C, Coppola G, Pierelli F. (2013). Use of Vitex agnus-castus in migrainous women with premenstrual syndrome: an open-label clinical observation. *Acta Neurol Belg.* 113(1):25–9.
71. Atmaca M, Kumru S, Tezcan E. (2003). Fluoxetine versus Vitex agnus castus extract in the treatment of premenstrual dysphoric disorder. *Hum Psychopharmacol.* 18(3):191–5.
72. Ciotta L, Pagano I, Stracquadanio M, Di Leo S, Andò A, Formuso C. (2011). Psychic aspects of the premenstrual dysphoric disorders. New therapeutic strategies: our experience with Vitex agnus castus. *Minerva Ginecol.* 63(3):237–45.
73. Cerqueira RO, Frey BN, Leclerc E, Brietzke E. (2017). Vitex agnus castus for premenstrual syndrome and premenstrual dysphoric disorder: a systematic review. *Arch Womens Ment Health.* 20(6):713–9.
74. Halaska M, Beles P, Gorkow C, Sieder C. (1999). Treatment of cyclical mastalgia with a solution containing a Vitex agnus castus extract: results of a placebo-controlled double-blind study. *Breast.* 8(4):175–81.
75. Dinç T, Coşkun F. (2014). Comparison of *Fructus agni casti* and flurbiprofen in the treatment of cyclic mastalgia in premenopausal women. *Ulus Cerrahi Derg.* 30(1):34–8.

76. Kilicdag EB, Tarim E, Bagis T, Erkanli S, Aslan E, Ozsahin K, et al. (2004). *Fructus agni casti* and bromocriptine for treatment of hyperprolactinemia and mastalgia. *Int J Gynaecol Obstet*. 85(3):292–3.
77. Yavarikia P, Shahnazi M, Hadavand Mirzaie S, Javadzadeh Y, Lutfi R. (2013). Comparing the effect of mefenamic Acid and *Vitex agnus* on intrauterine device induced bleeding. *J Caring Sci*. 31;2(3):245–54.
78. Zamani M, Mansour Ghanaei M, Farimany M, Nasrollahie SH. (2007). Efficacy of Mefenamic Acid and Vitex in Reduction of Menstrual Blood Loss and Hb Changes in Patients with a Complaint of Menorrhagia. *Iran J Obstet Gynecol Infertil*. 10(1):79–86.
79. Aksoy AN, Gözükara I, Kabil Kucur S. (2014). Evaluation of the efficacy of *Fructus agni casti* in women with severe primary dysmenorrhea: a prospective comparative Doppler study. *J Obstet Gynaecol Res*. 40(3):779–84.
80. Amann W. (1975). Acne vulgaris and Agnus castus (Agnolyt). *Z. Allgemeinmed*. 51;35:1645–8.
81. Christie S, Walker AF. (1998). Vitex agnus-castus L.:(1) A Review of its traditional and modern therapeutic use; current use from a survey of practitioners. *European Journal of Herbal Medicine*. 3;3:29–45.
82. Eltbogen R, Litschgi M, Gasser UE, Flueeli A, Nebel S, Zahner C. (2016). Vitex agnus-castus extract (ZE440) improves symptoms in women with menstrual cycle irregularities. *Reproductive Endocrinology*. 28.
83. Gerhard I, Patek A, Monga B, Blank A, Gorkow C. (1998). Mastodynon® for female infertility. Randomized placebo controlled, clinical double-blind study. *Forschende Komplementärmedizin/Res Compl Med*. 5(6):272–8.
84. Westphal LM, Polan ML, Trant AS. (2006). Double-blind, placebo-controlled study of Fertilityblend: a nutritional supplement for improving fertility in women. *Clin Exp Obstet Gynecol*. 33(4):205–8.
85. Brattström A, Kaiser WD. (2010). The restless leg syndrome – first experiences with an extract *From Vitex agnus-castus*. *Z Phytother*. 31(5): 247–50.
86. Eftekhari MH, Rostami ZH, Emami MJ, Tabatabaee HR. (2014). Effects of '*Vitex agnus castus*' extract and magnesium supplementation, alone and in combination, on osteogenic and angiogenic factors and fracture healing in women with long bone fracture. *J Res Med Sci*. 19:1–7.
87. Schellenberg R, Zimmermann C, Drewe J, Hoexter G, Zahner C. (2012). Dose-dependent efficacy of the Vitex agnus castus extract Ze 440 in patients suffering from premenstrual syndrome. *Phytomedicine*. 19(14):1325–31.

88. Weiss RF. (1988/2001). *Weiss's Herbal Medicine*. Stuttgart: Thieme.
89. Daniele C, Thompson Coon J, Pittler MH, Ernst E. (2005). Vitex agnus castus: a systematic review of adverse events. *Drug Saf.* 28(4):319–32.
90. Cahill DJ, Fox R, Wardle PG, Harlow CR. (1994). Multiple follicular development associated with herbal medicine. *Hum Reprod.* 9(8): 1469–70.

Chapter six

1. Parker S, May B, Zhang C, Zhang AL, Lu C, Xue CC. (2016). A Pharmacological Review of Bioactive Constituents of Paeonia lactiflora Pallas and Paeonia veitchii Lynch. *Phytother Res.* 30(9):1445–73.
2. Chen Z, Li XP, Li ZJ, Xu L, Li XM. (2013). Reduced hepatotoxicity by total glucosides of paeony in combination treatment with leflunomide and methotrexate for patients with active rheumatoid arthritis. *Int Immunopharmacol.* 15(3):474–7.
3. Zhang HF, Hou P, Xiao WG. (2007). Clinical observation on effect of total glucosides of paeony in treating patients with non-systemic involved Sjögren syndrome. *Zhongguo Zhong Xi Yi Jie He Za Zhi.* 27(7): 596–8.
4. Liang J, Chengyin Li, Yanping Li, Bin Wu. (2017). Clinical efficacy and safety of total glucosides of paeony for primary sjögren's syndrome: a systematic Review. *Evid Based Complement Alternat Med.* 3242301.
5. Zhu Q, Qi X, Wu Y, Wang K. (2016). Clinical study of total glucosides of paeony for the treatment of diabetic kidney disease in patients with diabetes mellitus. *Int Urol Nephrol.* 48(11):1873–80.
6. Jia YB, Tang TQ. (1991). Paeonia Lactiflora injection in treating chronic cor pulmonale with pulmonary hypertension. *Zhong Xi Yi Jie He Za Zhi.* 11(4):199–202, 195.
7. Roshan A, Verma NK, Kumar CS, Kumar CS, Chandra V, Singh DP, et al. (2012). Phytochemical constituent, pharmacological activity and medicinal uses through the millennia of *Glycyrrhiza glabra* Linn: a review. *International Research Journal of Pharmacy.* 3(8):45–55.
8. Josephs RA, Guinn JS, Harper ML, Askari F. (2001). Liquorice consumption and salivary testosterone concentrations. *Lancet.* 10;358(9293): 1613–4.
9. Armanini D, Bonanni G, Palermo M. (1999). Reduction of serum testosterone in men by liquorice. *N Engl J Med.* 341(15):1158.

10. Armanini D, Mattarello MJ, Fiore C, Bonanni G, Scaroni C, Sartorato P, et al. (2004). Liquorice reduces serum testosterone in healthy women. *Steroids*. 69(11–2):763–6.
11. Sigurjonsdottir HA, Axelson M, Johannsson G, Manhem K, Nystrom E, Wallerstedt S. (2006). Liquorice in moderate doses does not affect sex steroid hormones of biological importance although the effect differs between the genders. *Horm Res*. 65(2):106–10.
12. Mattarello MJ, Benedini S, Fiore C, Camozzi V, Sartorato P, Luisetto G, Armanini D. (2006). Effect of liquorice on PTH levels in healthy women. Steroids. 71(5):403–8.
13. Armanini D, Castello R, Scaroni C, Bonanni G, Faccini G, Pellati D, et al. (2007). Treatment of polycystic ovary syndrome with spironolactone plus liquorice. *Eur J Obstet Gynecol Reprod Biol*. 131(1):61–7.
14. Armanini D, De Palo CB, Mattarello MJ, Spinella P, Zaccaria M, Ermolao A, et al. (2003). Effect of liquorice on the reduction of body fat mass in healthy subjects. *J Endocrinol Invest*. 26(7):646–50.
15. Nahidi F, Zare E, Mojab F, Alavi-Majd H. (2012). Effects of liquorice on relief and recurrence of menopausal hot flashes. *Iran J Pharm Res*. 11(2):541–8.
16. Kimura M, Kimura I, Takahashi K, Muroi M, Yoshizaki M, Kanaoka M, et al. (1984). Blocking effects of blended paeoniflorin or its related compounds with glycyrrhizin on neuromuscular junctions in frogs and mice. *Jpn J Pharmacol*. 36:275–82.
17. Maeda T, Shinozuka K, Baba K, Hayashi M, Hayashi E. (1983). Effect of shakuyaku-kanzoh-toh, a prescription composed of shakuyaku (*Paeoniae Radix*) and kanzoh (*Glycyrrhizae Radix*) on guinea pig ileum. *Journal of Pharmacobio-Dynamics*. 6(3):153–60.
18. Sumi G, Yasuda K, Tsuji S, Kanamori C, Tsuzuki T, Cho H, et al. (2015). Lipid-soluble fraction of Shakuyaku-kanzo-to inhibits myometrial contraction in pregnant women. *J Obstet Gynaecol Res*. 41(5):670–9.
19. Sumi G, Yasuda K, Kanamori C, Kajimoto M, Nishigaki A, Tsuzuki T, et al. (2014). Two-step inhibitory effect of kanzo on oxytocin-induced and prostaglandin F2α-induced uterine myometrial contractions. *J Nat Med*. 68(3):550–60.
20. Tsuji S, Yasuda K, Sumi G, Cho H, Tsuzuki T, Okada H, Kanzaki H. (2012). Shakuyaku-kanzo-to inhibits smooth muscle contractions of human pregnant uterine tissue in vitro. *J Obstet Gynaecol Res*. 38(7):1004–10.
21. Kumada T, Kumada H, Makoto Y. (1999). Effect of shakuyaku-kanzo-to (Tsumura TJ-68) on muscle cramps accompanying cirrhosis in a

placebo-controlled double-blind parallel study. *J Clin Ther Med.* 15: 499–523.
22. Yosida M. (1995). Effects of shakuyaku-kanzo-to on muscle cramp in diabetics. *Neurol Ther.* 12:529–34.
23. Hyodo T, Taira T, Kumakura M, Yamamoto S, Yoshida K, Uchida T, et al. (2002). The immediate effect of Shakuyaku-kanzo-to, traditional Japanese herbal medicine, for muscular cramps during maintenance hemodialysis. *Nephron.* 90(2):240.
24. Yamashita JI. (1992). Effect of Tsumura skakuyaku-kanzo-to on pain at muscle twitch during and after dialysis in the patients undergoing dialysis. *Pain & Kampo Medicine.* 2:18–20.
25. Maruyama K. (1996). Effectiveness of shakuyaku-kanzo-to on convulsion and pain associated with alcohol dependence. *Kampolgaku.* 20:81–4.
26. Sakamoto T, Hosino M. (1995). Effect of shakuyaku-kanzo-to extract granules on convulsion of gastrocnemius muscle in patients with cerebrovascular disorder. *Jpn J Oriental Med.* 45:563–8.
27. Takao Y, Takaoka Y, Sugano A, Sato H, Motoyama Y, Ohta M, et al. (2015). Shakuyaku-kanzo-to (Shao-Yao-Gan-Cao-Tang) as Treatment of painful muscle cramps in patients with lumbar spinal stenosis and its minimum effective dose. *Kobe J Med Sci.* 4;61(5):E132–7.
28. Yamamoto K, Hoshiai H, Noda K. (2001). Effects of shakuyaku-kanzo-to on muscle pain from combination chemotherapy with paclitaxel and carboplatin. *Gynecol Oncol.* 81:333–4.
29. Sakamoto S, Mitamura T, Iwasawa M, Kitsunai H, Shindou K, Yagishita Y, et al. (1998). Conservative management for perimenopausal women with uterine leiomyomas using Chinese herbal medicines and synthetic analogs of gonadotropin-releasing hormone. *In Vivo.* 12:333–7.
30. Wang D, Wang W, Zhou Y, Wang J, Jia D, Wong HK, et al. (2015). Studies on the regulatory effect of Peony-Glycyrrhiza Decoction on prolactin hyperactivity and underlying mechanism in hyperprolactinemia rat model. *Neurosci Lett.* 8;606:60–5.
31. Yamada K, Kanba S, Murata T, Fukuzawa M, Terashi B, Yagi G, et al. (1996). Effectiveness of shakuyaku-kanzo-to in neuroleptic-induced hyperprolactinemia: a preliminary report. *Psychiatry Clin Neurosci.* 50(6):341–2.
32. Man SC, Li XB, Wang HH, Yuan HN, Wang HN, Zhang RG, et al. (2016). Peony-glycyrrhiza decoction for antipsychotic-related hyperprolactinemia in women with schizophrenia: a randomized controlled trial. *J Clin Psychopharmacol.* 36(6):572–9.

33. Yamada K, Kanba S, Yagi G, & Asai M. (1997). Effectiveness of herbal medicine (Shakuyaku-kanzo-to) for neuroleptic-induced hyperprolactinemia. *Journal of Clinical Psychopharmacology.* 17(3):234–5.
34. Yuan HN, Wang CY, Sze CW, Tong Y, Tan QR, Feng XJ, et al. (2008). A randomized, crossover comparison of herbal medicine and bromocriptine against risperidone-induced hyperprolactinemia in patients with schizophrenia. *J Clin Psychopharmacol.* 28(3):264–370.
35. Yamada K, Kanba S, Yagi G, Asai M. (1999). Herbal medicine (skakuyaku-kanzo-to) in the treatment of risperidone-induced amenorrhea. *J Clin Psychopharmacol.* 19:380–1.
36. Aboraya A, Fullen JE, Ponieman BL, Makela EH, Latocha M. (2004). Hyperprolactinemia associated with risperidone. A case report and review of literature. *Psychiatry (Edgmont).* 1(3):29–31.
37. Yang P, Li L, Yang D, Wang C, Peng H, Huang H, et al. (2017). Effect of peony-glycyrrhiza decoction on amisulpride-induced hyperprolactinemia in women with schizophrenia: a preliminary study. *Evid Based Complement Alternat Med.* 7901670.
38. Takeuchi T, Nishii O, Okamura T, Yaginuma T. (1991). Effect of paeoniflorin, glycyrrhizin and glycyrrhetic acid on ovarian androgen production. *Am J Chin Med.* 19(1):73–8.
39. Takeuchi T. (1988). Effect of shakuyaku-kanzo-to, shakuyaku, kanzo, paeoniflorin, glycyrrhetinic acid and glycyrrhizin on ovarian function in rats. *Nihon Naibunpi Gakkai Zasshi.* 20;64(11):1124–39.
40. Takahashi K, Kitao M. (1994). Effect of TJ-68 (shakuyaku-kanzo-to) on polycystic ovarian disease. *Int J Fertil Menopausal Stud.* 39(2):69.
41. Yaginuma T, Izumi R, Yasui H, Arai T, Kawabata M. (1982). Effect of traditional herbal medicine on serum testosterone levels and its induction of regular ovulation in hyperandrogenic and oligomenorrheic women. *Nihon Sanka Fujinka Gakkai Zasshi.* 34(7):939–44.
42. Takahashi K, Yoshino K, Shirai T, Nishigaki A, Araki Y, Kitao M. (1988). Effects of traditional medicine (Shakuyaku-kanzo-to) on testosterone secretion in patients with polycystic ovarian syndrome detected by ultrasound. *Nihon Sanka Fujinka Gakkai Zasshi.* 40(6):789–92.
43. Aizawa H, Niimura M. (1996). Serum androgen levels in women with acne vulgaris: The effect of Shakuyaku-Kanzo-To (SK). 38:37–41.
44. Homma M, Ishihara M, Qian W, Kohda Y. (2006). Effects of long term administration of Shakuyaku-kanzo-To and Shosaiko-To on serum potassium levels. *Yakugaku Zasshi.* 126(10):973–8.

45. Sung CK, Kang GH, Yoon SS, Lee IS, Kim DH, Sankawa U, et al. (1996). Glycosidases that convert natural glycosides to bioactive compounds. In: Waller G, Yamasaki K, eds. *Saponins Used in Traditional and Modern Medicine.* New York: Plenum Press, p. 24.

Chapter seven

1. Ratka A. (2005). Menopausal hot flashes and development of cognitive impairment. *Annals of the New York Academy of Sciences.* 1052(1):11–26.
2. Pollycove R, Naftolin F, Simon JA. (2011). The evolutionary origin and significance of menopause. *Menopause (New York, N.Y.).* 18(3):336–42.
3. Carr M. (2003). The Emergence of the Metabolic Syndrome with Menopause. *The Journal of Clinical Endocrinology & Metabolism.* 88(6):2404–11.
4. Anisha A Gupte, Henry J Pownall, Dale J Hamilton. (2015). Estrogen: an emerging regulator of insulin action and mitochondrial function. *Journal of Diabetes Research.* Article ID 916585, 9 pages.
5. Shanafelt TD, Barton DL, Adjei AA, Loprinzi CL. (2002). Pathophysiology and treatment of hot flashes. *Mayo Clin Proc.* 77(11):1207–18.
6. Bretler DM, Hansen PR, Sørensen R, Lindhardsen J, Ahlehoff O, Andersson C, et al. (2012). Discontinuation of hormone replacement therapy after myocardial infarction and short term risk of adverse cardiovascular events: nationwide cohort study. *BMJ.* 344:e1802.
7. Josefson D. (2002). Oestrogen only HRT increases risk of ovarian cancer. *BMJ.* 27;325(7357):180.
8. Panay N. (2011). The reality is that the number of women with menopausal symptoms wanting to consider alternative therapies rather than hormone replacement therapy (HRT) has increased over the last decade. *Climacteric.* 14(Suppl 2):1.
9. Bennesch MA, Picard D. (2015). Minireview: Tipping the balance: ligand-independent activation of steroid receptors. *Mol Endocrinol.* 29(3):349–63.
10. Rossouw JE, Anderson GL, Prentice RL, LaCroix AZ, Kooperberg C, Stefanick ML, et al. (2002). Risks and benefits of estrogen plus progestin in healthy postmenopausal women: principal results From the Women's Health Initiative randomized controlled trial. *JAMA.* 288(3):321–33.
11. Zhou J, Chen Y, Huang Y, Long J, Wan F, Zhang S. (2013). Serum follicle-stimulating hormone level is associated with human epidermal growth factor receptor type 2 and Ki67 expression in post-menopausal females with breast cancer. *Oncology letters.* 6:1128–32. Doi: 10.3892/ol.2013.1516.

12. Windham GC, Mitchell P, Anderson M, Lasley BL. (2005). Cigarette smoking and effects on hormone function in premenopausal women. *Environmental Health Perspectives.* 113(10):1285–90.
13. Kargozar R, Azizi H, Salari R. (2017). A review of effective herbal medicines in controlling menopausal symptoms. *Electron Physician.* 9(11):5826–33.
14. DeLeo V, Lanzetta D, Cazzavacca R, Morgante G. (1998). Treatment of neurovegetative menopausal symptoms with a phytotherapeutic agent. *Minerva Ginecol.* 50(5):207–11.
15. Rahimikian F, Rahimi R, Golzareh P, Bekhradi R, Mehran A. (2017). Effect of Foeniculum vulgare Mill. (fennel) on menopausal symptoms in postmenopausal women: a randomized, triple-blind, placebo-controlled trial. *Menopause.* 24(9):1017–21.
16. Heyerick A, Vervarcke S, Depypere H, Bracke M, De Keukeleire D. (2006). A first prospective, randomized, double-blind, placebo-controlled study on the use of a standardized hop extract to alleviate menopausal discomforts. *Maturitas.* 20;54(2):164–75.
17. Erkkola R, Vervarcke S, Vansteelandt S, Rompotti P, De Keukeleire D, Heyerick A. (2010). A randomized, double-blind, placebo-controlled, cross-over pilot study on the use of a standardized hop extract to alleviate menopausal discomforts. *Phytomedicine.* 17(6):389–96.
18. Aghamiri V, Mirghafourvand M, Mohammad-Alizadeh-Charandabi S, Nazemiyeh H. (2016). The effect of hop (*Humulus lupulus* L.) on early menopausal symptoms and hot flashes: A randomized placebo-controlled trial. *Complement. Ther Clin Pract.* 23:130–5.
19. Myers SP, Vigar V. (2017). Effects of a standardised extract of *Trifolium pratense* (Promensil) at a dosage of 80mg in the treatment of menopausal hot flushes: A systematic review and meta-analysis. *Phytomedicine.* 15;24:141–7.
20. Dietz BM, Hajirahimkhan A, Dunlap TL, Bolton JL. (2016). Botanicals and Their Bioactive Phytochemicals for Women's Health. *Pharmacol Rev.* 68(4):1026–73.
21. Ghazanfarpour M, Sadeghi R, Latifnejad Roudsari R, et al. (2016). Effects of flaxseed and Hypericum perforatum on hot flash, vaginal atrophy and estrogen-dependent cancers in menopausal women: a systematic review and meta-analysis. *Avicenna J Phytomed.* 6(3):273–83.
22. Dietz BM, Mahady GB, Pauli GF, Farnsworth NR. (2005). Valerian extract and valerenic acid are partial agonists of the 5-HT5a receptor *in vitro. Brain Res Mol Brain Res.* 138(2):191–7.

23. Mirabi P, Mojab F. (2013). The effects of valerian root on hot flashes in menopausal women. *Iran J Pharm Res*. 12(1):217–22.
24. Jenabi E, Shobeiri F, Hazavehei S, Roshanaei G. (2018). The effect of Valerian on the severity and frequency of hot flashes: A triple-blind randomized clinical trial. *Women & Health*. 58(3):297–304.
25. Leach MJ, Moore V. (2012). Black cohosh (*Cimicifuga* spp.) for menopausal symptoms. *Cochrane Database of Systematic Reviews*. 9.
26. Haines CJ, Lam PM, Chung TK, Cheng KF, Leung PC. (2008). A randomized, double-blind, placebo-controlled study of the effect of a Chinese herbal medicine preparation (Dang Gui Buxue Tang) on menopausal symptoms in Hong Kong Chinese women. *Climacteric*. 11(3):244–51.
27. Wang CC, Cheng KF, Lo WM, Law C, Li L, Leung PC, et al. (2013). A randomized, double-blind, multiple-dose escalation study of a Chinese herbal medicine preparation (Dang Gui Buxue Tang) for moderate to severe menopausal symptoms and quality of life in postmenopausal women. *Menopause*. 20(2):223–31.
28. Menati L, Khaleghinezhad K, Tadayon M, Siahpoosh A. (2014). Evaluation of contextual and demographic factors on Liquorice effects on reducing hot flashes in postmenopause women. *Health Care Women Int*. 35(1):87–99.
29. Asgari P, Bahramnezhad F, Narenji F, Golitaleb M, Askari M. (2015). A clinical study of the effect of *Glycyrrhiza glabra* plant and exercise on the quality of life of menopausal women. *Chron Dis J*. 3(2):79–86.
30. Nahidi F, Kariman N, Simbar M, Mojab F. (2012). The study on the effects of Pimpinella anisum on relief and recurrence of menopausal hot flashes. *Iran J Pharm Res*. 11(4):1079–85.
31. Begum SS, Jayalakshmi HK, Vidyavathi HG, Nair GG, Issac A, Maliakel BP, Geetha K, Suresha SV, Vasundhara M. et al. (2016). A Novel Extract of Fenugreek Husk (FenuSMART™) Alleviates postmenopausal symptoms and helps to establish the hormonal balance: a randomized, double-blind, placebo-controlled study: effect of fenusmart on postmenopausal discomforts. *Phytotherapy Research*. 30(11).
32. Abbaspoor Z, Hajikhani NA, Afshari P. (2011). Effect of vitexagnuscactus on menopausal early symptoms in postmenopausal women: A randomized, double-blind, placebo-controlled study. *Br J Med Res*. 1:132–40.
33. Wiklund IK, Mattsson LA, Lindgren R, Limoni C. (1999). Effects of a standardized ginseng extract on quality of life and physiological parameters in symptomatic postmenopausal women: a double-blind,

placebo-controlled trial. Swedish Alternative Medicine Group. *Int J Clin Pharmacol Res.* 19:89–99.
34. Franco OH, Chowdhury R, Troup J, Voortman T, Kunutsor S, Kavousi M, et al. (2016). Use of Plant-Based Therapies and Menopausal Symptoms; A Systematic Review and Meta-analysis. *JAMA.* 315(23):2554–63.
35. Yaralizadeh M, Abedi P, Najar S, Namjoyan F, Saki A. (2016). Effect of Foeniculum vulgare (fennel) vaginal cream on vaginal atrophy in postmenopausal women: A double-blind randomized placebo-controlled trial. *Maturitas.* 84:75–80.
36. Mercier J, Morin M, Lemieux MC, Reichetzer B, Khalifé S, Dumoulin C. (2016). Pelvic floor muscles training to reduce symptoms and signs of vulvovaginal atrophy: a case study. *Menopause.* 23(7):816–20.
37. Kim JM, Park YJ. (2017). Probiotics in the Prevention and Treatment of Postmenopausal Vaginal Infections: Review. *J Menopausal Med.* 23(3):139–45.
38. Recine N, Palma E, Domenici L, Giorgini M, Imperiale L, Sassu C, et al. (2016). Restoring vaginal microbiota: biological control of bacterial vaginosis. A prospective case-control study using *Lactobacillus rhamnosus* BMX 54 as adjuvant treatment against bacterial vaginosis. *Arch Gynecol Obstet.* 293(1):101–7.
39. Petricevic L, Unger FM, Viernstein H, Kiss H. (2008). Randomized, double-blind, placebo-controlled study of oral lactobacilli to improve the vaginal flora of postmenopausal women. *Eur J Obstet Gynecol Reprod Biol.* 141(1):54–7.
40. Saffari E, Mohammad-Alizadeh-Charandabi S, Adibpour M Mirghafourvand M, Javadzadeh Y. (2017). Comparing the effects of Calendula officinalis and clotrimazole on vaginal Candidiasis: A randomized controlled trial. *Journal Women & Health.* 57:10.
41. Sheidaei S, Sadeghi T, Jafarnejad F, Rajabi O, Najafzadeh M. (2017). Herbal Medicine and Vaginal Candidiasis in Iran: A Review. *Evidenced Based Care Journal.* 7;2(7):71–7.
42. Grin PM, Kowalewska PM, Alhazzan W, Fox-Robichaud AE. (2013). Lactobacillus for preventing recurrent urinary tract infections in women: meta-analysis. *Can J Urol.* 20(1):6607–14.
43. Taavoni S, Nazem Ekbatani N, Haghani H. (2013). Valerian/lemon balm use for sleep disorders during menopause. *Complement Ther Clin Pract.* 19(4):193–6.

44. Dericks-Tan JS, Schwinn P, Hildt C. (2003). Dose-dependent stimulation of melatonin secretion after administration of Agnus castus. *Exp Clin Endocrinol Diabetes.* 111(1):44–6.
45. Xie Z, Chen F, Li WA, Geng X, Li C, Meng X, et al. (2017). A review of sleep disorders and melatonin. *Neurol Res.* 39(6):559–65.
46. Xu Q, Parks CG, DeRoo LA, Cawthon RM, Sandler DP, Chen H. (2009). Multivitamin use and telomere length in women. *Am J Clin Nutr.* 89(6):1857–63.
47. Phillips GS, Wise LA, Harlow BL. (2007). A prospective analysis of alcohol consumption and onset of perimenopause. *Maturitas.* 20:56(3): 263–72.
48. Calabrese G. (1999). Nonalcoholic compounds of wine: the phytoestrogen resveratrol and moderate red wine consumption during menopause. *Drugs Exp Clin Res.* 25(2–3):111–4.
49. Huntley AL. (2007). Grape flavonoids and menopausal health. *Menopause Int.* 13(4):165–9.
50. Cicero AF, Derosa G, Brillante R, Bernardi R, Nascetti S, Gaddi A. (2004). Effects of Siberian ginseng (*Eleutherococcus senticosus* maxim.) on elderly quality of life: a randomized clinical trial. *Arch Gerontol Geriatr Suppl.* (9):69–73.
51. Farnsworth NR, Kinghorn AD, Soejarto DD, Waller DP. (1985). *Siberian Ginseng (Eleutherococcus senticosus): Current Status as an Adaptogen. Economic and Medicinal Plant Research. Volume 1.* London, UK: Academic Press, pp. 156–209.
52. Lee S, Rhee DK. (2017). Effects of ginseng on stress-related depression, anxiety, and the hypothalamic–pituitary–adrenal axis. *J Ginseng Res.* 41(4):589–94.
53. Hallstrom C, Fulder S, Carruthers M. (1978). Effects of Ginseng on the Performance of Nurses on Night Duty. *Am J Chin Med.* 6:277.
54. Mishra LC, Singh BB, Dagenais S. (2000). Scientific basis for the therapeutic use of Withania somnifera (ashwagandha): a review. *Altern Med Rev.* 5(4):334–46.
55. Ofir R, Tamir S, Khatib S, Vaya J. (2003). Inhibition of serotonin reuptake by Liquorice constituents. *J Mol Neurosci.* 20(2):135–40.
56. Al-Akoum M, Maunsell E, Verreault R, Provencher L, Otis H, Dodin S. (2009). Effects of *Hypericum perforatum* (St. John's wort) on hot flashes and quality of life in perimenopausal women: a randomized pilot trial. *Menopause.* 16(2):307–14.

57. Lindgren R, Mattsson LA, Meier W, Wiklund I. (1997). Has Ginsana any estrogen effects when measured by maturity index, plasma FSH, and estradiol? *Menopause*. 4:248.
58. Henneicke-von Zepelin HH. (2017). 60 Jahre Arzneimittel aus Cimicifuga racemosa: Meilensteine klinischer Forschung, aktuelle Studienergebnisse und derzeitige Entwicklung. *Wiener medizinische Wochenschrift* (1946), 167(7–8):147–59.
59. Briese V, Stammwitz U, Friede M, Henneicke-von Zepelin HH. (2007). Black cohosh with or without St. John's wort for symptom-specific climacteric treatment—results of a large-scale, controlled, observational study. *Maturitas*. 20:57(4):405–14.
60. Chung DJ, Kim HY, Park KH, Jeong KA, Lee SK, Lee YI, et al. (2007). Black cohosh and St. John's wort (GYNO-Plus) for climacteric symptoms. *Yonsei Med J*. 30:48(2):289–94.
61. Laakmann E, Grajecki D, Doege K, zu Eulenburg C, Buhling KJ. (2012). Efficacy of Cimicifuga racemosa, Hypericum perforatum and Agnus castus in the treatment of climacteric complaints: a systematic review. *Gynecol Endocrinol*. 28(9):703–9.
62. van Die MD, Burger HG, Teede HJ, Bone KM. (2009). *Vitex agnus-castus* (Chaste-Tree/Berry) in the treatment of menopause-related complaints. *J Altern Complement Med*. 15(8):853–62.
63. Diaz BL, Llaneza PC. (2008). Endocrine regulation of the course of menopause by oral melatonin: first case report. *Menopause*. 15(2): 388–92.
64. Dericks-Tan JS, Schwinn P, Hildt C. (2003). Dose-dependent stimulation of melatonin secretion after administration of agnus castus. *Exp Clin Endocrinol Diabetes*. 111:44–6
65. van Die MD, Burger HG, Bone KM, Cohen MM, Teede HJ. (2009). *Hypericum perforatum* with *Vitex agnus-castus* in menopausal symptoms: a randomized, controlled trial. *Menopause*. 16(1):156–63.
66. van Die MD, Bone KM, Burger HG, Reece JE, Teede HJ. (2009). Effects of a combination of *Hypericum perforatum and Vitex agnus-castus* on PMS-like symptoms in late-perimenopausal women: findings from a subpopulation analysis. *J Altern Complement Med*. 15(9):1045–8.
67. Wilt T, Ishani A, MacDonald R, Stark G, Mulrow C, Lau J. (1999). Beta-sitosterols for benign prostatic hyperplasia. *Cochrane Database of Systematic Reviews*. 3:CD001043. Doi: 10.1002/14651858.CD001043.
68. Kumar S, Madaan R, Sharma A. (2008). Pharmacological evaluation of Bioactive Principle of Turnera aphrodisiaca. *Indian Journal of Pharmaceutical Sciences*. 70(6):740–4.

69. Zhao J, Dasmahapatra AK, Khan SI, Khan IA. (2008). Anti-aromatase activity of the constituents from damiana (Turnera diffusa). *Journal of Ethnopharmacology.* 120(3):387–93.
70. Arletti R, Benelli A, Cavazzuti E, Scarpetta G, Bertolini A. (1999). Stimulating property of *Turnera diffusa* and *Pfaffia paniculata* extracts on the sexual-behavior of male rats. *Psychopharmacology.* 143(1):15–9.
71. Ito TY, Polan ML, Whipple B, Trant AS. (2006). The enhancement of female sexual function with ArginMax, a nutritional supplement, among women differing in menopausal status. *J Sex Marital Ther.* 32(5):369–78.
72. Greven KM, Case LD, Nycum LR, Zekan PJ, Hurd DD, Balcueva EP, et al. (2015). Effect of ArginMax on sexual functioning and quality of life among female cancer survivors: results of the WFU CCOP Research Base Protocol 97106. *J Community Support Oncol.* 13(3):87–94.
73. Oh KJ, Chae MJ, Lee HS, Hong HD, Park K. (2010). Effects of Korean red ginseng on sexual arousal in menopausal women: placebo-controlled, double-blind crossover clinical study. *J Sex Med.* 7(4 Pt 1):1469–77
74. Liu YR, Jiang YL, Huang RQ, Yang JY, Xiao BK, Dong JX. (2014). *Hypericum perforatum* L. preparations for menopause: a meta-analysis of efficacy and safety. *Climacteric.* 17(4):325–35.
75. Abedi P, Najafian M, Yaralizadeh M, Namjoyan F. (2018). Effect of fennel vaginal cream on sexual function in postmenopausal women: A double blind randomized controlled trial. *J Med Life.* 11(1):24–8.
76. Ibrahim RM, Hamdan NS, Ismail M, Saini SM, Abd Rashid SN, Abd Latiff L, et al. (2014). Protective Effects of Nigella sativa on Metabolic Syndrome in Menopausal Women. *Adv Pharm Bull.* 4(1):29–33.
77. Kim SY, Seo SK, Choi YM, Jeon YE, Lim KJ, Cho S, et al. (2012). Effects of red ginseng supplementation on menopausal symptoms and cardiovascular risk factors in postmenopausal women: a double-blind randomized controlled trial. *Menopause.* 19(4):461–6.
78. Freye E, Gleske G. (2013). Siberian ginseng results in beneficial effects on glucose metabolism in diabetes type 2 patients: a double blind placebo-controlled study in comparison to *Panax Ginseng. International Journal of Clinical Nutrition.* 1(1):11–7.
79. Lee YJ, Chung HY, Kwak HK, Yoon S. (2008). The effects of A. senticosus supplementation on serum lipid profiles, biomarkers of oxidative stress, and lymphocyte DNA damage in postmenopausal women. *Biochem Biophys Res Commun.* 10:375(1):44–8.

80. Zheng X, Lee S K, Chun O K. (2016). Soy Isoflavones and Osteoporotic Bone Loss: A Review with an Emphasis on Modulation of Bone Remodeling. *Journal of medicinal food*. 19(1):1–14.
81. Marini H, Bitto A, Altavilla D, Burnett BP, Polito F, Di Stefano V, et al. (2008). Breast safety and efficacy of genistein aglycone for postmenopausal bone loss: a follow-up study. *J Clin Endocrinol Metab*. 93:4787–96.
82. Morabito N, Crisafulli A, Vergara C, Gaudio A, Lasco A, Frisina N, et al. (2002). Effects of genistein and hormone-replacement therapy on bone loss in early postmenopausal women: a randomized double-blind placebo-controlled study. *J Bone Miner Res*. 17:1904–12.
83. Hwang YC, Jeong IK, Ahn KJ, Chung HY. (2009). The effects of Acanthopanax senticosus extract on bone turnover and bone mineral density in Korean postmenopausal women. *J Bone Miner Metab*. 27(5):584–90.
84. Mattarello MJ, Benedini S, Fiore C, Camozzi V, Sartorato P, Luisetto G, Armanini D. (2006). Effect of liquorice on PTH levels in healthy women. *Steroids*. 71(5):403–8.
85. Somjen D, Katzburg S, Vaya J, Kaye AM, Hendel D, Posner GH, Tamir S. (2004). Oestrogenic activity of glabridin and glabrene from liquorice roots on human osteoblasts and prepubertal rat skeletal tissues. *J Steroid Biochem Mol Biol*. 91(4–5):241–6.

Chapter eight

1. Barth C, Villringer A, Sacher J. (2015). Sex hormones affect neurotransmitters and shape the adult female brain during hormonal transition periods. *Front Neurosci*. 20;9:37.
2. Potter J, Bouyer J, Trussell J, Moreau C. (2009). Premenstrual syndrome prevalence and fluctuation over time: results from a French population-based survey. *J Womens Health (Larchmt)*. 18(1):31–9.
3. Silva, Celene Maria Longo da, et al. (2006). '[Population study of premenstrual syndrome]'. Revista de saude publica. 40(1):47–56.
4. Deuster P, Adera T, South-Paul J. (1999). Biological, social, and behavioral factors associated with premenstrual syndrome. *Arch Fam Med*. 8:122–8.
5. Poiană C, Muşat M, Carsote M, Chiriţă C. (2009). Premenstrual dysphoric disorder: neuroendocrine interferences. *Rev Med Chir Soc Med Nat Iasi*. 113(4):996–1000.
6. Masho SW, Adera T, South-Paul J. (2005). Obesity as a risk factor for premenstrual syndrome. *J Psychosom Obstet Gynaecol*. 26:33–9.

7. Perkonigg A, Yonkers K, Pfister H, Lieb R, Wittchen HU. (2004). Risk factors for premenstrual dysphoric disorder in a community sample of young women: The role of traumatic events and posttraumatic stress disorder. *J Clin Psychiatry.* 65:1314–22.
8. Bianco V, Cestari AM, Casati D, Cipriani S, Radici G, Valente I. (2014). Premenstrual syndrome and beyond: lifestyle, nutrition, and personal facts. *Minerva Ginecol.* 66(4):365–75.
9. Hashemi S, Tehrani FR, Mohammadi N, Dovom MR, Torkestani F, Simbar M, et al. (2016). Comparison of Metabolic and Hormonal Profiles of Women With and Without Premenstrual Syndrome: A Community Based Cross-Sectional Study. *Int J Endocrinol Metab.* 14(2): e28422.
10. İşik H, Ergöl Ş, Aynioğlu Ö, Şahbaz A, Kuzu A, Uzun M. (2016). Premenstrual syndrome and life quality in Turkish health science students. *Turk J Med Sci.* 19:46(3):695–701.
11. MacDonald PC, Dombroski RA, Casey ML. (1991). Recurrent secretion of progesterone in large amounts: An endocrine/metabolic disorder unique to young women? *Endocrine Rev.* 12:372–401.
12. Yonkers KA, O'Brien PM, Eriksson E. (2008). Premenstrual syndrome. *Lancet.* 5:371(9619):1200–10.
13. Bäckström T, Bixo M, Johansson M, Nyberg S, Ossewaarde L, Ragagnin G, et al. (2014). Allopregnanolone and mood disorders. *Prog Neurobiol.* 113:88–94.
14. Girdler SS, Klatzkin R, Morrow AL. (2007). Neurosteroids in the context of stress: Implications for depressive disorders. *Pharmacol Ther.* 116(1): 125–139.
15. Timby E, Bäckström T, Nyberg S, Stenlund H, Wihlbäck AC, Bixo M. (2016). Women with premenstrual dysphoric disorder have altered sensitivity to allopregnanolone over the menstrual cycle compared to controls-a pilot study. *Psychopharmacology (Berl).* 233(11):2109–17.
16. van Wingen GA, van Broekhoven F, Verkes RJ, Petersson KM, Backstrom T, Buitelaar JK, et al. (2008). Progesterone selectively increases amygdala reactivity in women. *Molecular Psychiatry.* 13(3):325–33.
17. Gingnell M, Morell A, Bannbers E, Wikström J, Sundström Poromaa I. (2012). Menstrual cycle effects on amygdala reactivity to emotional stimulation in premenstrual dysphoric disorder. *Horm Behav.* 62(4):400–6.
18. Studd J1, Nappi RE. (2012). Reproductive depression. *Gynecol Endocrinol.* 28 Suppl 1:42–5.
19. Schmidt PJ. (2005). Depression, the perimenopause, and estrogen therapy. *Ann NY Acad Sci.* 1052:27–40.

20. Almey A, Milner TA, Brake WG. (2015). Estrogen receptors in the central nervous system and their implication for dopamine-dependent cognition in females. *Hormones and behavior*. 74:125–38.
21. Menkes DB, Coates DC, Fawcett JP. (1994). Acute tryptophan depletion aggravates premenstrual syndrome. *J Affect Disord*. 32(1):37–44.
22. Melke J, Westberg L, Landén M, Sundblad C, Eriksson O, Baghei F, et al. (2003). Serotonin transporter gene polymorphisms and platelet [3H] paroxetine binding in premenstrual dysphoria. *Psychoneuroendocrinology*. 28(3):446–58.
23. Higgins A, Nash M, Lynch AM. (2010). Antidepressant-associated sexual dysfunction: impact, effects, and treatment. *Drug, healthcare and patient safety*. 2:141–50.
24. Baker FC, Driver HS. (2007). Circadian rhythms, sleep, and the menstrual cycle. *Sleep Med*. 8(6):613–22.
25. Jehan S, Auguste E, Hussain M, Pandi-Perumal SR, Brzezinski A, Gupta R, et al. (2016). Sleep and Premenstrual Syndrome. *J Sleep Med Disord*. 3(5):1061.
26. Shechter A, Lespérance P, Ying Kin NMKNg, Boivin DB. (2012). Pilot Investigation of the Circadian Plasma Melatonin Rhythm across the Menstrual Cycle in a Small Group of Women with Premenstrual Dysphoric Disorder. *PLoS One*. 7(12):e51929.
27. Jarry H, Leonhardt S, Wuttke W. (1995). The inhibitory effect of beta-endorphin on LH release in ovariectomized rats does not involve the preoptic GABAergic system. *Exp Clin Endocrinol Diabetes*. 103(5):317–23.
28. Chuong CJ, Hsi BP, Gibbons WE. (1994). Periovulatory beta-endorphin levels in premenstrual syndrome. *Obstet Gynecol*. 83(5 Pt 1):755–60.
29. Huang Y, Zhou R, Wu M, Wang Q, Zhao Y. (2015). Premenstrual syndrome is associated with blunted cortisol reactivity to the TSST. *Stress*. 18(2):160–8.
30. Facchinetti F, Fioroni L, Martignoni E, Sances G, Costa A, Genazzani AR. (1994). Changes of opioid modulation of the hypothalamo-pituitary-adrenal axis in patients with severe premenstrual syndrome. *Psychosom Med*. 56(5):418–22.
31. Cunningham J, Yonkers KA, O'Brien S, Eriksson E. (2009). Update on Research and Treatment of Premenstrual Dysphoric Disorder. *Harv Rev Psychiatry*. 17(2):120–137.
32. Kiesner J, Granger DA. (2016). A lack of consistent evidence for cortisol dysregulation in premenstrual syndrome/premenstrual dysphoric disorder. *Psychoneuroendocrinology*. 65:149–64.

33. Andersch B. (1983). Bromocriptine and premenstrual symptoms: a survey of double blind trials. *Obstet Gynecol Surv.* 38:643–6.
34. Wuttke W, Jarry H, Christoffel V, Spengler B, Seidlova-Wuttke D. (2003). Chaste tree (Vitex agnus-castus) – pharmacology and clinical indications. *Phytomedicine.* 10:348–57.
35. O'Brien P, Abukhalil I. (1999). Randomized controlled trial of the management of premenstrual syndrome and premenstrual mastalgia using luteal phase-only danazol. *Am J Obstet Gynecol.* 180:18–23.
36. Oksa S, Luukkaala T, Maenpaa J. (2006). Toremifene for premenstrual mastalgia: a randomised, placebo-controlled crossover study. *BJOG.* 113: 713–8.
37. Fink G. (1988). Oestrogen and progesterone interactions in the control of gonadotrophin and prolactin secretion. *J Steroid Biochem.* 30(1–6):169–78.
38. Sobrinho LG. (2003). Prolactin, psychological stress and environment in humans: adaptation and maladaptation. *Pituitary.* 6(1):35–9.
39. Walker SE, Miller D, Hill DL, Komatireddy GR. (1998). Prolactin, a pituitary hormone that modifies immune responses. Proceedings of the Mini-symposium on Prolactin and SLE, held at the 5th International Conference on Systemic Lupus Erythematosus, Cancun, Mexico. *Lupus.* 7:371–5.
40. Sharma LK, Sharma N, Gadpayle AK, Dutta D. (2016). Prevalence and predictors of hyperprolactinemia in subclinical hypothyroidism. *Eur J Intern Med.* 26. pii: S0953-6205(16)30219-9.
41. Nikolai TF, Mulligan GM, Gribble RK, Harkins PG, Meier PR, Roberts RC. (1990). Thyroid function and treatment in premenstrual syndrome. *J Clin Endocrinol Metab.* 70(4):1108–13.
42. Schmidt PJ, Grover GN, Roy-Byrne PP, Rubinow DR. (1993). Thyroid function in women with premenstrual syndrome. *J Clin Endocrinol Metab.* 76(3):671–4.
43. Rosenfeld R, Livne D, Nevo O, Dayan L, Milloul V, Lavi S, et al. (2008). Hormonal and volume dysregulation in women with premenstrual syndrome. *Hypertension.* 51(4):1225–30.
44. Bertone-Johnson ER, Houghton SC, Whitcomb BW, Sievert LL, Zagarins SE, Ronnenberg AG. (2016). Association of Premenstrual Syndrome with Blood Pressure in Young Adult Women. *J Womens Health (Larchmt).* 25(11):1122–8.
45. Bertone-Johnson ER, Ronnenberg AG, Houghton SC, Nobles C, Zagarins SE, Takashima-Uebelhoer BB, et al. (1987). Association of inflammation markers with menstrual symptom severity and premenstrual syndrome in young women. *Hum Reprod.* 29(9):1987–94.

46. Mulak A, Taché Y, Larauche M. (2014). Sex hormones in the modulation of irritable bowel syndrome. *World J Gastroenterol.* 14:20(10): 2433–48.
47. Vetvik KG, Russell MB. (2008). Menstrual migraine. *Tidsskr Nor Laegeforen.* 20:128(22):2575–8.
48. Imai A, Ichigo S, Matsunami K, Takagi H. (2015). Premenstrual syndrome: management and pathophysiology. *Clin Exp Obstet Gynecol.* 42(2):123–8.
49. Yonkers KA, Simoni MK. Premenstrual disorders. (2018). *Am J Obstet Gynecol.* 218(1):68–74
50. Deuster P, Adera T, South-Paul J. (1999). Biological, social, and behavioral factors associated with premenstrual syndrome. *Arch Fam Med.* 8:122–8.
51. Masho SW, Adera T, South-Paul J. (2005). Obesity as a risk factor for premenstrual syndrome. *J Psychosom Obstet Gynaecol.* 26:33–9.
52. Bianco V, Cestari AM, Casati D, Cipriani S, Radici G, Valente I. (2014). Premenstrual syndrome and beyond: lifestyle, nutrition, and personal facts. *Minerva Ginecol.* 66(4):365–75.
53. Hashemi S, Tehrani FR, Mohammadi N, Dovom MR, Torkestani F, Simbar M, et al. (2016). Comparison of Metabolic and Hormonal Profiles of Women With and Without Premenstrual Syndrome: A Community Based Cross-Sectional Study. *Int J Endocrinol Metab.* 14(2):e28422.
54. İşik H, Ergöl Ş, Aynioğlu Ö, Şahbaz A, Kuzu A, Uzun M. (2016). Premenstrual syndrome and life quality in Turkish health science students. *Turk J Med Sci.* 19:46(3):695–701.
55. İşik H, Ergöl Ş, Aynioğlu Ö, Şahbaz A, Kuzu A, Uzun M. (2016). Premenstrual syndrome and life quality in Turkish health science students. *Turk J Med Sci.* 19;46(3):695–701.

    Bianco V, Cestari AM, Casati D, Cipriani S, Radici G, Valente I. (2014). Premenstrual syndrome and beyond: lifestyle, nutrition, and personal facts. *Minerva Ginecol.* 66(4):365–75.
56. Purdue-Smithe AC, Manson JE, Hankinson SE, Bertone-Johnson ER. (2016). A prospective study of caffeine and coffee intake and premenstrual syndrome. *Am J Clin Nutr.* 104(2):499–507.
57. Heyden S, Fodor JG. (1986). Coffee consumption and fibrocystic breasts: an unlikely association. *Can J Surg.* 29(3):208–11.
58. Hashemi S, Tehrani FR, Mohammadi N, Dovom MR, Torkestani F, Simbar M, et al. (2016). Comparison of Metabolic and Hormonal Profiles of Women With and Without Premenstrual Syndrome: A Community Based Cross-Sectional Study. *Int J Endocrinol Metab.* 14(2): e28422.

59. Fernández MM, Saulyte J, Inskip HM, Takkouche B. (2018). Premenstrual syndrome and alcohol consumption: a systematic review and meta-analysis. *BMJ Open.* 8(3).
60. Jennifer L. Steiner JL, Crowell KT, Lang CH. (2015). Impact of Alcohol on Glycemic Control and Insulin Action. *Biomolecules.* 5(4):2223–46.
61. El-Lithy A, El-Mazny A, Sabbour A, El-Deeb A. (2015). Effect of aerobic exercise on premenstrual symptoms, haematological and hormonal parameters in young women. *J Obstet Gynaecol.* 35(4):389–92.
62. Bansal A, Kaushik A, Singh CM, Sharma V, Singh H. (2015). The effect of regular physical exercise on the thyroid function of treated hypothyroid patients: An interventional study at a tertiary care center in Bastar region of India. *Arch Med Health Sci.* 3:244–6.
63. Fischer LM, da Costa K, Kwock L, Galanko J, Zeisel. (2010). SH Dietary choline requirements of women: effects of estrogen and genetic variation. *Am J Clin Nutr.* 92(5):1113–9.
64. Allais G, Castagnoli Gabellari I, Burzio C, Rolando S, De Lorenzo C, Mana O, et al. (2012). Premenstrual syndrome and migraine. *Neurol Sci.* 33(Suppl 1):S111–5.
65. Akbarzadeh M, Dehghani M, Moshfeghy Z, Emamghoreishi M, Tavakoli P, Zare N. (2015). Effect of Melissa officinalis Capsule on the Intensity of Premenstrual Syndrome Symptoms in High School Girl Students. *Nurs Midwifery Stud.* 4(2):e27001.
66. Sharifi F, Simbar M, Mojab F, Majd HA. (2014). Comparison of the effects of Matricaria chamomila (Chamomile) extract and mefenamic acid on the intensity of premenstrual syndrome. *Complement Ther Clin Pract.* 20:81–8.
67. Becker A, Felgentreff F, Schröder H, Meier B, Brattström A. (2014). The anxiolytic effects of a Valerian extract is based on Valerenic acid. *BMC Complement Altern Med.* 14:267.
68. Rauwald H-W, Kuchta K, Savtschenko A, Brückner A, Rusch C, Appel K. (2013). GABA[A] Receptor Binding Assays of Standardized *Leonurus cardiaca* and *Leonurus japonicus* Extracts as Well as Their Isolated Constituents. *Planta Medica.* 79. 10.
69. Behboodi Moghadam Z, Rezaei E, Shirood Gholami R, Kheirkhah M, Haghani H. (2016). The effect of Valerian root extract on the severity of premenstrual syndrome symptoms. *J Tradit Complement Med.* 19;6(3): 309–15.

70. Delaram M, Heydarnejad MS. (2011). Herbal Remedy for Premenstrual Syndrome with Fennel (Foeniculum vulgare) – Randomized. Placebo-Controlled Study. 55:57–3.
71. Khayat S, Fanaei H, Kheirkhah M, Moghadam ZB, Kasaeian A, Javadimehr M. (2015). Curcumin attenuates severity of premenstrual syndrome symptoms: A randomized, double-blind, placebo-controlled trial. *Complement Ther Med*. 23(3):318–24.
72. Monteil-Seurin J, Ladure PH. (1991). Efficacy of Ruscus extract in the treatment of the premenstrual syndrome. *Return Circulation and Norepinephrine: An Update*. Paris, France: John Libbey, pp. 43–53.
73. Lagrue G, Behar A, Kazandjian M, Rahbar K. (1986). Idiopathic cyclic edema. The role of capillary hyperpermeability and its correction by Ginkgo biloba extract. *Presse Med*. 25;15(31):1550–3.
74. Tamborini A, Taurelle R. (1993). Value of standardized Ginkgo biloba extract (EGb 761) in the management of congestive symptoms of premenstrual syndrome. *Rev Fr Gynecol Obstet*. 88(7–9):447–57.
75. Ozgoli G, Selselei EA, Mojab F, Majd HA. (2009). A randomized, placebo-controlled trial of *Ginkgo biloba* L. in treatment of premenstrual syndrome. *J Altern Complement Med*. 15(8):845–51.
76. Chocano-Bedoya PO, Manson JE, Hankinson SE, Willett WC, Johnson SR, Chasan-Taber L, et al. (2011). Dietary B vitamin intake and incident premenstrual syndrome. *Am J Clin Nutr*. 93(5):1080–6.
77. Saeedian Kia A, Amani R, Cheraghian B. (2015). The Association between the Risk of Premenstrual Syndrome and Vitamin D, Calcium, and Magnesium Status among University Students: A Case Control Study. *Health Promot Perspect*. 25;5(3):225–30.
78. Abdollahifard S, Rahmanian Koshkaki A, Moazamiyanfar R. (2014). The effects of vitamin B1 on ameliorating the premenstrual syndrome symptoms. *Glob J Health Sci*. 29;6(6):144–53.
79. Soheila S, Faezeh K, Sayehmiri K, Bahmani M. (2016). Effects of vitamin B6 on premenstrual syndrome: A systematic review and meta-Analysis. *Journal of Chemical and Pharmaceutical Science*. 9(3).
80. Abraham GE, Rumley RE. (1987). Role of nutrition in managing the premenstrual tension syndromes. *J Reprod Med*. 32(6):405–22.
81. Ebrahimi E, Motlagh SK, Nemati S, Tavakoli Z. (2012). Effects of Magnesium and Vitamin B6 on the Severity of Premenstrual Syndrome Symptoms. *J Caring Sci*. 1(4):183–9.

82. Wilson SM, Bivins BN, Russell KA, Bailey LB. (2011). Oral contraceptive use: impact on folate, vitamin B_6, and vitamin B_{12} status. *Nutr Rev.* 69(10):572–83.

83. Bermond P. (1982). Therapy of side effects of oral contraceptive agents with vitamin B6. *Acta Vitaminol Enzymol.* 4(1–2):45–54.

84. Holley J, Bender DA, Coulson WF, Symes EK. (1983). Effects of vitamin B6 nutritional status on the uptake of [3H]-oestradiol into the uterus, liver and hypothalamus of the rat. *J Steroid Biochem.* 18(2):161–5.

85. Wyatt KM, Dimmock PW, Jones PW, Shaughn O'Brien PM. (1999). Efficacy of vitamin B-6 in the treatment of premenstrual syndrome: Systematic review. *Br Med J.* 318:1375–81.

86. Thys-Jacobs S. (2000). Micronutrients and the premenstrual syndrome: The case for calcium. *J Am Coll Nutr.* 19:220–7.

87. Bertone-Johnson ER, Chocano-Bedoya PO, Zagarins SE, Micka AE, Ronnenberg AG. (2010). Dietary vitamin D intake, 25-hydroxyvitamin D3 levels and premenstrual syndrome in a college-aged population. *J Steroid Biochem Mol Biol.* 121(1–2):434–7.

88. Bertone-johnson ER, Hankinson SE, Bendich A, Johnson SR, Willett WC, Manson JE. (2005). Calcium and vitamin D intake and risk of incident premenstrual syndrome. *Arch Intern Med.* 165:1264–52.

89. Eyles DW, Burne TH, McGrath JJ. (2012). Vitamin D, effects on brain development, adult brain function and the links between low levels of vitamin D and neuropsychiatric disease. *Front Neuroendocrinol.* 34: 47–64.

90. Forman JP, Williams JS, Fisher ND. (2010). Plasma 25-hydroxyvitamin D and regulation of the renin-angiotensin system in humans. *Hypertension.* 55:1283–8.

91. Lee SJ, Kanis JA. (1994). An association between osteoporosis and premenstrual symptoms and postmenopausal symptoms. *Bone Miner.* 24: 127–34.

92. Mandana Z, Azar A. (2014). Comparison of the effect of vitamin E, VitB6, calcium and Omega-3 on the treatment of premenstrual syndrome: A clinical randomized trial. *Annual Research and Review in Biology.* 4:1141–9.

93. Dadkhah H, Ebrahimi E, Fathizadeh N. (2016). Evaluating the effects of vitamin D and vitamin E supplement on premenstrual syndrome: A randomized, double-blind, controlled trial. *Iran J Nurs Midwifery Res.* 21(2):159–64.

94. Ataollahi M, Akbari SA, Mojab F, Alavi Majd H. (2015). The effect of wheat germ extract on premenstrual syndrome symptoms. *Iran J Pharm Res.* 14(1):159-66.
95. Su HM. (2010). Mechanisms of n-3 fatty acid-mediated development and maintenance of learning memory performance. *J Nutr Biochem.* 21(5):364–73.
96. Behboudi-Gandevani S, Hariri FZ, Moghaddam-Banaem L. (2017). The effect of omega 3 fatty acid supplementation on premenstrual syndrome and health-related quality of life: a randomized clinical trial. *Journal of Psychosomatic Obstetrics & Gynecology.* 14:1–7.
97. Sohrabi N, Kashanian M, Ghafoori SS, Malakouti SK. (2013). Evaluation of the effect of omega-3 fatty acids in the treatment of premenstrual syndrome: syndrome: 'a pilot trial'. *Complement Ther Med.* 21:141–6.
98. Rocha Filho EA, Lima JC, Pinho Neto JS, Montarroyos U. (2011). Essential fatty acids for premenstrual syndrome and their effect on prolactin and total cholesterol levels: a randomized, double blind, placebo-controlled study. *Reprod Health.* 8:2.
99. Collins A, Cerin A, Coleman G, Landgren BM. (1983). Essential fatty acids in the treatment of premenstrual syndrome. *Obstet Gynecol.* 81:93–8.
100. Innis SM. (2007). Dietary (n-3) fatty acids and brain development. *J Nutr.* 137:855–9.
101. Shamberger RJ. (2003). Calcium, magnesium, and other elements in the red blood cells and hair of normals and patients with premenstrual syndrome. *Biol Trace Elem Res.* 94:123–29.
102. Thys-Jacobs S, McMahon D, Bilezikian JP. (2007). Cyclical changes in calcium metabolism across the menstrual cycle in women with premenstrual dysphoric disorder. *J Clin Endocrinol Metab.* 92(8):2952–9.
103. Shobeiri F, Araste FE, Ebrahimi R, Jenabi E, Nazari M. (2017). Effect of calcium on premenstrual syndrome: A double-blind randomized clinical trial. *Obstet Gynecol Sci.* 60(1):100–5.
104. Ghanbari Z, Haghollahi F, Shariat M, Foroshani AR, Ashrafi M. (2009). Effects of calcium supplement therapy in women with premenstrual syndrome. *Taiwan J Obstet Gynecol.* 48:124–9.
105. Whelan AM, Jurgens TM, Naylor H. (2009). Herbs, vitamins and minerals in the treatment of premenstrual syndrome: a systematic review. *Can J Clin Pharmacol.* 16(3):e407–e429.
106. Jahnen-Dechent W, Ketteler M. (2012). Magnesium basics. *Clin Kidney J.* 5(Suppl 1):i3–i14.

107. Tarleton EK, Littenberg B. (2015). Magnesium intake and depression in adults. *J Am Board Fam Med.* 28(2):249–56.
108. Gröber U, Schmidt J, Kisters K. (2015). Magnesium in Prevention and Therapy. *Nutrients.* 7(9):8199–226.
109. Hermes Sales C, Azevedo Nascimento D, Queiroz Medeiros AC, et al. (2014). There is chronic latent magnesium deficiency in apparently healthy university students. *Nutr Hosp.* 30:200–4.
110. Fathizadeh N, Ebrahimi E, Valiani M, Tavakoli N, Yar MH. (2010). Evaluating the effect of magnesium and magnesium plus vitamin B6 supplement on the severity of premenstrual syndrome. *Iran J Nurs Midwifery Res.* 15(Suppl1):401–5.
111. Walker AF, De Souza MC, Vickers MF, Abeyasekera S, Collins ML, Trinca LA. (1998). Magnesium supplementation alleviates premenstrual symptoms of fluid retention. *J Womens Health.* 7(9):1157–65.
112. Khine K, Rosenstein DL, Elin RJ, Niemela JE, Schmidt PJ, Rubinow DR. (2006). Magnesium (Mg) retention and mood effects after intravenous mg infusion in premenstrual dysphoric disorder. *Biol Psychiatry.* 15; 59(4):327–33.
113. De Souza MC, Walker AF, Robinson PA, Bolland K. (2000). A synergistic effect of a daily supplement for 1 month of 200 mg magnesium plus 50 mg vitamin B6 for the relief of anxiety-related premenstrual symptoms: a randomized, double-blind, crossover study. *J Womens Health Gend Based Med.* 9(2):131–9.
114. Markou A, Sertedaki A, Kaltsas G, Androulakis II, Marakaki C, Pappa T, et al. (2015). Stress-induced aldosterone hyper-secretion in a substantial subset of patients with essential hypertension. *J Clin Endocrinol Metab.* 100(8):2857–64.
115. Matsuoka H. (2005). Aldosterone and magnesium. *Clin Calcium.* 15(2): 187–91.
116. Maret W. (2017). Zinc in cellular regulation: the nature and significance of 'zinc signals'. *Int J Mol Sci.* 18(11):2285.
117. Siahbazi S, Behboudi-Gandevani S, Moghaddam-Banaem L, Montazeri A. (2017). Effect of zinc sulfate supplementation on premenstrual syndrome and health-related quality of life: Clinical randomized controlled trial. *J Obstet Gynaecol Res.* 43(5):887–94.
118. Chocano-Bedoya PO, Manson JE, Hankinson SE, Johnson SR, Chasan-Taber L, Ronnenberg AG, et al. (2013). Intake of selected minerals and risk of premenstrual syndrome. *Am J Epidemiol.* 15;177(10):1118–27.

119. Caticha O, Norato DY, Tambascia MA, Santana A, Stephanou A, Sarlis NJ. (1996). Total body zinc depletion and its relationship to the development of hyperprolactinemia in chronic renal insufficiency. *J Endocrinol Invest.* 19(7):441–8.
120. Yehuda S, Mostofsky D. (2010). Iron Deficiency and Overload: From Basic Biology to Clinical Medicine. Totowa, NJ: Humana Press.
121. Albacar G, Sans T, Martn-Santos R. (2010). An association between plasma ferritin concentrations measured 48 h after delivery and postpartum depression. *J Affect Disord.* 131(1–3):136–42.
122. Chocano-Bedoya PO, Manson JE, Hankinson SE, Johnson SR, Chasan-Taber L, Ronnenberg AG, et al. (2013). Intake of selected minerals and risk of premenstrual syndrome. *Am J Epidemiol.* 15;177(10):1118–27.
123. Valussi M. (2012). Functional foods with digestion-enhancing properties. *International Journal of Food Sciences and Nutrition.* 63 Suppl 1(S1):82–9.
124. Panossian A, Wikman G. (2010). Effects of Adaptogens on the Central Nervous System and the Molecular Mechanisms Associated with Their Stress – Protective Activity. *Pharmaceuticals (Basel).* 3(1):188–224.
125. Yarnell E, Abascal K. (2006). Botanical Medicine for Thyroid Regulation. *Alternative and Complementary Therapies.* 12(3).
126. Wuttke W, Jarry H, Christoffel V, Spengler B, Seidlová-Wuttke D. (2003). Chaste tree (Vitex agnus-castus) – pharmacology and clinical indications. *Phytomedicine.* 10(4):348–57.
127. Loch EG, Selle, Boblitz N. (2000). Treatment of premenstrual syndrome with a phytopharmaceutical formulation containing Vitex agnus castus. *Journal of Women's Health & Gender-Based Medicine.* 3(9):315–20.
128. Mirghafourvand M, Mohammad Alizadeh Charandabi S, Javadzadeh Y, Ahmadpour P. (2015). Comparing the effects of Vitexagnus and flaxseed on premenstrual symptoms: a randomized controlled trial. *Journal of Hayat.* 21:68–78.
129. Dante G, Facchinetti F. (2011). Herbal treatments for alleviating premenstrual symptoms: a systematic review. *J Psychosom Obstet Gynaecol.* 32(1):42–51.
130. Atmaca M, Kumru S, Tezcan E. (2003). Fluoxetine versus *Vitex agnus castus* extract in the treatment of premenstrual dysphoric disorder. *Hum Psychopharmacol.* 18(3):191–5.
131. Ciotta L, Pagano I, Stracquadanio M, Di Leo S, Andò A, Formuso C. (2011). Psychic aspects of the premenstrual dysphoric disorders. New

therapeutic strategies: our experience with Vitex agnus castus. *Minerva Ginecol.* 63(3):237–45.
132. Rani A and Sharma A. (2013). The genus Vitex: A review. *Pharmacogn Rev.* 7(14):188–198.
133. van Die MD, Burger HG, Teede HJ, Bone KM. (2013). Vitex agnus-castus extracts for female reproductive disorders: a systematic review of clinical trials. *Planta Med.* 79(7):562–75.
134. Verkaik S, Kamperman AM, van Westrhenen R, Schulte PFJ. (2017). The treatment of premenstrual syndrome with preparations of Vitex agnus castus: a systematic review and meta-analysis. *Am J Obstet Gynecol.* 217(2):150–66.
135. Halaska M, Beles P, Gorkow C, Sieder C. (1999). Treatment of cyclical mastalgia with a solution containing a Vitex agnus castus extract: results of a placebo-controlled double-blind study. *Breast.* 8(4):175–81.
136. Dinç T, Coşkun F. (2014). Comparison of *Fructus agni casti* and flurbiprofen in the treatment of cyclic mastalgia in premenopausal women. *Ulus Cerrahi Derg.* 1;30(1):34–8.
137. Ambrosini A, Di Lorenzo C, Coppola G, Pierelli F. (2013). Use of Vitex agnus-castus in migrainous women with premenstrual syndrome: an open-label clinical observation. *Acta Neurol Belg.* 113(1):25–9.
138. Berger D, Schaffner W, Schrader E, Meier B, Brattström A. (2000). Efficacy of Vitex agnus castus L. extract Ze 440 in patients with premenstrual syndrome (PMS). *Arch Gynecol Obstet.* 264(3):150–3.
139. Rhyu RMR, Lu J, Webster DE, Fabricant DS, Farnsworth NR, Wang J. (2006). Black cohosh (Actaea racemosa, Cimicifuga racemosa) behaves as a mixed competitive ligand and partial agonist at the human mu opiate receptor. *J Agric Food Chem.* 27;54(26):9852–7.
140. Burdette JE, Liu J, Chen SN, Fabricant DS, Piersen CE, Barker EL, et al. (2003). Black cohosh acts as a mixed competitive ligand and partial agonist of the serotonin receptor. *J Agric Food Chem.* 10;51(19):5661–70.
141. Huang YX, Song L, Zhang X, Lun WW, Pan C, Huang YS. (2013). Clinical study of combined treatment of remifemin and paroxetine for perimenopausal depression. *Zhonghua Yi Xue Za Zhi.* 26;93(8):600–2.
142. Canning S, Waterman M, Orsi N, Ayres J, Simpson N, Dye L. (2010). The efficacy of Hypericum perforatum (St John's wort) for the treatment of premenstrual syndrome: a randomized, double-blind, placebo-controlled trial. *CNS Drugs.* 24(3):207–25.
143. Stevinson C1, Ernst E. (2000). A pilot study of *Hypericum perforatum* for the treatment of premenstrual syndrome. *BJOG.* 107(7):870–6.

144. Hicks SM, Walker AF, Gallagher J, Middleton RW, Wright J. (2004). The significance of 'nonsignificance' in randomized controlled studies: a discussion inspired by a double-blinded study on St. John's wort (*Hypericum perforatum* L.) for premenstrual symptoms. *J Altern Complement Med*. 10(6):925–32.
145. RyooJ JG, Chun SI, Lee YJ, Suh HS. (2010). The Effects of St. John's Wort on Premenstrual Syndrome in Single Women: A Randomized Double-Blind, Placebo-Controlled Study. *Clinical Psychopharmacology and Neuroscience*. 8(1):30–7.
146. van Die MD, Bone KM, Burger HG, Reece JE, Teede HJ. (2009). Effects of a combination of Hypericum perforatum and Vitex agnus-castus on PMS-like symptoms in late-perimenopausal women: findings from a subpopulation analysis. *J Altern Complement Med*. 15(9):1045–8.

Chapter nine

1. Reis FM, Petraglia F, Taylor RN. (2013). Endometriosis: hormone regulation and clinical consequences of chemotaxis and apoptosis. *Human Reproduction Update*. 19(4), 406–18.
2. Barthelmess EK, Rajesh KN. (2014). Polycystic ovary syndrome: current status and future perspective *Frontiers in Bioscience (Elite Edition)*. 6:104–19.
3. Mader, LS. (2013). Treating PCOS Naturally. *American Botanical Council HerbalEGram*. 10(3).
4. Javidnia K, Dastgheib L, Mohammadi Samani S, Nasiri A. (2003). Antihirsutism activity of Fennel (fruits of Foeniculum vulgare) extract. A double-blind placebo controlled study. *Phytomedicine: International Journal Of Phytotherapy and Phytopharmacology*. 10. 455–8. Doi: 10.1078/094471103322331386.

INDEX

Achillea millefolium, 128–129
Actaea racemosa L. *See* black cohosh
ACTH. *See* adrenocorticotrophic hormone
ADHD. *See* attention-deficit hyperactivity disorder
adrenal
    cortex, 4
    support, 200, 210–211
adrenarchy, 5
adrenocorticotrophic hormone (ACTH), 4
ageing, signs of, 96
AhR. *See* aryl hydrocarbon receptor
ALA. *See* α-linolenic acid
Alchemilla vulgaris, 129
aldosterone, 230
allopregnanolone, 43, 225
α-linolenic acid (ALA), 71, 75
amygdala, 60
androstenedione, 4–5, 7
Angelica sinensis, 193

anti-inflammatory herbs, 236
anti-tumour activity of flaxseeds, 74–75, 76
apigenin, 206
apolipoproteins, 77
ArginMax®, 206–207
aromatase, 21
    factors affecting activity in tissues, 22
aromatization, 4–5
aryl hydrocarbon receptor (AhR), 144
Ashwagandha, 202
Asparagus racemosus, 129. *See also* herbs
    actions and indications for, 133–134
    antiulcer activity, 132
    clinical studies, 131
    constituents, 130
    digestive system, 132
    galactagogue effect, 131–132
    in vivo effects for, 132–133
    promotion of gastric emptying, 132
    steroidal saponins, 131

Astragalus membranaceus, 193, 202
attention-deficit hyperactivity disorder (ADHD), 242
Avicenna, 99

bacterial vaginosis, 195–196
barefoot medical tradition, 165
benign prostatic hyperplasia (BPH), 97
benzodiazepines, 59
β-bitter acids, 103
bilateral oophorectomy, 183
biome and general health, 54. *See also* digestive system
bitter herbs, 56
black cohosh (*Actaea racemosa* L.), 135. *See also Vitex agnus-castus*
    actions and indications for, 144–145
    anti-proliferative effects, 143–144
    clinical trials, 141
    constituents, 139
    dosage, 146–147
    Eclectic physicians, 138–139
    effect on hepatic and lipid metabolism, 144
    effect on pituitary hormones, 140
    first people use, 138
    importance whole plant, 141
    in infertility, 142
    in vivo and *in vitro* research, 143
    menopausal symptom reduction, 143
    menopausal symptoms following breast cancer, 143
    mis-identification of herbs, 146
    mode of action, 139–140
    myths, 135
    neurotransmitter activity, 140–141
    no changes in endometrium, 142
    osteoprotective effects, 141
    pharmacokinetics, 141
    popularity, 135
    safety, 145–146
    side effects, 146
    urinary bladder muscle tone, 141
    vaginal pH lowering, 142
    for women with fibroids, 143

black cohosh, 193, 203, 247
BMD. *See* bone mineral density
BMI. *See* body mass index
body mass index (BMI), 96
bone mineral density (BMD), 74
bone-specific alkaline phosphatase, 141
BPH. *See* benign prostatic hyperplasia
brain. *See also* nervous system
    dopaminergic tracts in, 59–60
    neurotransmitters, 58–59
breast cancer, 75, 76
    risk, 84–85
    treatment and prognosis, 85

calcium antagonist, 242
casticin, 153–154
catechol-O-methyltransferase (COMT), 17
central nervous system (CNS), 172
Chamaelirium luteum, 125. *See also* herbs
    Achillea millefolium, 128–129
    actions and indications, 127
    Alchemilla vulgaris, 129
    alternatives to, 128
    constituents, 126
    pharmacology, 126
    traditional use, 126–127
chasteberry, 163
cholesterol, 3
Cimicifuga racemosa (L.) Nutt. *See* black cohosh
circulation, 87
circulatory and immune systems, 63, 66–67
    circulatory herbs, 64
    general wellbeing, 65
    importance of exercise and sleep, 64–65
    psychological health, 65
    specific indications and systematic therapeutics, 65–66
clerodadienols, 152–153
clomiphene, 142
clover disease, 92
CNS. *See* central nervous system
colorectal cancer, 76

INDEX   329

combination product (*Paeonia* and *Glycyrrhiza*), 172
   actions and indications of, 174
   adverse effects, 175
   clinical indications, 175
   clinical studies on PCOS patients, 174
   clinical trial on prolactin levels, 173
   clinical trials with, 172
   dosage, 175
   effects of herbs on hormonally-related functions, 176–179
   prolactin inhibition, 173
   reduces testosterone levels, 173
   spasmolytic effect of, 172
common peony (*Paeonia officinalis*), 166. *See also* combination product
   clinical studies, 167–168
   constituents, 166
   preclinical studies, 166–167
   traditional use, 165
COMT. *See* catechol-O-methyltransferase
conjugated oestrogens, 11, 19
cortisone, 62, 228
Crataegus laevigata, 207
C-reactive protein (CRP), 63
cross-talk, 2, 63
   between steroid hormones and immune system effects, 62–63
CRP. *See* C-reactive protein
cytochrome
   CYP3A4, 43
   CYP450, 11
   CYP450 1A1 and 1A2, 13–14
   CYP450 1B1, 15
   CYP450 3A4, 16

damiana, 206
Dang Gui Buxue Tang (DBT), 193
DBT. *See* Dang Gui Buxue Tang
dehydroepiandrostenedione sulphate (DHEAS), 171
dehydroepiandrosterone (DHEA), 43
depression, 86–87
DHA. *See* docosahexaenoic acid

DHEA. *See* dehydroepiandrosterone
DHEAS. *See* dehydroepiandrostenedione sulphate
digestive system, 52, 66–67
   biome and general health, 54
   EFAs, 58
   endocannabinoids, 57
   healthy gut epithelium and hormonal balance, 53–54
   L-cells and GLP-1, 55–57
   microbiome, 52
   role of liver, 57
Dioscorea villosa, 119. *See also* herbs
   clinical studies of menopause, 122–123
   clinical studies on cholesterol metabolism, 123
   constituents, 120
   effects found, 124
   historical use, 119
   modern times, 119–120
   pharmacology, 120–122
   research findings for, 124–125
   Tribestan® and diosgenin actions, 121–122
Dioscorides, 150
diosgenin, 123
   rich herbs, 41
diterpenes, 205
docosahexaenoic acid (DHA), 58
dopamine, 59–62, 222–225, 228–229. *See also* nervous system
dopaminergic tracts in brain, 59–60

EFAs, 58
EFSA. *See* European Food Safety Authority
eicosapentaenoic acid (EPA), 58
Eleutherococcus senticosus, 201
Ellingwood, F., 119
endocannabinoids, 57. *See also* digestive system
endocrine system, 2
endogenous opioids, 62, 228
endometrial cancer, 85

endometriosis, adenomyosis, 255.
    See also gynaecological
    conditions
  diet, 256
  exercise and lifestyle, 256
  herbal treatment, 256–257
  hormonal picture, 255
  management principles, 255–256
ENS. *See* enteric nervous system
enteric nervous system (ENS), 55
EPA. *See* eicosapentaenoic acid
EPSEs. *See* extra-pyramidal side effects
ER. *See* oestrogen receptors
European Food Safety Authority
    (EFSA), 87
exercise and sleep, 64–65
extra-pyramidal side effects
    (EPSEs), 172

Female Sexual Function Index
    (FSFI), 207
FertilityBlend®, 159
fibrocystic breasts, 259. *See also*
      gynaecological conditions
  hormonal health management, 260
  hormonal picture, 259
  tissue health management, 259–260
flavonoids, 153–154
flaxseed (*Linum usitatissum*), 63, 68, 78–79
  anti-tumour activity, 74–75, 76
  benefits in hypercholesterolaemia, 77
  breast cancer, 75
  colorectal cancer, 76
  constituents of, 71–73
  haemodialysis patients, 78
  history, 69
  hypoglycaemic effect, 77
  lignans, 72
  obesity, 77
  osteoporosis, 78
  prostate cancer, 76
  results of lignans, 73
  systemic lupus erythematosus
      nephritis, 78
  tamoxifen, 75
Foeniculum vulgare, 192

follicle-stimulating hormone (FSH),
    5, 6, 152
FSFI. *See* Female Sexual Function
    Index
FSH. *See* follicle-stimulating hormone
functional medicine, 51

GA. *See* glycyrrhetinic acid
GABA. *See* gamma-amino butyric acid
gamma-amino butyric acid (GABA),
    43, 58–59, 222–225, 237.
    See also nervous system
  progesterone sensitivity and,
      225–226
genistein, 85, 86
glabridin, 202
GLP-1. *See* glucagon-like peptide
glucagon-like peptide (GLP-1), 55–57.
    See also digestive system
glutamine, 58–59. *See also* nervous
    system
Glycine max, 192. *See* soy
glycyrhizinic acid (GZA), 170
glycyrrhetinic acid (GA), 170, 172
Glycyrrhiza, 170. *See also* liquorice
    glabra, 165, 193–194, 200–201
glycyrrhizic acid. *See* glycyrrhizin
glycyrrhizin, 170
gut-brain axis, 56
gut microbiome, 19
gynaecological conditions, xiv, 253
  endometriosis, adenomyosis,
      255–257
  fibrocystic breasts, 259–260
  PCOS, 257–259
  uterine fibroids, 254–255
GZA. *See* glycyrhizinic acid

habituation, 59
haem iron, 243
haemoglobin A1C (HbA1C), 77
HbA1C. *See* haemoglobin A1C
HCG. *See* human chorionic
    gonadotrophin injection
HDL-C. *See* high density lipoprotein
    cholesterol

healthy gut epithelium and hormonal
   balance, 53–54. *See also*
   digestive system
hepatic stimulants, 236
herbal treatment, 196
   circulatory and immune
      systems, 63–67
   digestive system, 52–58
   flaxseed, 68–79
   of gynaecological problems, 49
   of menopausal symptoms, 190
   nervous system, 58–63
   neuroimmunoendocrinology and
      systematic treatment, 50–51
   principles, xiii–xiv
   psycho-neuro-endocrino-
      immunology, 51–52
   soy, 79–89
   traditional indications, 222
herbs, 181, 207. *See also*
      phyto-oestrogens
   Asparagus racemosus, 129–134
   bitters, 255
   Chamaelirium luteum, 125–129
   Dioscorea villosa, 119–125
   fibroid management, 256
   gut flora, 255, 256
   hops, 99–107
   isoflavones and flavonoids, 91
   laxatives, 255
   liver, 255
   for menopause treatment, 209–210
   nervous and hormonal support, 206
   oestrogen clearance, 256
   progesterone myth, 117
   red clover, 91–98
   sage, 107–115
   steroidal saponins, 40–41, 117
   for stress, 258
   wild yam, 117
   Withania, 259
high density lipoprotein cholesterol
      (HDL-C), 208
high magnesium foods, 242
Hippocrates, 150
hMOR. *See* human μ-opiate receptors

holobionts, 54
hops (*Humulus lupulus*), 99. *See also*
      herbs
   anti-cancer, 105
   anti microbial uses, 103–104
   antioxidant, 104–105
   constituents, 100–101
   contraindications, 106
   general actions, 101
   hepatoprotective, 105–106
   for insomnia, 101–102
   for menopausal symptoms, 103
   oestrogenic effects, 102–103
   sedative and hypnotic action, 101
hormone replacement therapy (HRT),
      181, 186–187
   withdrawal and herbal support,
      198–199
hormones
   findings about hormonal
      herbs, 34–35
   metabolism of, 12
hormone therapy (HT), 221
hot flushes, 192
Hoxsey formula, 92
HPA axis. *See* hypothalamic-pituitary-
      adrenal axis
HPG. *See* hypothalamus-pituitary-
      gonadal
HRT. *See* hormone replacement therapy
HT. *See* hormone therapy
human chorionic gonadotrophin
      injection (HCG), 142
human μ-opiate receptors (hMOR), 247
humoral medicine, 50
Humulus lupulus, 192. *See* hops
Hypericum
   and Cimicifuga combination,
      203–204
   and Vitex combination, 248
Hypericum perforatum, 203, 247
   with *Vitex agnus-castus*, 205
hyperprolactinaemia, latent, 228–229
hypothalamic-pituitary-adrenal axis
      (HPA axis), 62, 226, 228.
      See also nervous system

hypothalamus-pituitary-gonadal (HPG), 245
hypothyroidism, 230

Ibn-Al Baitar, 99
insomnia, 197
  herbs for, 197–198
insulin-like growth factor 1 (IGF-1), 63, 75, 76, 185
interferon (IFN)-γ, 230
Islamic Golden Age, 150
isoflavone. *See also* soy
  and cancer protection, 84
  and fertility, 83
  hormonal effect of, 82–83
  pharmacodynamics, 82
  processed/unprocessed soybeans, 81
  soy-based foods, 81–82
isoflavonoids, 80

lacto-ferments, 52
latent hyperprolactinaemia, 228–229
laxatives, 255
L-cells, 55–57. *See also* digestive system
LDL. *See* low-density lipoprotein
LDL-C. *See* low-density lipoprotein cholesterol
leptin, 77
LH. *See* luteinizing hormone
lignans, 72. *See also* flaxseed
  flaxseed, 72
  hormonal effects, 73
  results of human trials using, 73
Linum usitatissimum, 193. *See* flaxseed
lipopolysaccharides (LPS), 55
lipotrophic factors, 236, 258
liquorice, 168, 200–201, 202–203.
    See also combination product
  actions, 170
  clinical trials of sex hormones, 171–172
  constituents, 170
  effect on endocrine system, 171
  traditional use, 165
liver
  herbs, 255

restoratives, 57
role of, 57
low-density lipoprotein (LDL), 77, 112
low-density lipoprotein cholesterol (LDL-C), 208
LPS. *See* lipopolysaccharides
luteal insufficiency, 215
luteinizing hormone (LH), 5, 6, 140, 152

Macrotys. *See* black cohosh
Madaus, G., 151
magnesium foods, high, 242
Medicago sativa, 192
medical herbalists, xi
medicine, functional, 51
melatonin, 226–227
  and PMDD, 227–228
menopause, 181, 210–211
  adrenal support, 200, 210–211
  ArginMax®, 206–207
  Astragalus membranaceus, 202
  Astragalus membranaceus and *Angelica sinensis*, 193
  cardiovascular disease and insulin resistance, 207
  characteristics of, 181
  Cimicifuga racemosa, 193, 203
  clinical trials of Hypericum and Cimicifuga combination, 203–204
  Crataegus laevigata, 207
  diet and lifestyle, 189
  Eleutherococcus senticosus, 201
  Foeniculum vulgare, 192
  Glycine max, 192
  Glycyrrhiza glabra, 193–194, 200–201
  herbal treatment, 196
  herbs, 207
  herbs for insomnia, 197–198
  herbs for treatment, 209–210
  hot flushes and night sweats, 192
  HRT, 186–187
  HRT withdrawal and herbal support, 198–199
  Humulus lupulus, 192
  Hypericum perforatum, 203

INDEX   333

Hypericum perforatum with *Vitex agnus-castus*, 205
Linum usitatissimum, 193
liquorice, 202–203
nervous and hormonal support herbs, 206
nervous function in menopause, 202
Nigella sativa, 208
nutrition, 199
oestrogen metabolism and lifestyle advice, 188–189
osteoporosis, 208–209
Panax ginseng, 194–195, 201–202, 208
perimenopause events, 183–184
Pimpinella anisum, 194
postmenopause events, 184–186
recurrent urinary tract infections, 196–197
reduced sexual desire, 206
resveratrol, 199–200
Salvia officinalis and *Medicago sativa*, 192
sexual desire reduction, 206
Siberian ginseng, 208
symptomatic treatment, 190
symptom management and trigger removal, 188
thrush and vaginal infections, 195–196
timing and incidence of natural and artificial, 183
treatment, 190, 212–213
treatment and physiological support for transition, 198
Trifolium pratense, 192
Trigonella foenum-graecum, 194
Turnera diffusa, 206
uterine prolapse, 198
vaginal dryness and vulvar atrophy, 195
Valeriana officinalis, 193
Vitex agnus-castus, 194, 204–205
Vitex and melatonin release, 205
Withania somnifera, 202
women's health initiative study, 186
Zizyphus spinosa, 195

Menopause Rating Scale (MRS), 111
menorrhagia, 27
menstrual cycle, 215, 216–217
menstruation, 2
metabolic syndrome, 234–235
microbiome, 52. *See also* digestive system
  healthy, 53
microgenderome, 230
monoamines, 59
MRS. *See* Menopause Rating Scale
multivitamin supplements, 199

nervine tonics, 247
nervous system, 58, 66–67
  brain neurotransmitters, 58–59
  cross-talk between steroid hormones and immune system effects, 62–63
  dopamine and prolactin, 62
  dopaminergic tracts in brain, 59–60
  endogenous opioids, 62
  oestrogen and progesterone receptors, 61
neuroimmunoendocrinology, 50–51
neuropsychological symptoms, 238
neurosteroids, 43
neurotransmitters associated with menstrual cycle, 222. *See also* premenstrual syndrome
  aetiological factors, 231–232
  aldosterone, 230
  conventional treatment, 231
  dopamine and latent hyperprolactinaemia, 228–229
  emotional component, 229–230
  endogenous opioids, 228
  GABA, dopamine, serotonin and opiates, 222–225
  gut flora, 230
  hormonal transition, 223–224
  hypothyroidism, 230
  melatonin and PMDD, 227–228
  oestrogen, serotonin, and melatonin, 226–227
  progesterone sensitivity and GABA, 225–226

symptoms, 230–231
variation of serotonin levels, 227
Nigella sativa, 208
night sweats, 192
nonsteroidal anti-inflammatory drugs (NSAIDs), 231
noradrenaline, 59–62. *See also* nervous system
NSAIDs. *See* nonsteroidal anti-inflammatory drugs

oestradiol, 4
oestrogen, 1, 47–48, 226–227.
  See also phyto-oestrogens; progesterone; progestogens
  androstenedione and aromatization, 4–5
  aromatase, 21–22
  availability of, 20
  COMT affecting nutrients, 17
  CYP450 1A1 and 1A2 affecting nutrients, 13–14
  CYP450 1B1 affecting nutrients, 15
  CYP450 3A4 affecting nutrients, 16
  deficiency, 112
  -dependent cancers, 9
  dietary influences on metabolism, 23–24
  diet for oestrogen conjugation and clearance, 25–26
  effects of, 8
  environmental, 27–33
  excess oestrogen symptoms, 27, 33–34
  herbal research, 34–35
  levels and effects, 7
  lifestyle and metabolism, 26
  after menopause, 6
  menstrual cycle, endometrium, mucus, and temperature, 6
  metabolising food, 53–54
  metabolism, 10–11
  metabolism and lifestyle advice, 188–189
  metabolism of hormones, 12
  misconceptions, 9
  myths about oestrogenic herbs, 1–2
  oestrogen receptors, 35–36
  2-OH oestrogens, 13
  16-OH oestrogens, 15
  4-OH oestrogens, 15
  ovarian hormones, 6
  and phyto-oestrogens, 34
  production of, 4
  and progesterone receptors, 61
  roles in body, 7–8
  sex hormone binding globulin, 20–21
  sex hormones, 2–3
  sources, 7
  SULT affecting nutrients, 18
  UGT and β glucuronidase affecting nutrients, 19
oestrogenic herbs, 1–2
oestrogenicity, 139
oestrogen receptors (ER), 35, 75
  ERα and ERβ, 36
  2-OH oestrogens, 13
  16-OH oestrogens, 15
  4-OH oestrogens, 15
omega 3 EFAs, 58, 71
OPG. *See* osteoprotegerin
opiates, 222–225
osteoporosis, 78, 208–209
osteoprotegerin (OPG), 140
ovarian hormones, 6

P450 aromatase, 5
Paeonia officinalis. See common peony
Panax ginseng, 194–195, 201–202, 208
Paracelsus, 99
PCOS. *See* polycystic ovary syndrome
Peony-Glycyrrhiza Decoction (PGD), 165
perimenopause, 183–184
Persian Medicine, 150
PGD. *See* Peony-Glycyrrhiza Decoction
PGE1. *See* prostaglandin E1
pharmaceutical oestrogens, 28
phyto-oestrogens, 36, 37–39. *See also* oestrogen; progesterone; progestogens
  herbs containing steroidal saponins, 40–41

myths about, 36–37
nutritional and herbal sources
of, 38–39
phenolic, 39–40
phenolic phyto-oestrogens, 39–40
phyto-oestrogenic compounds,
37–39
phytoSERMs, 37
as phytoserms, 37, 40
plants with, 2
resorcylic acid lactones, 41
-rich loaf, 68
steroidal saponins, 40
triterpenoid saponins, 41
pilocarpine, 112
Pimpinella anisum, 194
PIN. *See* prostatic intraepithelial
neoplasia
PMS. *See* premenstrual syndrome
PNEI. *See* psycho-neuro-endocrino-
immunology
polycystic ovary syndrome (PCOS),
257. *See also* gynaecological
conditions
diet, 258
exercise, 258
herbal treatment, 258–259
hormonal picture, 257
management, 257
postmenopause, 184–186
prebiotics, 52
pregnenolone, 4
premenstrual dysphoric disorder
(PMDD), 157. *See also*
premenstrual syndrome
diagnosis, 217
diet, lifestyle and herbal treatment
for, 250–251
melatonin and, 227–228
premenstrual syndrome (PMS),
215, 246, 248–249. *See also*
neurotransmitters associated
with menstrual cycle;
premenstrual dysphoric
disorder; supportive herbal
therapeutics
anti-inflammatory herbs, 236

calcium, 241–242
causes, 220–222
clinical trials, 237–238
diagnosis, 217
diet, lifestyle and herbal treatment
for, 250–251
elimination, 236
exercise, 235
intestinal health, 236
iron, 243–244
lifestyle, 234–235
magnesium, 242–243
omega 3, 241
PMS-like symptoms, 227
prevalence and distribution, 219
restoring function, 239
risk factors, 220
science, medicine, and menstrual
cycle, 216–217
symptomatic relief, 236–237
symptoms, 219
third phase of treatment
treatment, 232, 234, 238, 248
US Dept of Health PMS symptom
tracker, 218
vitamin B1 and B6, 239–240
vitamin D, 240
vitamin E, 241
zinc, 243
8-prenylnaringenin (8-PN), 102, 192
probiotics, 52
progesterone, 1, 225. *See also*
oestrogen; phyto-oestrogens;
progestogens
androstenedione and
aromatization, 4–5
deficiency, 45–46
deficiency treatment,
46–47
myths about progestogenic
herbs, 1–2
phase 2 conjugation,
16–20
production of, 4
receptors and oestrogen, 61
sex hormones, 2–3
progestogenic herbs, 1–2

progestogens, 41. *See also* oestrogen; phyto-oestrogens; progesterone
   actions of, 42–45
   laboratory tests, 46
pro-inflammatory cytokine, 63
prolactin, 62. *See also* nervous system
   control for, 245
   emotional component of, 229–230
   inhibiting factor, 230
Promensil®, 95
prostaglandin E1 (PGE1), 62, 229
prostate cancer, 76, 85–86
prostate specific antigen (PSA), 76
prostatic intraepithelial neoplasia (PIN), 76
PSA. *See* prostate specific antigen
pseudoaldosteronism, 175
psycho-neuro-endocrino-immunology (PNEI), 51–52, 221

RA. *See* rheumatoid arthritis
reactive oxygen species (ROS), 199
recurrent urinary tract infections, 196–197
red clover (*Trifolium pratense*), 91, 98. *See also* herbs
   anti-proliferative effects, 97
   benign prostatic hyperplasia and prostate cancer, 97
   bone density, 96
   clinical trials, 98
   clover disease, 92
   constituents, 94
   contraindications and adverse effects, 97
   coronary vascular disease risk reduction, 96
   dosage, preparations, usage, 98
   endometrial effects, 97
   extracts, 94
   history, 91–94
   indications, 94
   menopausal symptoms, 95–96
   pharmacokinetics, 94–95
   research findings for, 98
   skin, 96

Remifemin®, 147
renal disease, 86
resorcylic acid lactones, 41. *See also* phyto-oestrogens
restless leg syndrome (RLS), 159–160
resveratrol, 199–200
rheumatoid arthritis (RA), 161
rhizobium, 91
rhizome, 168
RLS. *See* restless leg syndrome
ROS. *See* reactive oxygen species

sage (*Salvia officinalis*), 107, 192. *See also* herbs
   acute pharyngitis, 113
   anti-inflammatory and antinociceptive properties, 113
   antimicrobial, 113–114
   antioxidant, 113
   anti-tumour activity, 113
   bone resorption inhibition, 113
   constituents, 109
   history, 107–109
   hot flushes, 111–112
   indications, 109–110
   memory and cognition clinical studies, 110–111
   menopause, 111
   metabolic effects on glycaemic control and lipid profile, 112
   perspiration-inhibiting effect studies, 112
   studies on, 110
   traditional and modern use, 114–115
Salvia officinalis. *See* sage
saponins, 117
SCFAs. *See* short chain fatty acids
SDG. *See* secoisolariciresinol diglucoside
secoisolariciresinol diglucoside (SDG), 72
selective oestrogen receptor modulators (SERMs), 37
selective serotonin reuptake inhibitors (SSRIs), 60, 185, 227

SERMs. *See* selective oestrogen receptor modulators
serotonergic pathways, 60
serotonin, 59–62, 222–225, 226–227. *See also* nervous system
sex hormone binding globulin (SHBG), 11, 122
   diet and lifestyle, 20–21
   endogenous factors affecting level of, 20, 21
sex hormone binding globulin (SHBG), 73
sex hormones, 2–3
Shatavari, 129
SHBG. *See* sex hormone binding globulin
short chain fatty acids (SCFAs), 55
Siberian ginseng, 208
SLE. *See* systemic lupus erythematosus
soy (glycine max), 63, 79, 88–89
   allergy to soy, 88
   bone density protection, 83–84
   breast cancer, 84–85
   cancer protection, 84
   circulation, 87
   consumption history, 80
   depression, 86–87
   endometrial cancer, 85
   epidemiology, 80
   hormonal effect of isoflavones, 82–83
   isoflavone contents, 81–82
   isoflavone pharmacodynamics, 82
   isoflavones and fertility, 83
   isoflavonoids, 80
   menopause and menarche, 87–88
   mineral uptake, 88
   myths about, 79–80
   prostate cancer, 85–86
   renal disease, 86
   side effects, 87
   soybean constituents, 81
   thyroid function, 88
squawroot. *See* black cohosh
SSRIs. *See* selective serotonin reuptake inhibitors

steroid
   hormones, 3, 63
   receptors, 63
steroidal saponins, 40. *See also* phyto-oestrogens
steroidogenesis, 4
St. John's wort, 247
sulphotransferases (SULTs), 10, 17
   nutrients affecting, 18
supportive herbal therapeutics, 244. *See also* premenstrual syndrome
   Cimicifuga racemosa, 247
   circulation, 244
   clinical studies on Vitex in PMS, 246–247
   digestive system, 244
   endocrine function, 244
   Hypericum and Vitex combination trial in perimenopausal women, 248
   Hypericum perforatum, 247
   hypothalamic-pituitary-adrenal axis, 245
   low oestrogen in perimenopause, 245
   nervines, 247
   neuroendocrine herbs, 246
   prolactin levels, 245
   thyroid support, 245
   Vitex agnus-castus, 246
symptomatic herbal treatment, 190
systematic treatment, 50–51
systemic lupus erythematosus (SLE), 78, 161

T3. *See* triiodothyronine
tamoxifen, 75. *See also* flaxseed
TC. *See* total cholesterol
testosterone production, 4
TG. *See* triglycerides
TGP. *See* total glycosides of peony
Theophrastus, 91, 168
thyroid function, 88
thyroid stimulating hormone (TSH), 111
thyrotropin-releasing hormone (TRH), 111

total cholesterol (TC), 208
total glycosides of peony (TGP), 167
transcription factor, 187
TRH. *See* thyrotropin-releasing hormone
Tribestan®, 121–122
Tribulus terrestris, 121. *See also Dioscorea villosa*
Trifolium pratense. *See* red clover
Trifolium pratense, 192
triglycerides (TG), 208
Trigonella foenum-graecum, 194
triiodothyronine (T3), 185
  receptors, 63
triterpenoid saponins, 41. *See also* phyto-oestrogens
tryptamine, 61
tryptophan-rich foods, 61
TSH. *See* thyroid stimulating hormone
Turnera diffusa, 206

UDP-glucuronosyltransferases (UGTs), 18
  nutrients affecting, 19
UGTs. *See* UDP-glucuronosyltransferases
uterine fibroids, 254. *See also* gynaecological conditions
  diet, 254
  exercise and lifestyle, 254
  herbal treatment, 255
  hormonal picture, 254
  management principles, 254
uterine prolapse, 198

vaginal
  dryness, 195
  infections, 195–196
vaginosis, bacterial, 195–196
valerenic acid, 193
Valeriana officinalis, 193
vascular cognitive impairment but no dementia (VCIND), 123
VCIND. *See* vascular cognitive impairment but no dementia

very low-density lipoproteins (VLDL), 112
Vitex agnus-castus, 62, 140, 147, 194, 204–205. *See also* black cohosh
  acne vulgaris, 158
  actions and indications, 160
  antiquity, 149–150
  casticin and other flavonoids, 153–154
  clinical trials, 156
  constituents, 152
  cyclic mastalgia, 157
  dopaminergic activity and clerodadienols, 152–153
  dosage, 162
  dysmenorrhoea, 158
  effect on prolactin, 153
  effects on fracture healing, 160
  FertilityBlend®, 159
  Hypericum perforatum with, 205
  hyperprolactinaemia, 157, 161
  intake timing, 161–162
  intrauterine device induced bleeding, and menorrhagia, 157–158
  in vivo and *in vitro* studies, 155–156
  in vivo reduction in LH and testosterone, 155
  melatonin release, 155
  menstrual cycle irregularities, 158–159
  menstruation problems, 161
  from middle ages to enlightenment, 150–151
  myths, 147, 149
  oestrogenic activity, 154
  opioid receptors, 155
  pharmacology, 152
  PMS, 156–157
  research, 151–152
  restless leg syndrome, 159–160
  studies on Vitex in PMS, 246–247
  traditions, 149
  Vitex and melatonin release, 205

VLDL. *See* very low-density
        lipoproteins
von Bingen, H., 99
vulvar atrophy, 195

whole person treatment, xiv–xvi
wild yam, 117
Withania, 259
    somnifera, 202
women's health initiative study, 186

xanthohumol, 103
xenoestrogens, 27

yams, 117
yarrow, 128

Zizyphus spinosa, 195